# THE PROSTAGLANDINS
## Pharmacological and Therapeutic Advances

# THE PROSTAGLANDINS
## Pharmacological
## and Therapeutic Advances

*Edited by*

M. F. Cuthbert, M.B., Ph.D.(London)

*Department of Pharmacology and Therapeutics*
*London Hospital Medical College.*

J. B. Lippincott Company

PHILADELPHIA

First published 1973

© M. F. Cuthbert, 1973

ISBN 0 397 58119 X

Printed in Great Britain

# Contributors

R. W. Butcher, Ph.D.
Department of Biochemistry, University of Massachusetts.

M. P. L. Caton, B.Sc., Ph.D.
Research Laboratories, May and Baker Ltd., Dagenham, Essex.

M. F. Cuthbert, M.B., Ph.D.
Department of Pharmacology and Therapeutics, London Hospital Medical College, University of London.

K. Hillier, B.Sc., Ph.D.
Nuffield Department of Obstetrics and Gynaecology, University of Oxford.

K. J. Hittelman, Ph.D.
Department of Biochemistry, University of Massachusetts.

S. M. M. Karim, B.Pharm., M.Sc., Ph.D.
Department of Pharmacology and Therapeutics, Makerere University Medical School, Kampala.

I. H. M. Main, B.Pharm., Ph.D.
Department of Pharmacology, School of Pharmacy, University of London.

E. E. Muirhead, M.D.
Department of Pathology, University of Tennessee.

J. Nakano, M.D.
Departments of Pharmacology and Medicine, University of Oklahoma.

Priscilla J. Piper, B.Pharm., Ph.D.
Department of Pharmacology, Institute of Basic Medical Sciences, Royal College of Surgeons of England.

# Contents

Preface     ix

Acknowledgements     xi

Chapter I   Chemistry Structure and Availability     1
M. P. L. CATON

II   General Pharmacology of Prostaglandins     23
J. NAKANO

III   Distribution and Metabolism     125
PRISCILLA J. PIPER

IV   Cyclic AMP and the Mechanism of Action of the Prostaglandins     151
K. J. HITTELMAN AND R. W. BUTCHER

V   Pharmacology and Therapeutic Applications of Prostaglandins in the Human Reproductive System     167
S. M. M. KARIM AND K. HILLIER

VI   Vasoactive and Anti-hypertensive Effects of Prostaglandins and other Renomedullary Lipids     201
E. E. MUIRHEAD

VII   Prostaglandins and Respiratory Smooth Muscle     253
M. F. CUTHBERT

VIII   Prostaglandins and the Gastro-intestinal Tract     287
I. H. M. MAIN

Index     324

# Preface

During the past three years there has been a remarkable growth of interest in the prostaglandins. There would appear to be two main reasons for this. Firstly, methods of biosynthesis and more recently total synthesis, have advanced sufficiently to enable adequate quantities of pure material to be made available for both fundamental research and for clinical investigation; secondly, the prostaglandins have been found to be potent uterine stimulants and to be effective in the induction of labour and therapeutic abortion.

The prostaglandins are very widely distributed in animal and human tissues and they have powerful effects on almost every physiological process which has been studied, as is evident from a brief examination of their pharmacological properties. These findings have suggested that the prostaglandins may regulate or be involved in many physiological processes. A function as 'local hormones' has been suggested but there is as yet little evidence to support this concept.

The possible therapeutic applications of the prostaglandins have not yet been extensively explored. On the present evidence it seems likely that they will have an established place in the induction of labour and therapeutic abortion. It is quite possible that the induction of abortion will prove to be practicable at any stage of pregnancy and the widespread use of the prostaglandins for this purpose may well give rise to social and ethical problems. There are also important implications in the control of fertility. Other potential applications, such as the control of blood pressure and the treatment of bronchial asthma and peptic ulceration, are at a very exploratory stage.

Extensive research into the properties of the prostaglandins has inevitably led to an overwhelming number of publications. Although reviews and the proceedings of some symposia have been published, most of the information on the prostaglandins is distributed in the specialist journals. The justification and aim of this book is to provide the interested medical and scientific reader with a concise account of the more important theoretical developments and also to outline those areas in which the prostaglandins are being introduced into clinical practice or have potential clinical application.

In chapters one to four the chemistry and classification, distribution and metabolism, general pharmacology and mechanism of action are considered. The second part of the book contains chapters on the relationship of the prostaglandins to the reproductive, cardiovascular, respiratory and gastro-intestinal systems with an emphasis on the human pharmacology and potential therapeutic applications. In the latter context, contributors have been encouraged to be speculative and although some of their suggestions regarding the possible use of the prostaglandins may in the future prove untenable it is likely that the next few years will see important developments in the clinical application of the prostaglandins.

*September 1972*                                                  M.F.C.

# Acknowledgements

I should like to take this opportunity to thank my wife, Mrs Margaret Cuthbert, BA and Mrs Ann Shannon (British Medical Association House) for valuable assistance in checking the manuscripts and references, and also Mr Geoffrey Jones for compiling the index. I am also indebted to Mr R. F. Ruddick, Photographic Department and Mrs Pat Hannaford, Medical Artist, both of the London Hospital, for help with the illustrations, and to Dr Raymond Greene and to Mr Owen R. Evans of William Heinemann Medical Books Ltd, for their consistent interest and encouragement.

*September 1972*                                          M. F. CUTHBERT

# Chemistry Structure and Availability

M. P. L. Caton

## 1. NOMENCLATURE

Prostaglandins are a group of closely related carboxylic acids containing a cyclopentane ring with two adjacent carbon side chains, one of which bears the carboxyl group at the terminal position. Most of the naturally occurring prostaglandins may be regarded as derivatives of the parent structure prostanoic acid (Fig. 1), the carbon atoms being numbered as shown. Individual members of the series are then distinguished by the number, type and arrangement of oxygen functions and double bonds which are built into this basic system.

Natural prostaglandins are divided into four groups and although these may be named in accordance with their relationship to prostanoic acid, they are more conveniently referred to by the letters E, F, A and B (Fig. 1).† All four groups have in common a *trans* double bond at the 13, 14 position and a hydroxyl group at $C_{15}$. The E and F series, often referred to as the primary prostaglandins, both possess an additional hydroxyl at $C_{11}$ and are distinguished from each other by the presence of a carbonyl function at $C_9$ in the E series and a $C_9$ hydroxyl in the F series. The A and B series may be regarded as dehydration products of the E compounds whereby loss of water has occurred with removal of the $C_{11}$ hydroxyl and formation of a double bond in the ring. This dehydration is readily effected chemically and it is considered that some of the A prostaglandins derived from natural sources are in reality artifacts formed from the E prostaglandins during the isolation procedure.

The A prostaglandins, in which this additional double bond is at $C_{10, 11}$, are the primary products of the dehydration but are relatively unstable and readily rearrange under alkaline conditions to the B

† Very recently two members of a fifth series have been isolated in small quantities. These are isomers of the A and B series, having the ring double bond at $C_{11, 12}$ and they have been designated by the letter C (Jones, 1972).

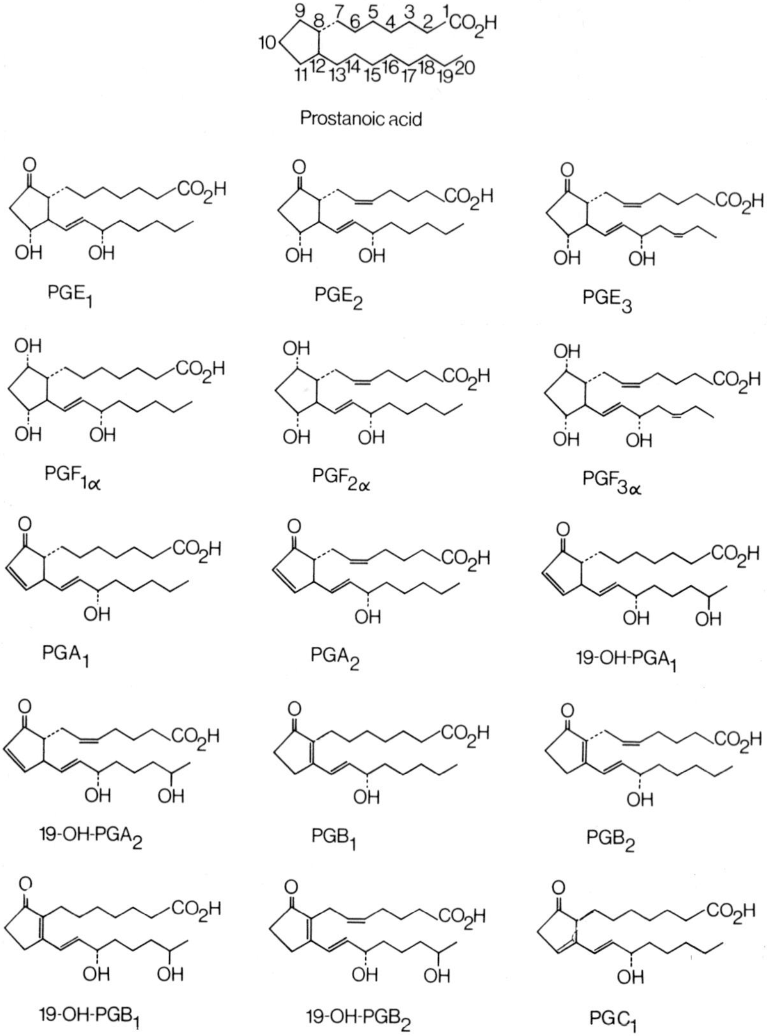

Prostanoic acid

PGE$_1$        PGE$_2$        PGE$_3$

PGF$_{1\alpha}$        PGF$_{2\alpha}$        PGF$_{3\alpha}$

PGA$_1$        PGA$_2$        19-OH-PGA$_1$

19-OH-PGA$_2$        PGB$_1$        PGB$_2$

19-OH-PGB$_1$        19-OH-PGB$_2$        PGC$_1$

Fig. 1. Prostanoic acid and some naturally occurring prostaglandins.

prostaglandins where the ring double bond lies between the two side chains, i.e. at $C_{8,\,12}$. Because A and B prostaglandins are conveniently characterized by their ultra-violet spectra they were formally known respectively as prostaglandins 217 and prostaglandin 278, the numbers referring to their U.V. absorption maxima (m$\mu$).

Each of these four principal series are subdivided according to whether one or two additional side chain double bonds are present. The total number of such double bonds is referred to by a subscript numeral after the letter, thus prostaglandin $E_1$ ($PGE_1$) has only the $C_{13,14}$ double bond, $PGE_2$ has a further (*cis*) double bond at $C_{5,6}$ and $PGE_3$ a third (*cis*) double bond at $C_{17,18}$. These double bonds occur in the same positions in all four groups, although $PGA_3$ and $PGB_3$ have not yet been isolated. Members of the A and B series are also known with an additional hydroxyl group at $C_{19}$.

Prostaglandins possess several asymmetric centres which give rise to a number of possible stereoisomeric forms. Most prostaglandins from natural sources have the stereochemistry shown for the examples in Fig. 1, where the side chains are *trans* to each other, i.e. they are oriented on opposite sides of the ring. $C_9$ and $C_{11}$ hydroxyl groups are in the α-configuration, i.e. on the same side of the ring as the carboxylic acid side chain. The $C_{15}$ hydroxyl is also designated α but that at $C_{19}$ has the opposite configuration. (For this purpose substituents attached below the plane of the ring are indicated in the formulae with a dotted line and those above with a continuous line). The absolute stereochemistry was determined in 1966, before which some publications showed the side chains in the opposite configuration (Nugteren, Van Dorp, Bergström, Hamberg and Samuelsson, 1966; Hamberg, 1968).

Stereochemical variants of these natural forms arise in three different ways, some examples of which are given for $PGE_1$ in Fig. 2. First, the side chains may lie in the alternative i.e. *cis* relationship to one another; these are termed 8-isoprostaglandins (e.g. 8-iso-$PGE_1$) and may be considered as based upon the parent isoprostanoic acid, analogous to prostanoic acid. Secondly, one or more hydroxyl groups may have the β configuration. Here the $C_{11}$ and $C_{15}$ β hydroxyls are sometimes referred to by the term *epi*, alternatively the $C_{15}$ hydroxyl group can also be named after the Cahn-Ingold-Prelog Convention, i.e. S for the α and R for the *epi* or β form. Thirdly, all prostaglandins are also capable of existing in two optically active forms because of the asymmetry of the

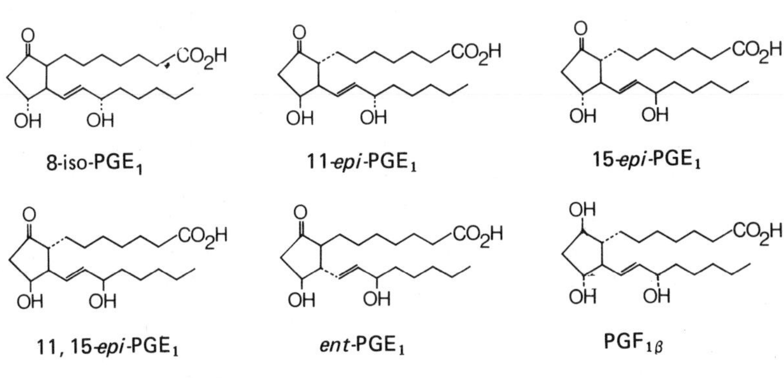

8-iso-PGE$_1$          11-*epi*-PGE$_1$          15-*epi*-PGE$_1$

11, 15-*epi*-PGE$_1$          *ent*-PGE$_1$          PGF$_{1β}$

Fig. 2. Some stereoisomers of prostaglandin $E_1$.

molecule. Natural prostaglandins are laevorotatory and their mirror images, which are dextrorotatory and have the side chains transposed are referred to as the *ent* forms. All these stereochemical variants may of course be combined with each other and it is therefore possible to envisage a very large number of different isomers.

It should be pointed out that the stereochemistry is understood and reference to it is therefore omitted in the abbreviated forms (PGE$_1$ etc.) used for the principal natural prostaglandins. However, with the F series the term $\alpha$ or $\beta$ (e.g. PGF$_{1\alpha}$, PGF$_{1\beta}$) is always added to denote the configuration of the C$_9$ hydroxyl group. This is because the PGF$_\beta$ compounds (Fig. 2), although not occurring naturally, have long been known together with the F$_\alpha$ compounds as reduction products of the E prostaglandins and it has become established practice to distinguish them in this way.

When it is desired to describe prostaglandins in terms of their full systematic nomenclature, a method based on the structure of prostanoic acid is adopted, details of which are given by Nugteren *et al.* (1966). Thus the full systematic name of PGE$_1$ is (−)-11$\alpha$, 15(S)-dihydroxy-9-oxo-13-*trans*-prostenoic acid, where the (−) sign refers to the laevorotation and the *'trans'* to the C$_{13,14}$ double bond.

A number of derivatives and structural variants of these natural prostaglandins occur as metabolites and other types have been prepared by biosynthesis and chemical synthetic methods. These have been conveniently named after the natural group to which they are most closely related or they may be described in terms of their relationship to prostanoic acid. Prostaglandins where the side chains are one or more methylene units shorter than normal are described by the terms nor, dinor, trinor etc. and the corresponding longer chain compounds are referred to as homo (Fig. 3). The letters $\alpha$ or $\omega$ are used here to signify whether the terms apply to the carboxyhexyl i.e. $\alpha$, or the hydroxyoctyl

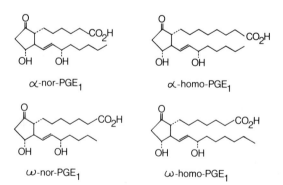

Fig. 3. Prostaglandin E$_1$ —side chain variants.

i.e. ω chain, the use of α here must not be confused with its stereochemical significance. Prostaglandins where one methylene unit is replaced by an oxygen atom are known as oxaprostaglandins and those deficient in one of the substituent oxygen functions present in the natural compounds are named deoxyprostaglandins. Examples of these and other types are given in subsequent sections.

## 2. SOURCES OF SUPPLY

There are fundamentally three sources from which prostaglandins may be obtained—direct extraction from tissues, laboratory biosynthesis and total chemical synthesis. A number of prostaglandins have also been obtained by chemical modification of other members of the series. In describing these methods some attempt is made to assess the relative merits of each and their usefulness for obtaining sufficient material for extensive biological testing and ultimate clinical use.

### Direct Extraction from Tissues

Although prostaglandins have been detected in a wide variety of mammalian tissues, owing to the very low concentrations in which they occur, direct extraction from these sources does not constitute a practical means of obtaining significant quantities. However, one prostaglandin—15-*epi*-PGA$_2$—has been discovered in relatively large quantities in a marine invertebrate, the Gorgonian (*Plexaura homomalla*), a species of coral found in the Caribbean region. This compound and the 15-acetyl derivative of its methyl ester are present in the air-dried cortex of that species to the extent of 0.2 and 1.3% respectively from which they have been isolated by solvent extraction and chromatography. Although the 15-*epi* prostaglandins are themselves of relatively low biological activity they can be converted chemically into other more useful members of the series and hence their availability from this widely distributed species constitutes a source of considerable potential value (Weinheimer and Spraggins, 1969; Bundy, Lincoln, Nelson, Pike and Schneider, 1971).

### Biosynthesis

Prostaglandins are biosynthesized from C$_{20}$ straight chain carboxylic acids which undergo ring closure and addition of the requisite number of oxygen atoms by a complex process, the overall result of which is shown in Fig. 4. This conversion has been demonstrated in a number of different animal tissues but its importance as a preparative method lies in the fact that extracts of the enzyme can be used to convert the substrate

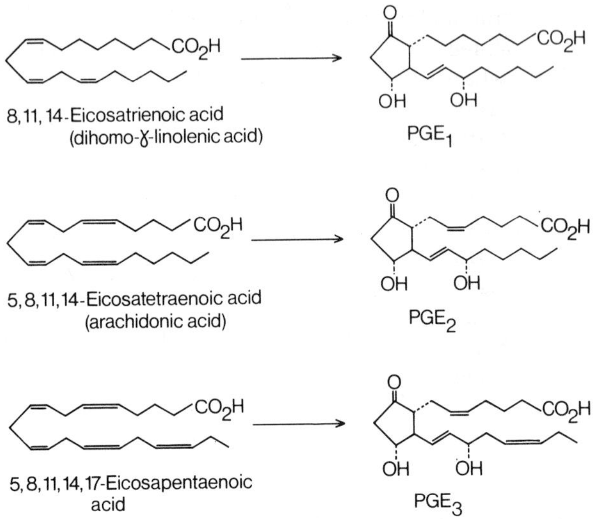

8,11,14-Eicosatrienoic acid
(dihomo-ɣ-linolenic acid)

PGE$_1$

5,8,11,14-Eicosatetraenoic acid
(arachidonic acid)

PGE$_2$

5,8,11,14,17-Eicosapentaenoic
acid

PGE$_3$

Fig. 4. Prostaglandins-Biosynthesis.

acids into prostaglandins on the laboratory scale (Van Dorp, Beerthuis, Nugteren and Vonkeman, 1964; Bergström, Danielsson and Samuelsson, 1964a; Bergström, Danielsson, Klenberg and Samuelsson, 1964b).

The process has been developed for some of the principal prostaglandins to enable the production of gram quantities and until chemical synthesis became available this was the only practical means of obtaining supplies of these compounds for biological investigation.

The enzyme system is most commonly derived from homogenates of the vesicular gland of the sheep, although acetone powders from bull seminal vesicle have also been used (Wallach, 1965). The homogenate is incubated with the substrate acid, usually in the presence of glutathione and an antioxidant such as hydroquinone which have been shown to produce favourable effects on the yield (Samuelsson, 1967; Nugteren, Beerthuis and Van Dorp, 1967).

The prostaglandins formed are purified by solvent extraction and by chromatography or a procedure based on dialysis. Yields of up to 60% are obtainable (Daniels and Pike, 1968; Lapidus, Grant and Alburn, 1968a; Lapidus, Grant and Alburn, 1968b).

Biosyntheses using vesicular gland homogenates give mainly prostaglandins of the E series and PGE$_1$, PGE$_2$ and PGE$_3$ are derived respectively from all cis-8,11,14-eicosatrienoic (dihomo-γ-linolenic), 5,8,11,14-eicosatetraenoic (arachidonic) and 5,8,11,14,17-eicosapentaenoic acids (Fig. 4). However, by using lung homogenates as the enzymic source, F$_\alpha$ compounds are also formed (Änggård and Samuelsson, 1965). Recent work has shown that certain bicyclo [2.2.1] heptane derivatives, which bear a structural resemblance to a key intermediate in the biosynthesis, inhibited the formation of $PGE_1$ by the enzyme from vesicular gland; whereas conversion to $PGF_{1\alpha}$ was slightly increased (Wlodawer, Samuelsson, Albonico and Corey, 1971). A few isomers of the principal natural prostaglandins have been obtained from these incubations. Thus 8-iso-$PGE_1$, (Fig. 2) has been isolated in low yield as a by-product from the dihomo-γ-linolenic acid incubation, although it may have arisen by isomerization of $PGE_1$ (Daniels, Krueger, Kupiecki, Pike and Schneider, 1968). 11-Dehydro-$PGF_{1\alpha}$ (Fig. 5) has been obtained as the major product from dihomo-γ-linolenic acid when the conversion was carried out with a purified microsomal enzyme fraction from sheep vesicular gland (Granström, Lands and Samuelsson, 1968).

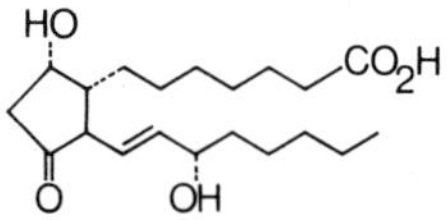

11-Dehydro-$PGF_{1\alpha}$

Fig. 5.

Prostaglandins with an oxygen function at $C_{18}$ and $C_{19}$ have been obtained by enzymatic ring closure with bull seminal vesicle microsomes of the appropriate oxygenated fatty acid prepared via microbiological hydroxylation of 5,8,11,14-eicosatetraenoic acid with *Ophiobolus graminis*. This is claimed to provide a relatively convenient route for the synthesis of oxygenated prostaglandin E derivatives which would be exceedingly difficult to prepare by conventional partial or total chemical synthesis; (Sih, Ambrus, Foss and Lai, 1969). Derivatives of $PGA_1$ hydroxylated at $C_{19}$ and $C_{20}$ are obtained on incubation of $PGA_1$ with a preparation of guinea-pig liver. Yields of 10-18% are obtainable and the product contains 65% of the 20-OH and 35% of the 19-OH compound (Israelsson, Hamberg and Samuelsson, 1969).

By using lower and higher homologues of the $C_{20}$ starting acids, certain nor- and homo-prostaglandins have been prepared. However, the substrate specificity of the enzyme imposes limitations on the success of this conversion which is dependent not only upon the total chain length of the acid but more particularly on the position of the double bond system relative to the carboxyl group. Nevertheless a series of prostaglandin homologues have been prepared by this method which has enabled their biological activity to be compared with that of the natural compounds (Bergström *et al.*, 1964b; Struijk, Beerthuis, Pabon and Van Dorp, 1966; Beerthuis, Nugteren, Pabon and Van Dorp, 1968; Struijk,

Beerthuis and Van Dorp, 1967; Beerthuis, Nugteren, Pabon, Steenhoek and Van Dorp, 1971).

Biosynthesis then, has proved useful as a means of producing limited quantities of prostaglandins in a single overall conversion step from starting materials which are either commercially available or are readily synthesized by chemical means. However, it suffers from the severe limitation of being dependent upon supplies of an enzyme available only in limited amounts at considerable cost. Moreover, with the few exceptions referred to above, biosynthesis is only able to provide natural prostaglandins and is not suitable for the preparation of prostaglandin analogues.

## Total Chemical Synthesis

In recent years total chemical synthesis has assumed major importance as a means of obtaining supplies of prostaglandins for which it is now the method of choice. Unlike biosynthesis, it is not subject to the limitations imposed by availability of an enzyme and it is capable of scaling up to produce substantial quantities of material. However, owing to the presence of several different functional groups which must be built into the correct positions of the molecule, together with the need to arrive at the required stereochemistry, these syntheses require a large number of stages and many of them are somewhat tedious to carry out. Nevertheless certain of the routes currently available are suitable for the preparation of hundred gram quantities of material.

Another advantage of total synthesis is its flexibility which enables the preparation of unnatural stereoisomers and novel structural variants unobtainable by any other means. Some of these have been prepared in an attempt to overcome clinical shortcomings of the natural forms such as their brief duration of action resulting from rapid metabolic inactivation or the presence of side effects consequent of their wide spectrum of biological activity. Other novel synthetic forms have the advantage over the natural compounds of greater ease of access owing to the possibility of preparation by shorter synthetic procedures.

Here an attempt is made first to list routes currently available to each of the main groups of natural prostaglandins and their stereoisomers and then to describe the novel structural variants. Details of the syntheses themselves have been reviewed elsewhere (Caton, 1971); although many of them have so far been published only in preliminary form and full experimental details are not yet available. The final products are usually purified by chromatography and solvent systems are available for separation of most of the principal prostaglandins and their stereo-isomers (Ramwell and Daniels, 1969; Andersen, 1969). In a number of

cases crystalline compounds have been obtained and recrystallized from suitable solvents.
*Natural Prostaglandins and Stereoisomers.* A number of routes are now available to the natural prostaglandins. It should be pointed out that the majority of these give rise to racemic mixtures, variously referred to as '*rac*', (±) or '*dl*', which consist of equal proportions of the natural and the corresponding '*ent*' forms; the '*ent*' compounds are often biologically relatively inactive and therefore merely serve to reduce the potency of the material to 50% of that obtained with the pure natural form. Since the racemic mixtures are more readily obtained, for some purposes it may be more economically desirable overall to utilize these despite this lower potency rather than to embark upon the additional effort and expenditure required to obtain the natural stereoisomers.

Prostaglandin $E_1$ (±)–$PGE_1$ has been synthesized by groups at Harvard University (Corey, Noyori and Schaaf, 1970a; Corey, Andersen, Carlson, Paust, Vedejs, Vlattas and Winter, 1968a; Corey, Vlattas, Andersen and Harding, 1968b; Corey, Vlattas and Harding, 1969a); McGill University and the Upjohn Laboratories (Schneider, Axen, Lincoln, Pike and Thompson, 1968; Schneider, Axen, Lincoln, Pike and Thompson, 1969; Axen, Lincoln and Thompson, 1969); the Ciba Laboratories (Ciba, 1969; Finch and Fitt, 1969) and the Merck, Sharp and Dohme Laboratories (Taub, Hoffsommer, Kuo, Slates, Zelawski and Wendler, 1970; Slates, Zelawski, Taub and Wendler, 1972). These syntheses involve some 15-30 stages; full experimental details are available for the Upjohn and Ciba routes; the latter afforded $PGE_1$ as the methoxime derivative.

The Harvard work has been adapted to give the pure natural stereoisomer. This has been achieved by two different routes, resolution being effected on an intermediate amine in the first, and a carboxylic acid in the second, affording in each case the optically active (laevo) forms of these compounds which are then carried through to the final products by the same sequence of reactions used for the synthesis of racemic $E_1$ (Corey *et al.*, 1969a; 1970a).

The second route has the advantage that the optical resolution can be effected at an early stage. Moreover, reagents have been employed which bring about selective formation of the required hydroxy stereoisomers, thus eliminating the need to remove the unwanted '*epi*' forms by chromatography. This method, which has the further advantage of permitting the synthesis of all six primary prostaglandins from the same precursor, is currently being used on a substantial scale in several industrial laboratories. Recent work has effected several improvements in the procedure first published and has simplified operations for working on a large scale (Corey, Koelliker and Neuffer, 1971a; Corey, Albonico, Koelliker, Schaaf and Varma, 1971b). The pure natural stereoisomer of

PGE$_1$ has also been synthesized by the Merck group (Slates *et al.*, 1972).

PGE$_2$ and PGE$_3$ have been prepared by suitable modifications of the above Upjohn-McGill and Harvard syntheses, the latter affording the pure natural stereoisomers (Schneider, 1969; Axen, Thompson and Pike, 1970; Ferdinandi and Just, 1971; Corey, Weinshenker, Schaaf and Huber, 1969b; Corey, Arnold and Hutton, 1970b; Corey, Schaaf, Huber, Koelliker and Weinshenker, 1970c; Corey *et al.*, 1970a; Corey, Shirahama, Yamamoto, Terashima, Venkateswarlu and Schaaf, 1971c).

A number of unnatural stereoisomers of the E series have been synthesized. (±)-8-iso-PGE$_1$ is obtainable by a modification of the Upjohn E$_1$ process and this work has also afforded a preparation of (±)-15-*epi*-PGE$_1$ (Schneider *et al.*, 1968; Axen *et al.*, 1969). (±)-11-*Epi*-,(±)-15-*epi*- and (±)-11,15-*epi*-PGE$_1$ have been prepared by the Harvard procedures (Corey *et al.*, 1968a, b). Pure *ent* PGE$_1$ has been obtained via the dextro form of the same intermediate amine used to prepare the natural form (Corey *et al.*, 1969a).

The only unnatural stereoisomer of PGE$_2$ apparently so far reported is the (±)-15-*epi*-compound* (Schneider, 1969) and none are yet known for PGE$_3$. However members of this series could no doubt be synthesized by suitable modification of the methods used to prepare the corresponding forms of PGE$_1$.

Natural F prostaglandins, PGF$_{1\alpha}$, PGF$_{2\alpha}$, and PGF$_{3\alpha}$ have all been synthesized by the Harvard workers using the same key intermediates employed for the E series (Corey *et al.*, 1968a, b; Corey *et al.*, 1969b; Corey *et al.*, 1970a, b, c; Corey and Noyori, 1970 and Corey *et al.*, 1971c). (±) F prostaglandins are also available from Upjohn-McGill work (Schneider *et al.*, 1968; Just, Simonovitch, Lincoln, Schneider, Axen, Spero and Pike, 1969; Schneider, 1969). Unnatural stereoisomers of the F series which have been prepared by suitable modification of routes to corresponding E compounds include (±)-PGE$_{1\beta}$ (±)-PGF$_{2\beta}$, (±)15-*epi*-PGF$_{2\alpha}$, (±)-15-*epi*-PGF$_{1\alpha}$,* (±)-8-iso-PGF$_{1\alpha}$,* and (±)-8-iso-PGF$_{1\beta}$.*

PGF compounds are also conveniently prepared by reduction of the ring ketone of the E series with sodium borohydride. This reduction affords a 50 : 50 mixture of F$_\alpha$ and F$_\beta$ compounds which are separated by chromatography (Pike, Lincoln and Schneider, 1969); but recent work has shown that specific reduction to the F$_\alpha$ compound can be achieved using a bulky trialkyl borohydride reagent (Corey and Varma, 1971).

Prostaglandins of the A series are readily obtained by dehydration of the corresponding E compounds. This is effected under acidic conditions since the use of alkali results in rearrangement to the B series, hydrochloric acid (Corey *et al.*, 1968a) or acetic acid (Pike *et al.*, 1969)

* Product obtained as an ester.

have been used. Recently a direct synthesis of A prostaglandins has been reported (Corey and Grieco, 1972).

Prostaglandins of the B series may be obtained by the action of sodium hydroxide on those of the E series; full details are available (Pike *et al.*, 1969). Also, several independent synthetic routes are available to (±)-PGB$_1$ (Hardegger, Schenk and Broger, 1967; Klok, Pabon and Van Dorp, 1968; Yura and Ide, 1969; Collins, Jung and Pappo, 1968; Katsube and Matsui, 1969). These routes involve as few as 7-9 steps and are thus considerably shorter than those to the other series.

*Prostaglandin Metabolites.* Several routes are available to 13,14-dihydroprostaglandins and 15-dehydroprostaglandins (alternatively known as 15-ketoprostaglandins) some of which occur as prostaglandin metabolites (Fig. 6).

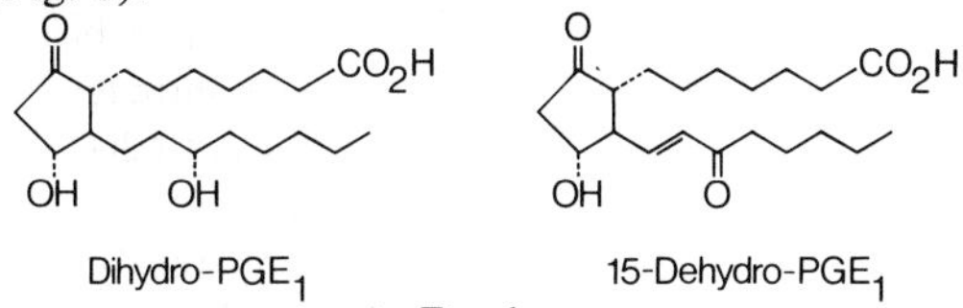

Dihydro-PGE$_1$      15-Dehydro-PGE$_1$

Fig. 6.

(±)-Dihydro-PGE$_1$* has been synthesized in 10 steps by Upjohn workers (Beal III, Babcock and Lincoln, 1966). A route by American Home Products afforded (±)-dihydro-PGA$_1$, which can in turn be converted to (±)-dihydro-PGE$_1$ (Strike and Smith, 1970). (±)-Dihydro-PGB$_1$ has also been synthesized and this has also been converted to the E compound, although in low yield (Klok, Pabon and Van Dorp, 1970). Another sequence afforded (±)-8-iso-dihydro-PGF$_{1\alpha}$ (Beal III, Babcock and Lincoln, 1967; Babcock and Beal III, 1967).

15-Dehydroprostaglandins can be prepared from the primary prostaglandins by selective oxidation of the 15-hydroxyl group (Pike *et al.*, 1969). Total syntheses are available to racemic 15-dehydro-PGE$_1$ and the corresponding PGB compound* (Miyano, 1969; 1970; Miyano and Dorn, 1969).

*Novel Synthetic Prostaglandins.* Whilst it is possible to envisage the preparation by chemical synthesis of many different classes of novel prostaglandins not found in nature, those reported so far fall mainly into four groups—methylprostaglandins, oxaprostaglandins, deoxyprostaglandins and cyclohexane analogues. Some examples of these are shown in Fig. 7.

Prostaglandins with one or two methyl substituents at the 2,3,19 and 20 positions in the side chains have been reported in the patent literature (Pike, 1970). 15-Methylprostaglandins have been synthesized with the object of blocking the enzymatic oxidation of the 15-hydroxyl by the prostaglandin dehydrogenase (Bundy *et al.*, 1971).

* Product obtained as an ester.

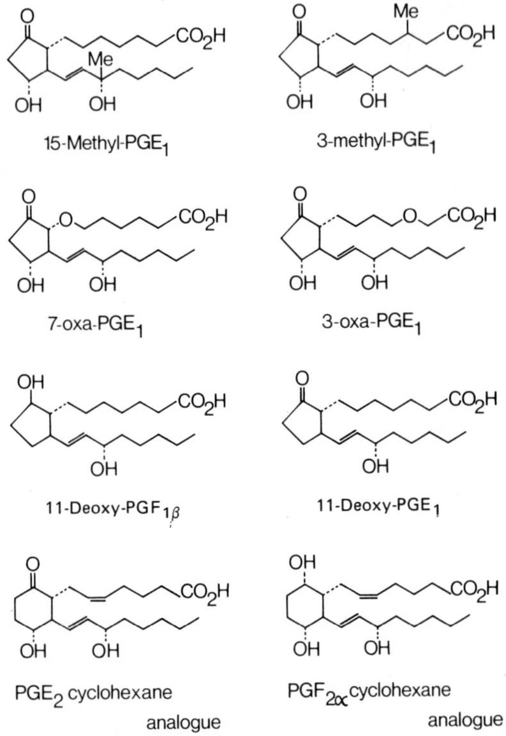

Fig. 7. Prostaglandin analogues.

3-Oxaprostaglandins, available by modification of Upjohn routes to the E, F and A series, have been prepared in order to block the metabolic breakdown of the carboxyhexyl side chain by $\beta$ oxidation (Nelson, 1971). ($\pm$)-7-Oxa-PGE$_1$, ($\pm$)-7-oxa-PGF$_{1\alpha}$ and a number of 7-oxa compounds of simpler structure have been synthesized by workers at the University of Chicago (Fried, Heim, Etheredge, Sunder-Plassmann, Santhanakrishnan, Himizu and Lin, 1968; Fried, Mehra, Kao and Lin, 1970; Fried, Santhanakrishnan, Himizu, Lin and Ford, 1969). Recent work has led to the synthesis of (+) and ($-$)-7-oxa-PGF$_{1\alpha}$ and their 15-epimers (Fried, Mehra and Kao, 1971).

Total syntheses are available to ($\pm$)-11-deoxyprostaglandins E$_1$, E$_2$ and the corresponding F compounds as well as to some of their 13,14-dihydro derivatives; some of these routes involving as few as 7-8 steps (Bagli, Bogri, Deghenghi and Wiesner, 1966; Bagli and Bogri, 1967; Bagli and Bogri, 1969a; Corey and Ravindranathan, 1971; Crabbé and Guzmán, 1972; Caton, Coffee and Watkins, 1972). ($\pm$)-15-Deoxyprostaglandin E$_1$ has also been synthesized (Sih, Salomon, Price, Peruzzoti and Sood, 1972).

11-Deoxyprostaglandins have also been obtained by hydrogenation of the natural A prostaglandins, of which they may be regarded as 10,11-dihydro derivatives (Beal III and Pike, 1967; Beal III, Lincoln and Pike, 1967).

Cyclohexane analogues of $PGE_2$ and $PGF_{2\alpha}$ have been synthesized by I.C.I. workers using a modification of the Harvard procedure to the natural prostaglandins (Crossley, 1971).

## 3. CHEMICAL PROPERTIES

The principal prostaglandins are crystalline solids with characteristic melting points. Physical constants, spectral data and solubilities in organic solvents are listed in reviews by Ramwell, Shaw, Clarke, Grostic, Kaiser and Pike (1968) and Shaw and Ramwell (1969) as well as many of the papers on chemical synthesis and biosynthesis referred to in preceding sections.

Since they are carboxylic acids, prostaglandins are soluble in alkali and form water soluble alkali metal salts. Derivatives of functional groups in the molecule are obtainable by standard methods and those which have been prepared include esters, oximes (Pike *et al.,* 1969), ureides, thiosemicarbazones (Lapidus *et al.,* 1968b), methyl ethers (Bergström, Krabisch, Samuelsson and Sjövall, 1962) and acetyl compounds (Samuelsson, 1965). Several of these have provided a convenient means of facilitating purification and identification of the parent prostaglandin.

The chemical stability of prostaglandins is of major importance in connection with their potential clinical utility since they must clearly be able to withstand preparation and storage of the required formulated products. Monoenoic prostaglandins ($E_1$ etc.) are relatively stable in the crystalline form if stored under nitrogen at $4°C$ but the di- and trienoic prostaglandins ($E_2$, $E_3$ etc.) are much less stable, gradually undergoing autoxidation on exposure to air at room temperature (Shaw and Ramwell, 1969).

Solutions of prostaglandins are much less stable than the crystalline solids, this is particularly so with the E series which, as already indicated, undergo facile loss of water to the A and B compounds. A systematic study has been carried out of the effects of different pH values on 100 ng/ml solutions of four prostaglandins ($E_1$, $E_2$, $F_{1\alpha}$, $F_{2\alpha}$), at room temperature, the extent of decomposition being determined by measuring the loss with time of smooth muscle stimulating activity (Karim, Devlin and Hillier, 1968). The E compounds are particularly unstable in the pH range 8-11; thus $PGE_1$ had lost 100% of its activity within 1 hour at pH 10-11 and 20% after 1 day at pH 8. By contrast, the F series were stable at these pH values and showed no loss of activity after 6 months. The F compounds were similarly stable at the pH 5-7 range whereas the E compounds had lost a substantial part of their activity at 60 days. However, at pH 1-4 the E series were more stable than the F series. F prostaglandins are better able to survive elevated temperatures in solution at pH 7 than do those of the E series. All four prostaglandins studied ($E_1$, $E_2$, $F_{1\alpha}$, $F_{2\alpha}$) may be stored in solution at a low temperature, thus 100 ng/ml solutions at pH 7 showed no loss of activity after 6 months at $-20°$ C.

Recent studies have shown that the potency of $PGE_2$ in saline solutions for clinical use deteriorate on storage. This can be prevented by preparing the compounds in concentrated alcoholic solutions in ampoules which can be kept for long periods at $-20°$ and diluted with sterile isotonic saline as required within 24 hours of use (Brummer, 1971).

## 4. STRUCTURE-ACTIVITY RELATIONSHIPS

Reference has already been made to the desirability of obtaining prostaglandins which show a greater specificity of biological action than some of the natural forms and indeed this is probably essential for certain of the clinical applications envisaged. Because of the use of different species and test systems by the various workers concerned and the fact that data are so far incomplete for some of the prostaglandin groups, direct comparisons of biological activity are often difficult to draw. However, an attempt is made here to indicate briefly, in broad terms, the present status of the structure-activity pattern of the natural and synthetic forms with particular reference to some of the cases where enhanced specificity has been most marked. The reader is referred to other reviews and individual papers for more detailed accounts.

The principal pharmacological activities shown by prostaglandins, where comparative data have been reported for representative members of the series, include stimulation of gastro-intestinal and reproductive smooth muscle, relaxation and contraction of respiratory smooth muscle, lowering of blood pressure and inhibition of the lipolysis of fatty acids, gastric acid secretion and blood platelet aggregation. $PGE_1$ is characterized by a high level of activity on all these systems and is frequently used as the standard for comparison with other prostaglandins. $PGE_2$ and $PGE_3$ generally have a similar spectrum of activity to $E_1$ with some quantitative differences, $E_3$ often being rather less active. An outstanding divergence between $PGE_1$ and $PGE_2$ is seen on blood platelet aggregation where $E_2$ has a much lower level of action and in some instances has caused a stimulation of aggregation (Kloeze, 1969; Sekhar, 1970).

Variations in the length of the side chains bring about certain changes in the degree of activity. $\alpha$-Nor and $\alpha$-homo E prostaglandins generally show substantially less activity than $PGE_1$ whereas the corresponding $\omega$ compounds still show high potency (Struijk *et al.,* 1967; Struijk *et al.,* 1966; Beerthuis *et al.,* 1968; Horton and Main, 1966). $\omega$-Homo $PGE_1$ shows a particularly high level of activity, approximately four times that of $PGE_1$, on blood platelet aggregation (Kloeze, 1969).

Marked specificity of action is found with 8-iso-$PGE_1$ where blood platelet aggregation activity is of a high order and comparable to that of $PGE_1$, whereas on smooth muscle, blood pressure and lipolysis, potency is very low. This indicates that the iso-compound would have clear advantages over the natural form if employed as an antithrombotic agent since unwanted side effects would be minimized (Sekhar, Weeks and Kupiecki, 1968; Weeks, Sekhar and Kupiecki, 1968).

Direct comparisons have been made of the activities of the synthetic prostaglandin stereoisomers on smooth muscle and on blood pressure (Ramwell, Shaw, Corey and Andersen, 1969). Reference has already been made to the low potency of *ent* forms which effectively halves the activity of the racemates and indeed *ent*-$PGE_1$ has only 1/1000th the activity of natural $PGE_1$ on smooth muscle. Natural and racemic 15-*epi*-$PGE_1$ and racemic 11-*epi*-$PGE_1$ are much less active than natural $PGE_1$, however, racemic 15-*epi*-$E_1$ is more active than natural 15-*epi*-$E_1$ indicating that here the *ent* form is more active than its natural counterpart. A very high level of activity has been recorded for racemic 11,15-*epi*-$PGE_1$ (approx. 5 times that of $PGE_1$ on rabbit jejunum) which is attributed to an even higher level of potency for the *ent* component.

The $PGF_\alpha$ compounds, like the E series, generally show high potency on smooth muscle although there are substantial species variations. An important divergence of action is noted on non-pregnant human uterus which is relaxed by E but stimulated by the F prostaglandins, whereas pregnant myometrium undergoes contraction with both series (Bygdeman, 1967). F prostaglandins are generally much less potent than the E compounds as relaxants of respiratory smooth muscle (Horton and Main, 1965; 1966) and on human bronchial muscle $PGF_{2\alpha}$ causes contraction (Sweatman and Collier, 1968). The F prostaglandins show considerable species variation in their effects on blood pressure, for example, in the rabbit and the cat they are depressor like the E compounds (Horton and Main, 1965) but in the dog and rat they are pressor (DuCharme and Weeks, 1967). F compounds are much less active than their E counterparts on the inhibition of blood platelet aggregation, lipolysis and gastric secretion (Kloeze, 1969; Steinberg and Vaughan, 1967; Robert, Nezamis and Phillips, 1967).

$PGF_\beta$ compounds have effects qualitatively similar to the $F_\alpha$ compounds although there are some substantial differences in the level of activity; thus $PGF_{1\alpha}$ is 30 times as active as $PGF_{1\beta}$ on the rabbit jejunum (Horton and Main, 1966). Data from racemic $PGF_{1\alpha}$ show that *ent*-$PGF_{1\alpha}$ appears to be virtually inactive, as is the corresponding E compound (Ramwell *et al.,* 1969).

The A prostaglandins are characterized by a high degree of hypotensive activity comparable to that of the E series, but they have only a weak effect on other systems (Weeks, Sekhar and DuCharme, 1969). This series thus offers the most promise for specific action in the hypotensive field. The B prostaglandins have only weak activity on all test systems (Bergström, Carlson and Orö, 1967).[†]

13,14-Dihydroprostaglandins retain most of the high activity on blood pressure and smooth muscle shown by the parent compounds but the 15-keto compounds are only weakly active (Änggård, 1966; Pike, Kupiecki and Weeks, 1967).

15-Methylprostaglandins have been shown to exhibit smooth muscle activity approaching that of their natural counterparts (Bundy *et al.,* 1971). Oxaprostaglandins are also active but at a much lower level; thus 3-oxa-$PGE_1$ ethyl ester has 0.039 of the potency of natural $PGE_1$ on isolated gerbil colon and smooth muscle data for the 7-oxa series all show activity at less than 0.5% of that of $PGE_1$. The 7-oxa series are interesting as antagonists of the action of the natural prostaglandins (Bundy *et al.,* 1971; Ford and Fried, 1969; Fried *et al.,* 1969, 1970) 11-Deoxyprostaglandins possess low potency on smooth muscle ($<$5% of $PGE_1$) but 11-deoxy-$PGE_1$ (methyl ester) approaches the activity of $PGE_1$ on blood pressure whereas 11-deoxy F prostaglandins are only weakly active (Pike *et al.,* 1967). Certain 11-deoxyprostaglandins are highly potent inhibitors of gastric secretion, ($\pm$)-11-deoxy-13,14-dihydro-$PGE_1$ in particular having been shown to possess half the activity of natural $PGE_1$ against gastric secretion in the rat (Lippmann, 1969; 1970). The cyclohexane analogues are stated to be active in several biological assays although they are less potent than the natural prostaglandins; details are not yet available (Crossley, 1971).

## REFERENCES

Andersen, N. H. (1969). Preparative thin-layer and column chromatography of prostaglandins. *Journal of Lipid Research,* **10,** 316.

Änggård, E. (1966). The biological activities of three metabolites of prostaglandin $E_1$. *Acta Physiologica Scandinavica,* **66,** 509.

Änggård, E. and Samuelsson, B. (1965). Biosynthesis of prostaglandins from arachidonic acid in guinea-pig lung. *The Journal of Biological Chemistry,* **240,** 3518.

[†] C Prostaglandins have been shown to possess a greater vasodepressor potency than the A series as well as a longer duration of action (Jones, 1972).

Axen, U., Lincoln, F. H. and Thompson, J. L. (1969). A total synthesis of prostaglandin $E_1$ and related substances via *endo*-bicyclohexane intermediates. *Chemical Communications*, 303.

Axen, U., Thompson, J. L. and Pike, J. E. (1970). A total synthesis of (±)-prostaglandin $E_3$ methyl ester via endo-bicyclohexane intermediates. *Chemical Communications*, 602.

Babcock, J. C. and Beal III, P. F. (1967). Process for making prostaglandins and compounds related to prostaglandins. *South African Patent* 66/7385.

Bagli, J. F. and Bogri, T. (1967). Prostaglandins II–An improved synthesis and structural proof of (±)-11-deoxyprostaglandin $F_{1\beta}$. *Tetrahedron Letters*, 5.

Bagli, J. F. and Bogri, T. (1969a). Hypotensive 15-hydroxy-9-oxo-13-prostenoic acid. German Patent, 1,810,824. *Chemical Abstracts*, 71, 70181z.

Bagli, J. F. and Bogri, T. (1969b). Prostaglandins III-(±) 11-deoxy-13,14,dihydroprostaglandin $F_{1\alpha}$ and $F_{1\beta}$–A novel synthesis of prostanoic acids. *Tetrahedron Letters*, 1639.

Bagli, J. F., Bogri, T., Deghenghi, R. and Wiesner, K. (1966). Prostaglandins I–Total synthesis of 9β, 15ξ-dihydroxyprost-13-enoic acid. *Tetrahedron Letters*, 465.

Beal III, P. F., Babcock, J. C. and Lincoln, F. H. (1966). A total synthesis of a natural prostaglandin. *Journal of the American Chemical Society*, 88, 3131.

Beal III, P. F., Babcock, J. C. and Lincoln, F. H. (1967). Synthetic approaches in the prostanoic acid series. Prostaglandins, Proceedings of the Second Nobel Symposium, Stockholm, p. 219. Almqvist and Wiksell, Stockholm.

Beal III, P. F., Lincoln, F. H. and Pike, J. E. (1967). Prostaglandin analogues and processes for preparing them. *South African Patent*, 67/2357.

Beal III, P. F. and Pike, J. E. (1967). Prostanoic acid derivatives and processes for preparing them. *South African Patent*, 66/3600.

Beerthuis, R. K., Nugteren, D. H., Pabon, H. J. J. and Van Dorp, D. A. (1968). Biologically active prostaglandins from some new odd-numbered essential fatty acids. *Recueil des Travaux Chimiques des Pays-Bas*, 87, 461.

Beerthius, R. K., Nugteren, D. H., Pabon, H. J. J., Steenhoek, A. and Van Dorp, D. A. (1971). Synthesis of a series of polyunsaturated fatty acids, their potencies as essential fatty acids and as precursors of prostaglandins. *Recueil des Travaux Chimiques des Pays-Bas*, 90, 943.

Bergström, S., Carlson, L. A. and Orö, L. (1967). A note on the cardiovascular and metabolic effects of prostaglandin $A_1$. *Life Sciences (Oxford)*, 6, Part I, 449.

Bergström, S., Danielsson, H., Klenberg, D. and Samuelsson, B. (1964b). The enzymatic conversion of essential fatty acids into prostaglandins. *The Journal of Biological Chemistry*, 239, PC 4006.

Bergström, S., Danielsson, H. and Samuelsson, B. (1964a). The enzymatic formation of prostaglandin $E_2$ from arachidonic acid. Prostaglandins and related factors 32. *Biochimica et Biophysica Acta*, 90, 207.

Bergström, S., Krabisch, L., Samuelsson, B. and Sjövall, J. (1962). Preparation of prostaglandin F from prostaglandin E. *Acta Chemica Scandinavica*, 16, 969.

Brummer, H. C. (1971). Storage life of prostaglandin $E_2$ in ethanol and saline. *Journal of Pharmacy and Pharmacology*, 23, 804.

Bundy, G., Lincoln, F., Nelson, N., Pike, J. and Schneider, W. (1971). Novel prostaglandin syntheses. *Annals of the New York Academy of Sciences*, 180, 76.

Bygdeman, M. (1967). Studies of the effects of prostaglandins in seminal plasma on human myometrium *in vitro*. Proceedings of the Second Nobel Symposium, Stockholm, p. 71. Almqvist and Wiksell, Stockholm.

Caton, M. P. L. (1971). The Prostaglandins. *Progress in Medicinal Chemistry* (G. P. Ellis and G. B. West, Eds.), Butterworth, London, 8, 317.

Caton, M. P. L., Coffee, E. C. J. and Watkins, G. L. (1972). Prostaglandins—A new total synthesis of (±)-11-deoxyprostaglandins. *Tetrahedron Letters*, 773.

Ciba (1969). Cyclopentyl alkane acids hypotensive. *Netherlands Patent*, 6807186.

Collins, P., Jung, C. J. and Pappo, R. (1968). Prostaglandin studies. The total synthesis of *dl*-prostaglandin $B_1$. *Israel Journal of Chemistry*, 6, 839.

Corey, E. J., Albonico, S. M., Koelliker, U., Schaaf, T. K. and Varma, R. K. (1971b). New reagents for stereoselective carbonyl reduction. An improved synthetic route to the primary prostaglandins. *Journal of the American Chemical Society*, 93, 1491.

Corey, E. J., Andersen, N. H., Carlson, R. M., Paust, J., Vedejs, E., Vlattas, I. and Winter, R. E. K. (1968a). Total synthesis of prostaglandins. Synthesis of the pure *dl*-$E_1$, -$F_{1\alpha}$ -$F_{1\beta}$, -$A_1$, and -$B_1$ hormones. *Journal of the American Chemical Society*, 90, 3245.

Corey, E. J., Arnold, Z. and Hutton, J. (1970b). Total synthesis of prostaglandins $E_2$ and $F_{2\alpha}$(*dl*) via a tricarbocyclic intermediate. *Tetrahedron Letters*, 307.

Corey, E. J. and Grieco, P. A. (1972). A highly efficient route to a key intermediate for the synthesis of A prostaglandins. *Tetrahedron Letters*, 107.

Corey, E. J., Koelliker, U. and Neuffer, J. (1971a). Methoxymethylation of thallous cyclopentadienide. A simplified preparation of a key intermediate for the synthesis of prostaglandins. *Journal of the American Chemical Society*, 93, 1489.

Corey, E. J. and Noyori, R. (1970). A total synthesis of prostaglandin $F_{2\alpha}$(*dl*) from 2-oxabicyclo{3.3.0}oct-6-en-3-one. *Tetrahedron Letters*, 311.

Corey, E. J., Noyori, R. and Schaaf, T. K. (1970a): Total synthesis of prostaglandins $F_{1\alpha}$, $E_1$, $F_{2\alpha}$ and $E_2$ (natural forms) from a common synthetic intermediate. *Journal of the American Chemical Society*, 92, 2586.

Corey, E. J. and Ravindranathan, T. (1971). A simple route to a key intermediate for the synthesis of 11-desoxyprostaglandins. *Tetrahedron Letters*, 4753.

Corey, E. J., Schaaf, T. K., Huber, W., Koelliker, U. and Weinshenker, N. M. (1970c). Total synthesis of prostaglandins $F_{2\alpha}$ and $E_2$ as the naturally occurring forms. *Journal of the American Chemical Society*, 92, 397.

Corey, E. J., Shirahama, H., Yamamoto, H., Terashima, S., Venkateswarlu, A. and Schaaf, T. K. (1971c). Stereospecific total synthesis of prostaglandins $E_3$ and $F_{3\alpha}$. *Journal of the American Chemical Society*, 93, 1490.

Corey, E. J. and Varma, R. K. (1971). Specific reduction of E prostaglandins to $F_\alpha$ prostaglandins and prostaglandin $E_2$ to prostaglandin $E_1$. *Journal of the American Chemical Society*, 93, 7319.

Corey, E. J., Vlattas, I., Andersen, N. H. and Harding, K. (1968b). A new total synthesis of prostaglandins of the $E_1$ and $F_1$ series including 11-epi prostaglandins. *Journal of the American Chemical Society*, 90, 3247.

Corey, E. J., Vlattas, I. and Harding, K. (1969a). Total synthesis of natural (laevo) and enantiomeric (dextro) forms of prostaglandin $E_1$. *Journal of the American Chemical Society*, 91, 535.

Corey, E. J., Weinshenker, N. M., Schaaf, T. K. and Huber, W. (1969b). Stereo-controlled synthesis of prostaglandins $F_{2\alpha}$ and $E_2$ (*dl*). *Journal of the American Chemical Society,* **91**, 5675.

Crossley, N. S. (1971). Cyclohexane analogues of the prostaglandins. *Tetrahedron Letters,* 3327.

Crabbé, P. and Guzmán, A. (1972). Synthesis of 11-desoxyprostaglandins. *Tetrahedron Letters.* 115.

Daniels, E. G., Krueger, W. C., Kupiecki, F. P., Pike, J. E. and Schneider, W. P. (1968). Isolation and characterisation of a new prostaglandin isomer. *Journal of the American Chemical Society,* **90**, 5894.

Daniels, E. G. and Pike, J. E. (1968). Isolation of prostaglandins. Prostaglandin Symposium of the Worcester Foundation for Experimental Biology, p. 379. Interscience, New York.

DuCharme, D. W, and Weeks, J. R. (1967). Cardiovascular pharmacology of prostaglandin $F_{2\alpha}$, a unique pressor agent. Prostaglandins, Proceedings of the Second Nobel Symposium, Stockholm, p. 173. Almqvist and Wiksell, Stockholm.

Ferdinandi, E. S. and Just, G. (1971). A synthesis of *dl*-prostaglandin $E_2$ methyl ester and related compounds. *Canadian Journal of Chemistry,* **49**, 1070.

Finch, N. and Fitt, J. (1969). The synthesis of *dl*-prostaglandin $E_1$ methoxime, *Tetrahedron Letters,* 4639.

Ford, S. H. and Fried, J. (1969). Smooth muscle activity of *rac* -7-oxaprostaglandin $F_{1\alpha}$ and related substances. *Life Sciences,* (Oxford), **8**, part 1, 983.

Fried, J., Heim, S., Etheredge, S. J., Sunder-Plassmann, P., Santhanakrishnan, T. S., Himizu, J. and Lin, C. H. (1968). Synthesis of (±)-7-oxaprostaglandin $F_{1\alpha}$. *Chemical Communications,* 634.

Fried, J., Mehra, M. M., Kao, W. L. and Lin, C. H. (1970). Synthesis of (±)-7-oxaprostaglandin $E_1$. *Tetrahedron Letters,* 2695.

Fried, J., Mehra, M. M. and Kao, W. L. (1971). Synthesis of (+)- and (−)-7-oxaprostaglandin $F_{1\alpha}$ and their 15-epimers. *Journal of the American Chemical Society,* **93**, 5594.

Fried, J., Santhanakrishnan, T. S., Himizu, J., Lin, C. H. and Ford, S. H. (1969). Prostaglandin antagonists: synthesis and smooth muscle activity. *Nature,* **223**, 208.

Granström, E., Lands, W. E. M. and Samuelsson, B. (1968). Biosynthesis of 9α, 15-dihydroxy-11-ketoprost-13-enoic acid. *The Journal of Biological Chemistry,* **243**, 4104.

Hamberg, M. (1968). On the absolute configuration of 19-hydroxy-prostaglandin $B_1$. *European Journal of Biochemistry,* **6**, 147.

Hardegger, E., Schenk, H. P. and Broger, E. (1967). Synthesese der DL-Form eines natürlichen Prostaglandins. *Helvetica Chimica Acta.,* **50**, 2501.

Horton, E. W. and Main, I. H. M. (1965). A comparison of the actions of prostaglandins $F_{2\alpha}$ and $E_1$ on smooth muscle. *British Journal of Pharmacology and Chemotherapy,* **24**, 470.

Horton, E. W. and Main, I. H. M. (1966). The relationship between the chemical structure of the prostaglandins and their biological activity. *Memoirs of the Society for Endocrinology No. 14, Endogenous Substances Affecting the Human Myometrium,* p. 29.

Israelsson, U., Hamberg, M. and Samuelsson, B. (1969). Biosynthesis of 19-hydroxy-prostaglandin $A_1$. *European Journal of Biochemistry,* **11**, 390.

Jones, R. L. (1972). Properties of a new prostaglandin. *British Journal of Pharmacology,* **45**, 144.

Just, G., Simonovitch, C., Lincoln, F. H., Schneider, W. P., Axen, U., Spero, G. B. and Pike, J. E. (1969). A synthesis of prostaglandin $F_{1\alpha}$ and related substances. *Journal of the American Chemical Society,* **91**, 5364.

Karim, S. M. M., Devlin, J. and Hillier, K. (1968). The stability of dilute solutions of prostaglandins $E_1$, $E_2$, $F_{1\alpha}$ and $F_{2\alpha}$. *European Journal of Pharmacology,* **4**, 416.

Katsube, J. and Matsui, M. (1969). Synthetic studies on cyclopentane derivatives, Part I. Alternative routes to *dl*-prostaglandin-$B_1$ and dihydrojasmone. *Agricultural Biological Chemistry (Tokyo),* **33**, 1078.

Kloeze, J. (1969). Relationship between chemical structure and platelet aggregation activity of prostaglandins. *Biochimica et Biophysica Acta.,* **187**, 285.

Klok, R., Pabon, H. J. J. and Van Dorp, D. A. (1968). Synthesis of *dl*-prostaglandin $B_1$ and its reduction product *dl*-prostaglandin $E_1$-237. *Recueil des Travaux Chimiques des Pays-Bas.,* **87**, 813.

Klok, R., Pabon, H. J. J. and Van Dorp, D. A. (1970). Synthesis of 2-(6'-carboxyhexyl)-4-hydroxy-3-(3'-hydroxyoctyl)-1-cyclopentanone (racemic dihydroprostaglandin $E_1$). *Recueil des Travaux Chimiques des Pays-Bas,* **89**, 1043.

Lapidus, M., Grant, N. H. and Alburn, H. E. (1968a). Enzymatic preparation and purification of prostaglandin $E_2$. *Journal of Lipid Research,* **9**, 371.

Lapidus, M., Grant, N. H. and Alburn, H. E. (1968b). Prostaglandin $E_2$: Biosynthesis purification and derivatives. Prostaglandin Symposium of the Worcester Foundation for Experimental Biology, p. 365, Interscience, New York.

Lipmann, W. (1969). Inhibition of gastric acid secretion in the rat by synthetic prostaglandins. *Journal of Pharmacy and Pharmacology,* **21**, 335.

Lipmann, W. (1970). Inhibition of gastric secretion by a potent synthetic prostaglandin. *Journal of Pharmacy and Pharmacology,* **22**, 65.

Miyano, M. (1969). Synthetic studies on prostaglandins II. A novel synthesis of methyl esters of 15-dehydro-$PGB_1$ and PGE 237. *Tetrahedron Letters,* 2771.

Miyano, M. (1970). Prostaglandins III. Synthesis of methyl esters of 15-dehydro-$PGB_1$, 15-dehydro-PGE 237 and *dl*-PGE 237. *Journal of Organic Chemistry,* **35**, 2314.

Miyano, M. and Dorn, C. R. (1969). Total synthesis of 15-dehydro-prostaglandin $E_1$. *Tetrahedron Letters,* 1615.

Nelson (1971). Nouveaux composés de la classe des prostaglandines et leur procédé de preparation. Belgian patent 754, 114.

Nugteren, D. H., Beerthuis, R. K. and Van Dorp, D. A. (1967). Biosynthesis of prostaglandins. Prostaglandins, Proceedings of the Second Nobel Symposium, Stockholm, p. 45, Almqvist and Wiksell, Stockholm.

Nugteren, D. H., Van Dorp, D. A., Bergström, S., Hamberg, M. and Samuelsson, B. (1966). Absolute configuration of the prostaglandins. *Nature,* **212**, 38.

Pike, J. E. (1970). Prostaglandin derivate. Netherlands Patent 1937, 675.

Pike, J. E., Kupiecki, F. P. and Weeks, J. R. (1967). Biological activity of the prostaglandins and related analogs. Prostaglandins, Proceedings of the Second Nobel Symposium, Stockholm, p. 161, Almqvist and Wiksell, Stockholm.

Pike, J. E., Lincoln, F. H. and Schneider, W. P. (1969). Prostanoic acid chemistry. *Journal of Organic Chemistry*, **34**, 3552.

Ramwell, P. W. and Daniels, E. G. (1969). Chromatography of the prostaglandins. *Lipid Chromatographic Analysis* (Ed. G. V. Marinetti), Marcel Decker, New York, **2**, 313.

Ramwell, P. W., Shaw, J. E., Clarke, G. B., Grostic, M. F., Kaiser, D. G. and Pike, J. E. (1968). Prostaglandins. *Progress in Chemistry of Fats and Other Lipids*, **9**, 233.

Ramwell, P. W., Shaw, J. E., Corey, E. J. and Andersen, N. (1969). Biological activity of synthetic prostaglandins. *Nature*, **221**, 1251.

Robert, A., Nezamis, J. E. and Phillips, J. P. (1967). Inhibition of gastric secretion by prostaglandins. *American Journal of Digestive Diseases*, **12**, 1073.

Samuelsson, B. (1965). The prostaglandins, *Angewandte Chemie International Edition in English*, **4**, 410.

Samuelsson, B. (1967). Biosynthesis and metabolism of prostaglandins. *Progress in Biochemical Pharmacology*, **3**, 59.

Schneider, W. P. (1969). The synthesis of (±)-prostaglandins $E_2$, $F_{2\alpha}$ and $F_{2\beta}$, *Chemical Communications*, 304.

Schneider, W. P., Axen, U., Lincoln, F. H., Pike, J. E. and Thompson, J. L. (1968). The total synthesis of prostaglandins. *Journal of the American Chemical Society*, **90**, 5895.

Schneider, W. P., Axen, U., Lincoln, F. H., Pike, J. E. and Thompson, J. L. (1969). The synthesis of prostaglandin $E_1$ and related substances. *Journal of the American Chemical Society*, **91**, 5372.

Sekhar, N. C. (1970). Effect of eight prostaglandins on platelet aggregation. *Journal of Medicinal Chemistry*, **13**, 39.

Sekhar, N. C., Weeks, J. R. and Kupiecki, F. P. (1968). Antithrombotic activity of a new prostaglandin, 8-iso-$PGE_1$. *Circulation*, **38**, Suppl. VI-23.

Shaw, J. E. and Ramwell, P. W. (1969). Separation, identification, and estimation of prostaglandins. *Methods of Biochemical Analysis*, **17**, 325.

Sih, C. J., Ambrus, G., Foss, P. and Lai, C. J. (1969). A general biochemical synthesis of oxygenated prostaglandins E. *Journal of the American Chemical Society*, **91**, 3685.

Sih, C. J., Salomon, R. G., Price, P., Peruzzoti, G. and Sood, R. (1972). Total synthesis of (±)-15-deoxyprostaglandin $E_1$. *Journal of the Chemical Society, Chemical Communications*, 240.

Slates, H. L., Zelawski, Z. S., Taub, D. and Wendler, N. L. (1972). A new stereoselective total synthesis of prostaglandin $E_1$ and its optical antipodes. *Journal of the Chemical Society, Chemical Communications*, 304.

Steinberg, D. and Vaughan, M. (1967). *In vitro* and *in vivo* effects of prostaglandins on free fatty acid metabolism. Prostaglandins, Proceedings of the Second Nobel Symposium, Stockholm, p. 109. Almqvist and Wiksell, Stockholm.

Strike, D. P. and Smith, H. (1970). A novel approach to the synthesis of prostaglandins. *Tetrahedron Letters*, 4393.

Struijk, C. B., Beerthuis, R. K. and Van Dorp, D. A. (1967). Specificity in the enzymatic conversion of poly-unsaturated fatty acids into prostaglandins. Prostaglandins, Proceedings of the Second Nobel Symposium, Stockholm, p. 51, Almqvist and Wiksell, Stockholm.

Struijk, C. B., Beerthuis, R. K., Pabon, H. J. J. and Van Dorp, D. A. (1966). Specificity in the enzymic conversion of polyunsaturated fatty acids into prostaglandins. *Recueil des Travaux Chimiques des Pays-Bas,* **85,** 1233.

Sweatman, W. J. F. and Collier, H. O. J. (1968). Effects of prostaglandins on human bronchial muscle. *Nature,* **217,** 69.

Taub, D., Hoffsommer, R. D., Kuo, C. H., Slates, H. L., Zelawski, Z. S. and Wendler, N. L. (1970). A stereoselective total synthesis of prostaglandin $E_1$. *Chemical Communications,* 1258.

Van Dorp, D. A. Beerthuis, R. K., Nugteren, D. H. and Vonkeman, H. (1964). The biosynthesis of prostaglandins. *Biochimica et Biophysica Acta,* **90,** 204.

Wallach, D. P. (1965). The enzymic conversion of arachidonic acid to prostaglandin $E_2$ with acetone powder preparations of bovine seminal vesicles. *Life Sciences, (Oxford),* **4,** 361.

Weeks, J. R., Sekhar, N. C. and DuCharme, D. W. (1969). Relative activity of prostaglandins $E_1$, $A_1$, $E_2$ and $A_2$ on lipolysis, platelet aggregation, smooth muscle and the cardiovascular system. *Journal of Pharmacy and Pharmacology,* **21,** 103.

Weeks, J. R., Sekhar, N. C. and Kupiecki, F. P. (1968). Pharmacological profile of a new prostaglandin, 8-iso-prostaglandin $E_1$. *Pharmacologist,* **10,** 212.

Weinheimer, A. J. and Spraggins, R. L. (1969). The occurrence of two new prostaglandin derivatives (15-*epi*-$PGA_2$ and its acetate, methyl ester) in the Gorgonian Plexaura Homomalla. *Chemistry of coelenterates XV. Tetrahedron Letters,* **59,** 5185.

Wlodawer, P., Samuelsson, B., Albonico, S. M. and Corey, E. J. (1971). Selective inhibition of prostaglandin synthetase by a bicyclo [2.2.1] heptene derivative. *Journal of the American Chemical Society,* **93,** 2815.

Yura, Y. and Ide, J. (1969). A total synthesis of a *dl*-prostaglandin $B_1$. *Chemical and Pharmaceutical Bulletin (Tokyo),* **17,** 408.

# CHAPTER II

# General Pharmacology of Prostaglandins

Jiro Nakano

Kurzrok and Lieb (1930) first reported that fresh human seminal fluid could cause both relaxation and potent contraction on the isolated human uterine strip. Later, Goldblatt (1933) and von Euler (1934a, 1934b) independently found that human seminal plasma and sheep seminal vesicle contain a potent lipid substance which exerts smooth muscle stimulating and depressor actions. However, thereafter little definitive information on the pharmacology of prostaglandins has been obtained until Bergström and his associates (Bergström and Sjövall, 1957; Bergström, Duner, von Euler, Pernow and Sjövall, 1959a; Bergström, Eliasson, von Euler and Sjövall, 1959b; Bergström, Carlson and Orö, 1964) isolated and synthesized different pure prostaglandins. For the past several years, especially for the last two or three years, great progress has been made on the elucidation of the precise pharmacodynamic and biochemical actions of each prostaglandin as larger quantities of pure prostaglandins became available for experimental and clinical studies. The pharmacological actions of prostaglandins are summarized in Table 1. As seen with vasoactive peptides and biogenic amines, there are considerable species and tissue differences in the pharmacological responses to a given prostaglandin and to different prostaglandins (Bergström, Carlson and Weeks, 1968; Vane, 1969). The purpose of this communication is to review the important developments in the pharmacology of prostaglandins in many species of animals. Because of the phenomenally rapid and extensive progress of the research on the prostaglandins, it is nearly impossible to cite all of the information available on the prostaglandins. The reader should refer to the recent monograms and reviews on prostaglandins for detailed

Table 1
Summary of the pharmacological actions of prostaglandins

---

1. Reproductive system
   *PGE₁ and PGE₂:* Inhibits the motility and tone of the non-pregnant uterus, and increases that of the pregnant uterus.
   *PGF₂ₐ:* Increases the motility and tone of both the non-pregnant and the pregnant uterus. Stimulates steroidogenesis on the corpus luteum *in vitro* but induces luteolysis *in vivo*. Induction of abortion and labour. Antifertility action. Increases tubal and sperm motility.

2. Cardiovascular system
   Positive chronotropic and inotropic actions. Increases cardiac output.
   Increases pulmonary arterial pressure. Increases capillary permeability.
   *PGEs and PGAs:* Decreases systemic arterial pressure and venous pressure.
   Increases coronary and regional arterial blood flow.
   *PGFs:* Increases systemic arterial and venous pressure. Decreases regional arterial blood flow.

3. Respiratory system
   *PGE₁ and PGE₂:* Bronchial dilatation.
   *PGF₂ₐ:* Bronchial constriction.

4. Nervous system
   Induces stupor, catatonia or excitement in some species of animals.
   Pulsating headache. Pyrexia by stimulating hypothalamus. Inhibits spinal reflexes.
   Inhibits noradrenaline release by sympathetic nerve stimulation.

5. Renal system
   Increases blood flow and induces natriuresis and water diuresis.
   Redistribution of blood flow from the outer renal medulla to the renal cortex, thereby antagonizing the elaboration of renin.
   Antagonizes vasopressin. Increases ureter and bladder motility.

6. Gastrointestinal system
   Decreases gastric acidity. Increases gastric and intestinal motility, and may induce vomiting and diarrhoea.

7. Endocrine system and metabolism
   Increases cyclic AMP levels and the secretion of the hormones in different endocrine organs (thyroid, adrenal cortex, ovary and parathyroid). Modulates the cyclic-AMP mediated actions of a variety of hormones or drugs at the target tissues. PGE₁ antagonizes hormone-stimulated lipolysis in adipose tissues. Hyperglycemia.

8. Hematological system
   *PGE₁:* Inhibition of platelet aggregation and adhesiveness and stimulation of platelet adenyl cyclase. Retardation of clot retraction.
   *PGE₂:* Stimulation of platelet aggregation.

9. Eye and nose
   Meiosis. Increases intraocular pressure.
   Decreases the airway resistance in the nasal cavity (vasoconstrictor).

10. Skin
    Hyperemia. Increases permeability. Stimulates epidermal proliferation and keratinization. Releases histamine.

information (Bergström *et al.*, 1968; von Euler and Eliasson, 1967; Horton, 1969; Speroff and Ramwell, 1970a; Ramwell and Shaw, 1970; Bennett and Fleshler, 1970).

## 1. STRUCTURE-ACTIVITY RELATIONSHIPS

Several investigators (Horton and Main, 1963, 1967; Pike, Kupiecki and Weeks, 1967; Weeks, Sekhar and DuCharme, 1969; Kloeze, 1969; Ramwell, Shaw, Corey and Andersen, 1969; Sekhar, 1970; Christ and Nugteren, 1970) have studied the relationship between the chemical structure and the biological activities of different prostaglandins, especially their depressor, smooth muscle stimulant, anti-lipolytic and platelet aggregation inhibitory actions. It should be cautioned that in most *in vivo* studies on the relationship between the structure and the circulatory effects, the effect of intravenously injected prostaglandins on blood pressure was made in anaesthetized rats, guinea pigs, rabbits and dogs. Since some prostaglandins are inactivated in the lungs, it is rather difficult to assess the precise structure-activity relationship in a given system of the intact animal. Recently, for this purpose, the vasoactivity of various prostaglandins injected intraarterially was studied using the dog hind limb preparation (Nakano, 1972a).

In a given biological system, the structure-activity relationship of prostaglandins can be analyzed by comparing the actions of the prototype and the most biologically potent prostaglandin $E_1$ ($PGE_1$) as a standard. The chemical modifications of the three major components of the structure of $PGE_1$, i.e., carboxyl side chain, cyclopentane ring and alkyl side chain can be discussed for this purpose.

### Carboxyl side chain variations

As seen with $PGE_2$ and prostaglandin $A_2$ ($PGA_2$), the unsaturation of C-5 does not modify significantly or increase the anti-lipolytic and vasodilator actions of $PGE_1$ or $PGA_1$ with the exception of the effect on platelet aggregation (Steinberg, Vaughan, Nestel, Strand and Bergström, 1964; Christ and Nugteren, 1970; Nakano, 1972a). The potency of the inhibitory effect of $PGE_1$ and $PGA_1$ on ADP-induced platelet aggregation is markedly greater than that of $PGE_2$ and $PGA_2$, respectively (Weeks *et al.*, 1969; Sekhar, 1970). Furthermore, Kloeze (1967) showed that $PGE_2$ may stimulate platelet aggregation. As seen with $PGE_1$-methyl and -ethyl esters, the esterification of the carboxyl radical in $PGE_1$ reduces slightly the smooth muscle stimulating, depressor and antilipolytic actions of $PGE_1$ (Pike, Kupiecki and Weeks, 1967). Likewise, the replacement of $CH_2$ at 3C with oxygen, as seen with 3-oxa-$PGE_1$, slightly decreases the smooth muscle stimulating action of $PGE_1$ (Bundy, Lincoln, Nelson, Pike and Schnieder, 1971). It appears that 3-oxa-$PGE_1$ is resistant to $\beta$-oxidation in the liver. In contrast, as seen with 7-oxa-$PGE_1$, 7-oxa-$PGF_{1\alpha}$ and 7-oxa-13, 14 prostynoic acid, the replacement of C-5 by an oxygen atom decreases considerably or abolishes the vasodilator and smooth muscle-stimulating actions of $PGE_1$. Furthermore, the non-vascular smooth muscle-stimulating action, adrenocorticoid-producing action, platelet aggregation inhibitory action of $PGE_1$ and $PGE_2$ are competitively or non-competitively antagonized by 7-oxa-13, 14-prostynoic acid (Fried, Santhanakrishnan, Himizar, Lin and Ford, 1969; Fried, Lin, Mehra, Kao and Dalven, 1971; Ramwell and Shaw, 1970), although no such inhibition is noticed with the other nonvascular as well as vascular smooth muscles (Ramwell and Shaw, 1970; Nakano, 1972a). As seen with 8-iso-$PGE_1$, when the entire trans-orientation of the carboxyl side chain of $PGE_1$ is altered to the cis-form relative to the cyclopentane ring plane, the vasodilator, depressor, antilipolytic and smooth muscle stimulating activity of $PGE_1$ are markedly diminished although the platelet inhibitory activity is essentially unimpaired (Weeks *et al.*, 1968; Sekhar, Weeks and Kupiecki, 1968; Nakano and Kessinger, 1970). In addition, 8-iso-$PGE_1$ is a mild vasodilator on the systemic circulation but exerts a vasoconstrictor action on the pulmonary vascular beds in dogs (Nakano and Kessinger, 1970). Recently, Nakano (unpublished data) also found that, as seen with the major urinary metabolites, dinor- or tetranor-$PGE_1$, the shortening of the carboxyl side chain in $PGE_1$ reduces markedly its vasodilator action in dogs. In addition, these metabolites are almost always oxidized at C-15 position and reduced at $\Delta^{13}$ double bond as 15-keto-dihydro-tetranor-$PGE_1$, or 11-hydroxy-11, 15-diketo-$\omega$-carboxy-tetranor prostanoic acid (Samuelsson, 1970; Samuelsson, Granström, Green and Hamberg, 1971), which would abolish completely their cardiovascular actions.

*Cyclopentane ring variations*

It is well established that E and A prostaglandins are powerful vasodilators in many species of animals, whereas $PGF_{1\alpha}$ and $PGF_{2\alpha}$ are moderately potent vasoconstrictor and/or pressor substances in dogs, rats and monkeys (Pike *et al.*, 1967; Nakano and McCurdy, 1967a, 1967b; DuCharme, Weeks and Montgomery, 1968; Weeks *et al.*, 1969; Nakano and Cole, 1969). The presence of a carbonyl group at C-9 must be essential for the vasodilator system and many other biological actions of $PGE_1$ including their effects on platelet aggregation, various smooth muscles and endocrine glands (Pike *et al.*, 1967; Bergström *et al.*, 1968; Kloetze, 1969, Crunkhorn and Willis, 1971; Nakano, 1972b).

Compounds AY-16809, AY-21669 and AY21670, which lack this radical or are replaced by a hydroxyl group at C-9 exert markedly weaker antacid and vasodilator actions than their 9-keto analogues, compounds AY-20524 and AY-22093 in rats and dogs (Lippmann, 1969, 1970; Nakano, 1972a). There are species differences in the vascular response to $PGF_{1\alpha}$ and $PGF_{2\alpha}$. They exert vasoconstrictor and pressor actions in dogs, rats and monkeys, and a vasodilator action in cats and rabbits (Pike *et al.*, 1967; Bergström *et al.*, 1968; DuCharme *et al.*, 1968; Nakano, 1968b; Nakano and Cole, 1969). Sanner, Rozek and Cammarata (1968) observed that the vasodilator and smooth muscle stimulating actions of $PGF_{2\alpha}$ are more potent than those of $PGF_{2\beta}$ in rats, indicating that the biological actions of $PGF_{2\alpha}$ depend significantly on the orientation of the hydroxyl group at C-9. On the other hand, the inhibitory action of $PGF_{1\beta}$ and $PGF_{2\beta}$ on the rat platelet aggregation is practically similar with that of $PGF_{1\alpha}$ and $PGF_{2\alpha}$. As seen with $PGA_1$, $PGA_2$, $PGB_1$, $PGB_2$ and synthetic 11 desoxy-prostaglandins (AY-20524 and AY-22093), the removal of a hydroxyl group at C-11 and formation of $\Delta^{10}$ double bond in the structure of $PGE_1$ and $PGE_2$ significantly reduce the vasodilator, antilipolytic, antacid and smooth muscle stimulating actions of $PGE_1$ and $PGE_2$ (Pike *et al.*, 1967; Robert, Nezamis and Phillips, 1968a; Nakano, Ishii and Gin, 1968b; Nakano, Perry and Denton, 1968c; Weeks *et al.*, 1969; Nakano, 1971, 1972a; Crunkhorn and Willis, 1971). Although the magnitude of the vasodilator action of intraarterially injected $PGA_1$ or $PGA_2$ is slightly smaller than that of intraarterially injected $PGE_1$ or $PGE_2$ in anaesthetized dogs (Nakano, 1968b, 1972a), the magnitude of the vasodilator and depressor actions of intravenously injected $PGA_1$ or $PGA_2$ is generally greater than that of intravenously injected $PGE_1$ or $PGE_2$. Weeks, Sekhar and DuCharme (1969) showed that, in conscious rats and dogs, $PGE_1$, $PGE_2$, $PGA_1$ and $PGA_2$ decrease systemic arterial pressure. $PGA_1$ and $PGA_2$ have an equipotent hypotensive action in rats and dogs, but $PGE_1$ exerts three times more hypotensive action than either $PGA_1$ or $PGA_2$, and ten times than $PGE_2$ in rats. On the other hand, both $PGA_1$ and $PGA_2$ exert 2.5 times more hypotensive action than $PGE_1$, whereas $PGE_1$ is 7-10 times less hypotensive than $PGE_2$ in dogs. Many investigators (Ferreira and Vane, 1967; Vane, 1969; Horton and Jones, 1969; McGiff, Terragno, Strand, Lee, Lonigro and Ng, 1969b) have attributed this difference in the depressor response to a greater metabolic degradation of intravenously injected $PGE_1$ or $PGE_2$ by 15-hydroxy-prostaglandin dehydrogenase (PGDH) in the lungs (Nakano, 1970a, b; Nakano and Prancan, 1971). In the isolated rabbit duodenum, the smooth muscle stimulant action of $PGA_1$ and $PGA_2$ is markedly weaker than that of $PGE_1$ and $PGE_2$ (Weeks *et al.*, 1969; Pike *et al.*, 1967) showed that both $PGB_1$ and $PGB_2$ cause very little or no effect on the systemic arterial pressure and intestinal motility in rats. Since the planar orientation of both the alkyl and the carboxyl side chains has been markedly altered in $PGB_1$ and $PGB_2$, it can be expected that both prostaglandins may exert little or no biological action with the exception of their effects on the thyroid gland (Field, Dekker, Zor and Kaneko, 1971) and skin (Kischer, 1967, 1969).

*Alkyl side chain variations*

One of the most important structural features of prostaglandins is that these fatty acids possess a hydroxyl group at C-15 position. A $PGE_1$ metabolite, 15-keto-$PGE_1$, which lacks a hydroxyl group at C-15 exerts very little or no biological action in dogs and rats (Änggård, 1966; Pike *et al.*, 1967; Nakano, 1971, 1972a). The stereochemical orientation of this hydroxyl group is critical for the biological actions of prostaglandins. Biologically active prostaglandins have a hydroxyl group at C-15 in the S-orientation by the conversion rule proposed by Cahn, Ingold and Prelog (1956). Ramwell *et al.* (1969) and Nakano (1970b, 1972a) found that $PGE_1$ (15-S-$PGE_1$), $PGA_1$ (15-S-$PGE_1$) and $PGA_2$ (15-S-$PGA_2$) are very potent vasodilator and depressor as well as smooth muscle stimulant agents, whereas their epimers, 15-R-$PGE_1$, 15-R-$PGA_1$ and 15-R-$PGA_2$, are very feeble pharmacological agents and do not exert vasodilator and smooth muscle stimulating actions in anesthetized rats and dogs and the isolated intestine and uterus. These observations suggest the receptor sites in the vascular smooth muscle for prostaglandins are stereospecific for their intrinsic action. It is of interest that, 15-hydroxy-prostaglandin dehydrogenase also has a similar stereospecificity for its substrates (Nakano, Änggård, Samuelsson, 1969; Shio, Plasse and Ramwell, 1970; Marrazzi and Matschinsky, 1971). $PGE_1$ (15-S-$PGE_1$) is the best substrate for this enzyme whereas its epimer 15-R-$PGE_1$, is not a substrate but an inhibitor for this enzyme with $PGE_1$ as a substrate *in vitro*. Recently, Bundy *et al.* (1971) showed that 15-methyl-$PGA_2$ and 15-methyl-$PGE_2$ are resistant to 15-hydroxy prostaglandin dehydrogenase (PGDH) but retain considerable biological actions. As seen with 19-hydroxy-$PGA_1$, hydroxylation of C-19 in $PGA_1$ significantly diminishes the depressor and smooth muscle stimulating actions of $PGA_1$ (Horton and Jones, 1969). Very feeble depressor activity observed with 19-hydroxy-$PGB_1$ is not due to its hydroxylation at C-19 but mostly to the structure of $PGB_1$ itself as mentioned above. As seen with $\omega$-nor-$PGE_1$, $\omega$-nor-$PGE_2$ and $\omega$-dinor-$PGE_2$, the shortening of the alkyl side chains of $PGE_1$ or $PGE_2$ also markedly reduces the antilipolytic action whereas its elongation ($\omega$-homo-$PGE_1$ and $\omega$-dihomo-$PGE_1$) has little change in the action (Böhle and May, 1968; Christ and Nugteren, 1970). Recently, large numbers of rac- and ent-$PGE_1$, -$PGA_1$ and $PGF_{1\alpha}$ were synthesized by

Corey *et al.* (see Ramwell *et al.* 1969). It has been shown that these analogues have very feeble or no biological actions in anaesthetized rats or isolated rat uterus, and guinea pig and rabbit intestines, as compared to natural or optically pure $PGE_1$, $PGA_1$ and $PGF_{1\alpha}$ (Ramwell *et al.,* 1969; Lippmann, 1969).

## 2. CELLULAR AND SUBCELLULAR MECHANISMS OF THE ACTIONS OF PROSTAGLANDINS

Prostaglandins have a large variety of biological actions in various systems of the body. Furthermore, different prostaglandins exert variable or sometimes opposite biological effects in the same system. Hence, it is difficult to establish a unitarian mechanism responsible for the actions of prostaglandins in different tissues. Although many hypotheses have been postulated (Bergström *et al.,* 1968; Horton, 1969), the precise physiological roles of prostaglandins in different systems remain controversial. The biological actions of prostaglandins appear to be closely associated with those of various hormones in the body. Several workers (Coceani, Pace-Asciak and Wolfe, 1968; Vogt, Meyer, Kunze, Luffte and Babilli, 1969; Änggård, 1970; Ramwell and Shaw, 1970; Kunze and Vogt, 1971) have suggested that as the circulating hormones and nerve action potentials reach the regional cell membranes and exert their biological actions, the phospholipase in the membranes are simultaneously activated to cleave the phospholipids to release polyunsaturated fatty acids, arachidonic acid and linolenic acid. These precursors of prostaglandins are converted by prostaglandin synthetase in the cell membranes to form prostaglandins (Samuelsson, 1970; Samuelsson *et al.,* 1971). Thus, it has been postulated that on nerve or hormonal stimulations prostaglandins play a role of a negative feed back mechanism in the peripheral tissues, such as adipose tissue (Ramwell and Shaw, 1969), stomach (Coceani and Wolfe, 1966; Horton, 1969) and CNS (Horton, 1969) and vascular smooth muscle (Hedqvist, 1970).

It has been observed that the electrolytes, especially, $Ca^{++}$, $Na^+$ and $K^+$, are very important for the biological actions of prostaglandins. The effects of prostaglandins on alimentary and reproductive smooth muscle, heart, vascular smooth muscle, CNS and hormonal target tissues could be linked to their ability to displace membrane $Ca^{++}$ (Bergström *et al.,* 1968; Horton, 1969; Ramwell and Shaw, 1970). In addition, the biological actions of prostaglandins are closely coupled with the activity of the cyclic AMP (second messenger) system in the body (Bergström *et al.,* 1968; Horton, 1969; Ramwell and Shaw, 1970). Both hormones and prostaglandins act on the adenyl cyclase system in the cell membranes, and modulate the biological actions in certain tissues. Since the close interrelation between prostaglandins and $Ca^{++}$ on the cyclic AMP system has been confirmed in certain homogenous tissues such as fat cells (Butcher and Baird, 1969; Fain, 1968b), platelets (Wolfe and Shulman, 1970; Marquis, Becker and Vigdahl, 1970) and frog skin (Fassina, Carpenedo and Santi, 1969; Ramwell and Shaw, 1970), rapid progress has been made on the better understanding of the sub-cellular mechanism of the prostaglandin actions at least in these tissues. However, a complexity of this problem requires more experimental observations to unify the theories. The interrelationship between the actions of prostaglandins and cyclic AMP system are discussed in Chapter IV.

## 3. SYSTEMIC ACTIONS OF PROSTAGLANDINS

The actions of the prostaglandins on the respiratory and gastro-intestinal systems are not considered here but are discussed in Chapters VII and VIII respectively.

### REPRODUCTIVE SYSTEM

It is well established that different prostaglandins are synthesized in the male and female reproductive organs including seminal vesicles, testicle, prostate, uterus and placenta. They are present in seminal plasma, menstrual fluid, utero-ovarian venous blood and amniotic fluid of human and many other species of animals (Karim, 1966; Bergström *et al.,* 1968; Speroff and Ramwell, 1970a). It is tempting to assume that naturally occurring prostaglandins may play physiological and pathophysiological roles in the reproductive organs. Several attractive hypotheses for physiological functions of prostaglandins have been postulated, but more definitive studies should be made to prove their validity.

**Actions on the uterus**

Since pure prostaglandins became available, extensive studies have been made on the motility and reactive pattern of the myometrium in responses to the prostaglandins in many species of animals including man at different stages of the reproductive cycle. Both E and F prostaglandins contract isolated uteri of rats and guinea pigs (Bergström, Duner, von Euler, Pernow and Sjövall, 1959a; Eliasson, 1959; Horton and Main, 1963, 1965; Ramwell and Shaw, 1966; Sullivan, 1966). In the guinea-pig uterus, the potency of the stimulant effect of $PGE_1$ and $PGE_2$ is greater than that of $PGF_{2\alpha}$ (Bergström *et al.,* 1959b; Sullivan, 1966). As seen in Fig. 1, all three PGE compounds decrease the tonus, frequency and amplitude of the spontaneous contractions of isolated, non-pregnant human uterine strips (Bygdeman and Eliasson, 1963b; Pickles and Hall, 1963; Sandberg, Ingelman-Sundberg and Ryden, 1963, 1964; Bygdeman,

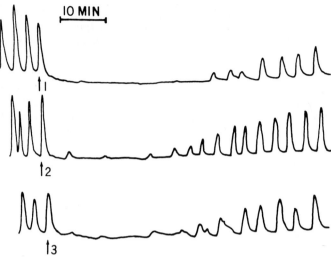

Fig. 1. Effect of $PGE_1$, $PGE_2$ and $PGE_3$ on human isolated myometrium. The strips are from an uterus in the middle secretory phase; $1 = PGE_1$ (30 ng/ml); $2 = PGE_2$ (30 ng/ml); $3 = PGE_3$ (30 ng/ml). Reproduced from Bygdeman and Eliasson (1963b) with permission of the authors and publishers.

1964). Human semen (predominantly E compounds) inhibits the spontaneous motility of isolated non-pregnant human myometrium (Kurzrok and Lieb, 1930; Cockrill, Miller and Kurzrok, 1935; Eliasson, 1959). The two main prostaglandins in human endometrium and menstrual fluid are $PGE_2$ and $PGF_{2\alpha}$ with the latter being the principal compound (Eglinton, Raphael, Smith, Hall and Pickles, 1963). $PGF_{1\alpha}$ and $PGF_{2\alpha}$ always stimulate both tone and amplitude of the myometrium (Pickles and Hall, 1963; Bygdeman and Eliasson, 1963a; Bygdeman, 1964; Sandberg, Ingelman-Sundberg and Ryden, 1965; Bygdeman and Hamberg, 1967). In the isolated nonpregnant human cervix, $PGE_2$ causes a marked relaxation while the effect of $PGF_{2\alpha}$ is variable (Najak, Hillier and Karim, 1970). PGA, PGB and 19-hydroxy-lated compounds exert an inhibitory action similar to PGE compounds but require higher concentrations (Bygdeman and Hamberg, 1967). In mixtures, the effect of the compounds are additive, and PGA- and PGB-compounds, and their hydroxylated compounds may make an appreciable contribution to the total effect of the human seminal plasma (Bygdeman and Hamberg, 1967).

The sensitivity of isolated human myometrial strips to prostaglandins is influenced by the menstrual cycle and thereby the hormonal state of individuals. Isolated human myometrial strips are 3- to 5 times more sensitive to $PGE_1$ at mid-cycle near ovulation time (Bygdeman and Eliasson, 1963a; Sandberg *et al.,* 1963; Bygdeman, 1964). In contrast, uterine strips are more sensitive to $PGF_{2\alpha}$ just before menstruation and during pregnancy (Pickles, 1959; Eglinton *et al.*, 1963; Bygdeman, 1964; Pickles, Hall, Best and Smith, 1965). *In vitro*, addition of progesterone depresses the responsiveness of both guinea pig and rat uterus to $PGE_1$ and $PGF_{2\alpha}$ (Sullivan, 1966). On the other hand, treatment of the animal with oestrogen or combined oestrogen and progesterone has been reported to have little effect (Eliasson, 1966; Sullivan, 1966) or to increase (Änggård and Bergström, 1963) or decrease (Pickles, Hall, Glegg and Sullivan, 1966); the sensitivity of the isolated uterus to prostaglandins. Hawkins, Jessup and Ramwell (1968) showed that all prostaglandins tested contract the isolated uterus from adrenalecto-mized-ovariectomized rats. However, pre-treatment of the rats with oestrogen, and to a lesser extent, progesterone, reduced the responsiveness of the tissues. Ovarian hormones added directly to the medium either inhibit or have no effect on oxytocic substances (Hawkins *et al.*, 1968).

The sensitivity of human myometrium is also influenced by oestrogen and progesterone *in vitro* (Bygdeman, 1964). Progesterone and/or oestradiol decrease the response to $PGE_1$ at mid-cycle. The effect of prostaglandins on human myometrial strips is decreased in specimens obtained from post-menopausal women (Bygdeman, 1964; Bygdeman and Eliasson, 1963a). The increased sensitivity of human myometrium at ovulation may be related to a physiological role for prostaglandins at coitus since uterine motility is inhibited by coitus (Bickers and Main, 1941). It has been postulated that the inhibitory effects of $PGE_1$ and $PGE_2$ in semen on human myometrium at the time of ovulation may facilitate sperm migration and/or play a role in captivation and fertilization of the ova.

Both E and F prostaglandins, applied to a guinea pig myometrium in sub-threshold amounts, diminish the effects of catecholamines (Clegg, 1966; Clegg, Hall and Pickles, 1966). Furthermore, the action of $PGE_1$ on the rat uterine horn is not abolished by cholinergic, adrenergic, histamine or serotonin antagonists (Paton and Daniel, 1967). Therefore, $PGE_1$ does not appear to produce contractions in the rat uterus by releasing noradrenaline, acetylcholine, histamine and serotonin. Neither vasopressin nor oxytocin influences the effect of $PGE_1$ on the isolated human myometrial strip (Eliasson, 1966). The effects of $PGE_1$ and $PGF_{1\alpha}$ on isolated human myometrium at mid-cycle can be changed by changes in the extra-cellular (bath fluid) $Ca^{++}$ and $K^+$ concentration (Bygdeman, 1964). A decreased concentration of $Ca^{++}$ increases the inhibitory effect of $PGE_1$ at mid-cycle. The inhibitory effect of $PGE_1$ is enhanced at low $K^+$ levels, while the sensitivity to the stimulatory effect of $PGF_{1\alpha}$ is increased at high potassium concentrations, suggesting a relationship between prostaglandins and membrane potential.

*In vivo*

PGE$_1$ (1 µg/kg) injected intravenously contracts guinea pig uteri but has no effect on cat and rat uteri (Eliasson, 1959; Berti, Lentati and Usardi, 1965). Various results have been reported for rabbit uteri (Asplund, 1947; Berti *et al.,* 1965; Eliasson, 1959; Horton and Main, 1965). In pregnant women, Bygdeman, Kwon and Wiqvist (1967) found that intravenous infusions of PGE$_1$ (0.6 µg/min or more) increase the amplitude and frequency of uterine contraction. Either stimulation or stimulation followed by inhibition of the non-pregnant human uterus is obtained after introducing human seminal fluid or its extract (HSF-PG) into the vagina (Cockrill *et al.,* 1935; Karlson, 1959; Eliasson and Posse, 1960). Likewise HSF-PG consistently inhibited uterine motility during intravenous infusion of posterior pituitary hormones. PGE$_1$ and PGE$_2$ infused intravenously increase the uterine motility in pregnant women (14-22 weeks). A low dose (4 µg/min or less) of PGE$_1$ increases tonus and contractile activity without inhibiting motility. Similar but less pronounced effects are obtained with PGF$_{2\alpha}$. On the other hand, the intravenous infusion of PGF$_{1\alpha}$, PGF$_{1\beta}$ and PGA$_1$ have no effect on motility, although much larger doses than of PGE$_1$ are given (Bygdeman *et al.,* 1967). Usually, the doses that exert the stimulant action on uterine motility are below the doses that cause a demonstrable fall in blood pressure.

In order to study a possible role of prostaglandins on fertility, Eliasson and Posse (1960) introduced prostaglandins into the posterior fornix of 8 normal fertile women volunteers, in amounts corresponding to those usually found in ejaculates. During menstruation and in the proliferative and secretory phases, prostaglandins had little effect whereas, at the time of ovulation, prostaglandins increased uterine activity which was followed by inhibition. This is attributed to a gradual increase in blood or tissue concentration, producing stimulation at low dosage and inhibition at high dosage as with *in vitro* experiments (Eliasson, 1959). In an attempt to mimic conditions during coitus, a slow continuous infusion of oxytocin was carried out in women at mid-cycle. During this period, simultaneous intravenous infusion of prostaglandins caused the initial stimulation followed by inhibition. Hence, Eliasson (1959) and Eliasson and Posse (1960) suggested that this inhibitory actions of prostaglandins *in vivo* may play a role in facilitating sperm migration.

*Pregnant Uterus*

In uterine strips obtained at Caesarean section, Embry and Morrison (1968) showed that both PGE$_2$ and PGF$_{2\alpha}$ contract the upper segment myometrium but are relatively inactive on lower segment strips. This stimulatory response of the pregnant uterus to PGE$_2$ contrasts with the usual inhibitory response to E compounds in the non-pregnant uterus.

$PGF_{2\alpha}$ interrupts early stages of pregnancy in rhesus monkeys (Kirton, Pharriss and Forbes, 1970; Kirton, Duncan, Oesterling and Forbes, 1971) (Fig. 2) and rodents (Gutknecht, Cornette and Pharris, 1969; Gutknecht, Wyngarden and Pharris, 1971). Kirton *et al.* (1970, 1971) subsequently reported that both $PGE_2$ and $PGF_{2\alpha}$ terminate pregnancy when administered to monkeys either subcutaneously or intravenously

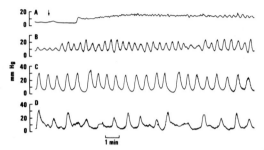

Fig. 2. Uterine contractility recorded following subcutaneous injection (2 mg) at a vertical arrow, (B) 20 min, (C) 40 min and (D) 240 min after drug application. Reproduced from Kirton *et al.* (1971) with permission of the authors and publisher.

between 30 and 41 days after conception. Increased uterine tonus and contractions of about 60 mm Hg occur at a frequency of three per min within 10 min after starting an infusion of $PGF_{2\alpha}$ (60 $\mu$g/min) or $PGE_2$ (8 $\mu$g/min). Plasma progestin concentrations decline 24-48 hr after initial administration. Fuchs, Prieto and Marcus (1971) showed that in pregnant rhesus monkeys at near term or in the mid-trimester, the intravenous infusion of $PGF_{2\alpha}$ (12.5-50 $\mu$g/min) or $PGE_2$ (2-9.5 $\mu$g/min) markedly increases uterine activity and labour-like pattern of contraction, but fails to produce abortion or delivery for 18 hrs.

### Actions on the placenta and umbilical cord

Karim and Devlin (1967) and Karim (1966) have identified four prostaglandins in human amniotic fluid obtained during normal labour and during spontaneous abortion. The concentrations of prostaglandins in amniotic fluid, placental vessels, umbilical cord and maternal uterine venous blood seem to be related to labour (Karim, 1967; Karim and Devlin, 1967). The concentrations of prostaglandins increased with the progression of labour. $PGE_2$, $PGF_{1\alpha}$ and $PGF_{2\alpha}$ each caused contraction of the isolated umbilical artery at term, but $PGE_1$ caused dilation (Hillier and Karim, 1968). Contraction of the arterial smooth muscle was caused by a mixture of all four prostaglandins in the same proportion in which they were present in the cord although specimens obtained early in gestation generally did not respond. A striking correlation between $PGF_{2\alpha}$ concentration and the contraction was noted. It has been demonstrated that neural fibers in the human umbilical cord give off branches to form a plexus in the walls of the umbilical vessels. Hence, it is tempting to speculate that a relationship exists between prostaglandins, neural activity in the umbilical cord, and the important changes which occur in the umbilical vessels at birth.

## Actions on the Fallopian tubes

*In vitro*

Sandberg, Ingelman-Sundberg, Lindgren and Ryden (1962) and Sandberg *et al.*, 1963, 1964, 1965) studied the effect of prostaglandins on the human Fallopian tube by dividing its longitudinal muscle into four equal parts. As seen in Fig. 3, $PGE_1$ caused contraction in the segment proximal to the uterus and relaxation in the distal three segments, regardless of the phase of the cycle (Sandberg *et al.*, 1963). $PGE_2$ increased the tone and maximum amplitude of the proximal segment and relaxed the remaining segments. The stimulatory effect was more pronounced in the secretory phase. $PGE_2$ inhibited all four segments in both proliferative and secretory phases (Sandberg *et al.*, 1964). $PGF_{2\alpha}$

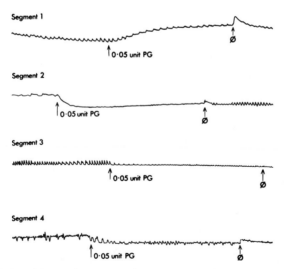

Fig. 3. Effect of prostaglandin $E_1$ on the longitudinal musculature of four segments from the human Fallopian tube in the ovulatory phase. Reproduced from Sandberg *et al.* (1963) with permission of the authors and publisher.

induced a potent contraction in all segments of tubes even greater than its effect on uterine muscle (Sandberg *et al.,* 1965). $PGF_{1\alpha}$ also stimulated all four segments, but had a greater effect on the proximal segment. $PGF_{1\beta}$ caused a feeble contraction whereas $PGF_{2\beta}$ had a weak relaxing effect (Sandberg *et al.,* 1965). The E compounds were generally less effective than the F compounds. However, the effects of $PGE_1$ and $PGE_2$, i.e., contraction of the proximal segment and relaxation of the rest of the tube may have physiological significance since both $PGE_1$ and $PGE_2$ are predominant in human semen. Sandberg *et al.* (1962-1965) proposed that seminal prostaglandins might function to retain the ovum in the Fallopian tube to allow fertilization. In the isolated human tube, Zetler and Wiechell (1969) found that the magnitude of the contractile action of $PGF_{2\alpha}$ is considerably smaller than that of eledoisin, physalaemin and substance P but more potent than that of serotonin, histamine or acetylcholine.

*In vivo*

In rabbits, intravenous $PGE_1$ causes relaxation of the isthmic circular muscles and thereby reduces the opening pressure (Asplund, 1947; Brundin, 1968). $PGF_{1\alpha}$ and $PGF_{2\alpha}$ stimulate the rabbit Fallopian tube *in vivo* (Horton and Main, 1963, 1965). Intravenous or intravaginal administration of $PGE_1$ and $PGE_2$ reduces spontaneous contractions of the oviduct in the rabbit (Horton, Main and Thompson, 1965). Similar effects are obtained in pithed and with *in vitro* preparations, suggesting their direct effect on the tube. It is not certain, however, whether this is a physiological mechanism in the rabbit since the prostaglandin content of semen in this species is barely detectable. In sheep, in which the semen is rich in prostaglandins, intravenous or intraaortic administration of crude prostaglandin stimulates the oviduct of some animals but relaxes others (Horton and Main, 1965). The intravaginal threshold dose for an effect in the ewe oviduct is four times the total prostaglandin content present in a single ram ejaculate.

In Rubin's test (tubal insufflation) performed in women at mid-cycle, Eliasson and Posse (1965) showed that prostaglandins administered intravaginally have increased intratubal pressure. However, Hawkins (1968) has not been able to confirm this observation, and in fact has shown a fall in pressure in two patients. Nutting and Cammarata (1969) showed *in vivo* that subcutaneous administration of prostaglandins in pharmacological doses may delay transportation of the fertilized ovum through the rat oviduct thus producing an antifertility effect. This is demonstrated by obtaining blastocysts from oviductal and uterine washings on day seven of pregnancy. In the rabbit, electrical stimulation of the hypogastric nerve causes constriction in the uterine part of the oviduct. Brundin (1968) found that the intravenous administration of $PGE_1$ causes an inhibition of this response. After administration of $PGE_1$ there is a decreased response to noradrenaline, suggesting that the $PGE_1$ is involved in inhibition of adrenergic neural activity.

## Actions on the ovary

Although small amounts of prostaglandin-like material have been known to be present in the ovaries of cows and sheep (von Euler, 1936) and the possible correlation between prostaglandins and fertility has been suggested (Asplund, 1947), attention has been focused on the actions of prostaglandins on the ovary only recently because of their possible therapeutic use as luteolytic and antifertility agents. The development of the corpus luteum is known to be controlled by pituitary hormones, but the mechanism responsible for regression of the corpus luteum when pregnancy does not occur remains obscure. It has been suggested that an uncharacterized factor, luteolysin, is produced by the uterus. The search for luteolysin has been stimulated by the observation of an apparent luteolytic effect of the uterus in many mammals other than primates and marsupials (Fisher, 1967). For instance, in the rat, hamster and rabbit with a bicornate uterus, hemi-hysterectomy during pseudopregnancy results in a prolonged life-span of the ipsilateral corpus luteum. In the guinea pig, sheep, pig and cow, hysterectomy extends the normal oestrus cycle to apparently that of gestation. Neill, Johansson and Knobil (1969) showed that hysterectomy in rhesus monkeys does not lengthen ovulatory cycles. In pseudopregnant rats, $PGF_{2\alpha}$ given subcutaneously shortens the mean length of pseudopregnancy to seven days from a normal of 14 days (Pharriss and Wyngarden, 1969). Likewise, Gutknecht *et al.* (1971) showed that in pregnant hamsters, $PGF_{2\alpha}$ decreases both plasma and ovarian progesterone levels (Fig. 4). Subcutaneous injection of $PGA_2$ or $PGF_{2\beta}$ and intravenous injection of $PGE_1$ up to toxic levels are all without effect on the life-span of the corpus luteum. $PGF_{2\alpha}$, therefore, appears to exert a luteolytic action in the rat *in vivo.* Furthermore, when $PGF_{2\alpha}$ (1 mg/kg/day) is infused into the uterus or the right heart of pseudopregnant rats on days 5 and 6 of pseudopregnancy, progesterone levels are decreased and concentrations of its metabolite, 20α-dihydro-progesterone (20α-OHP), are increased in the ovaries of these rats. The pseudopregnant rat ovary produces primarily two steroids, progesterone and 20α-OHP, and a shift from progesterone production to 20α-OHP production has been reported to be one of the earliest signs of corpus luteum degeneration (Lindner and Zmigrod, 1967). This decrease in progesterone synthesis and secretion in the ovaries may be the

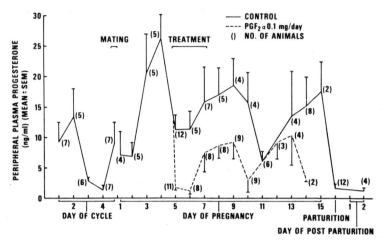

Fig. 4. Effect of $PGF_{2\alpha}$ on peripheral plasma progesterone levels in pregnant hamsters. Reproduced from Gutknecht *et al.* (1971) with permission of the authors and publisher.

mechanism by which $PGF_{2\alpha}$ terminates pseudopregnancy in rats. The biochemical mode of the action of the decreased progesterone synthesis by $PGF_{2\alpha}$ *in vivo* has been studied intensively but remains controversial. The pituitary does not seem to be involved because $PGF_{2\alpha}$ decreases the ratio of ovarian progesterone to its metabolite when pseudopregnancy is maintained in hypophysectomized rats by prolactin administration. Furthermore, $PGF_{2\alpha}$ (2 mg/day for 5 days) does not alter the pituitary LH content in rats (Pharriss *et al.*, 1968). Blatchley and Donovan (1969) also found that $PGF_{2\alpha}$ is luteolytic in the guinea pig, and that this effect does not require the presence of the uterus. In hysterectomized guinea pigs, the intraperitoneal injection of $PGF_{2\alpha}$ (0.5 mg twice a day for 7 days) increases a marked regression of corpus luteum. The question has been raised whether $PGF_{2\alpha}$ may exert a direct toxic effect on pseudopregnant rat ovaries. However, addition of $PGF_{2\alpha}$ to rat ovaries incubated *in vitro* does not decrease the rate of progesterone synthesis. Contrarily, $PGF_{2\alpha}$ is found to produce a dose-dependent increase in steroidogenesis in rats and cows (Pharriss *et al.*, 1968). On the other hand, Bedwani and Horton (1968) showed that during incubation of rabbit ovaries with $PGE_1$ and $PGE_2$, there is no consistent increase in ovarian steroidogenesis except for a substantial potentiation of the production of 20α-OHP in incubations with $PGE_2$ and gonadotropins in five out of six experiments. E and F prostaglandins are present in the bovine ovary, but only F activity is detectable in the bovine corpus luteum (Speroff and Ramwell, 1970a). Prostaglandins are apparently absent from human, rabbit, and bovine follicular fluid. $PGE_1$, $PGE_2$,

$PGF_{2\alpha}$ and $PGA_1$ stimulate steroidogenesis in bovine corpus luteum slices *in vitro* (Speroff and Ramwell, 1970a). The stimulatory action of $PGE_2$ on ovarian steroidogenesis is abolished by cyclohexamide. Marsh (1970, 1971), Kuehl, Humes, Tarnoff, Cirillo and Ham (1970a) also found that the stimulatory effect of LH, $PGF_{2\alpha}$, $PGE_1$ and $PGE_2$ on progesterone synthesis *in vitro* is coupled with that of adenyl cyclase activity and with the increased cyclic AMP levels in the ovarian homogenates, suggesting that prostaglandin-induced steroidogenesis is mediated by cyclic AMP *in vitro*. These effects of prostaglandins on the mouse ovary are competitively inhibited by the prostaglandin antagonist, 7-oxa-13-prostynoic acid (Kuehl *et al.*, 1970a).

The observations on the actions of prostaglandins on the ovaries seem to be paradoxical, i.e., stimulatory effect of $PGF_{2\alpha}$ *in vitro* and the inhibitory effect *in vivo* on progesterone synthesis. At least, these data exclude the toxic effect of $PGF_{2\alpha}$ on the ovaries *in vivo*, and hence, support the concept of an indirect mechanism for local luteal control by uterine tissue and an indirect effect of $PGF_{2\alpha}$ on the ovary. Since all animals which exhibit a local influence of the uterus on the corpus luteum also have a common venous pathway shared by the ovary and the nearby uterine horn, a substance which exerts a local venoconstrictive effect could regulate ovarian blood flow. Previously, DuCharme *et al.* (1968) showed that in the dog $PGF_{2\alpha}$ produces venous constriction. Pharriss (1970) suggested that restriction of venous outflow from the ovary by $PGF_{2\alpha}$ might lead to relative ovarian ischemia, limitation of substrates for progesterone synthesis and/or accumulation of metabolites. The concentrations of $PGF_{2\alpha}$ in endometrium seem to be synchronized with the activity of the corpus luteum, i.e., it is present in secretory endometrium in greater concentrations than in proliferative endometrium (Pickles and Hall, 1963; Pickles *et al.*, 1966). Pharriss (1970, 1971) confirmed his hypothesis by observing that $PGF_{2\alpha}$ reduces the blood flow in the utero-ovarian vein of rats and rabbits (Fig. 5). In hysterectomized guinea pigs however, Blatchley and Donovan (1969) showed that $PGF_{2\alpha}$ (1 mg daily for 7 days) induces an advanced regression of corpus luteum without any adverse histological effects on follicular development. This suggests no reduction in ovarian blood flow, although the precise sensitivity of the follicle and the corpus luteum to a reduction in ovarian blood flow is not known. Recently, contrary to the observations made by Pharriss, Cornette and Gutknecht (1970), MacCracken, Glew and Scaramuzzi (1970) and Behrman, Yoshinaga and Greep (1971) found that $PGF_{2\alpha}$ decreases progesterone secretion without changing the ovarian blood flow in rats. Although there is tissue specificity in the microcirculatory effect of many pharmacological agents, the hypothesis of Pharriss *et al.* appears to be a rather over-simplified one for such a complicated phenomenon as the

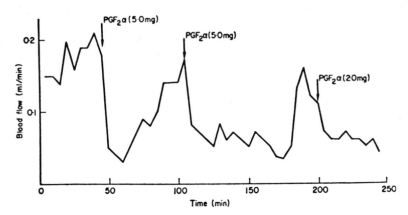

Fig. 5. Effect of intravenous injection of PGF$_{2\alpha}$ or vehicle on uteroovarian vein blood flow in the rat. Reproduced from Pharriss (1970) with permission of the author and publisher.

modulation of steroidogenesis. Very recently, McCracken (1971) found that the radioactive PGF$_{2\alpha}$ injected into the uterine vein is found to concentrate several fold in the ovarian artery. This indicates that a selective counter current transport of a luteolytic factor or PGF$_{2\alpha}$ released from the uterus takes place between the utero-ovarian vein and the ovarian artery. This is further evidenced by the observations that complete surgical separation of the ovarian artery from the surface of the utero-ovarian vein prevents luteal regression in all ewes.

### Antifertility Action

As discussed before, Nutting and Cammarata (1969) showed that in rats the subcutaneous injection of prostaglandin mixtures (predominantly either PGE$_2$ or PGF$_{2\alpha}$, 1 mg/day) on each of the first six to seven days of pregnancy produces inhibition of the implantations or its delay and tardy arrival of fertilized ova into the uterus or early reabsorption of the implantation. Prostaglandins, therefore, seem to exert an antifertility action, possibly by delaying nidation and/or an indirect or direct effect on the implantation site. The mixture containing predominantly PGE$_2$ exerts the same luteolytic effect as the mixture containing PGF$_{2\alpha}$ *in vivo* in the pseudopregnant rat, whereas PGE$_1$ has no such effect (Pharriss and Wyngarden, 1969). Because of the relatively large doses involved, side effects such as defoecation and signs of central nervous system disturbance occur in the animals, developing five minutes after injection and lasting three to four hours.

Since progesterone from a persistent corpus luteum is necessary for maintenance of early pregnancy, early regression of the corpus luteum would prevent nidation of fertilized ova and establishment of pregnancy. In rhesus monkeys Kirton *et al.* (1970, 1971) showed that $PGF_{2\alpha}$ (30 mg/day) given subcutaneously for five days starting on day 11 after ovulation markedly reduces circulating progestin levels. This effect is rapid, initiating menses on the second, third and fourth day of $PGF_{2\alpha}$ administration. However, no antifertility effect is observed in animals in which $PGF_{2\alpha}$ administration starts earlier in the luteal phase (on day 7 after ovulation). When $PGF_{2\alpha}$ is given at appropriate times after mating, it either prevents or reduces the incidence of pregnancy and plasma ovarian progesterone levels in rats, rabbits and hamsters (Gutknecht *et al.*, 1969; Gutknecht, *et al.*, 1971) and monkeys (Kirton *et al.*, 1970). Exogenous progesterone (medroxy-progesterone acetate) protects rats against the antinidatory action of $PGF_{2\alpha}$ (Gutknecht *et al.*, 1969) presumably because it replaces the progesterone which is lost by the regression of the corpus luteum. Early pregnancy in the monkey is associated with a sustained elevation of plasma progesterone. Wiqvist and Bygdeman (1970) reported that in non-pregnant women, vigorous uterine contractions and menstrual-like bleeding may be induced during the secretory phase of the cycle by infusion of $PGF_{2\alpha}$. The 18th to 19th day of the cycle, when implantation of the blastocyst takes place, or 2-4 days following the first missed menstrual period might even be more vulnerable periods to prostaglandin administration than later stages of pregnancy.

The therapeutic applications of the prostaglandins on the human reproductive system are discussed in detail in Chapter V.

## CARDIOVASCULAR SYSTEM

*Systemic circulation-Systemic arterial pressure, cardiac output and total peripheral resistance*

Goldblatt (1933, 1935) and von Euler (1934a, 1934b) independently showed that crude prostaglandin from sheep seminal vesicles causes a prolonged fall in systemic arterial pressure in anaesthetized cats and rabbits. Since Bergström *et al.* (1959b, 1968) isolated, identified and biosynthesized a family of prostaglandins, many investigators have studied the effect of different prostaglandins on the systemic circulation in animals and human subjects.

*$PGE_1$, $PGE_2$ and $PGE_3$*

The intravenous administration of $PGE_1$ (0.1-10 $\mu$g/kg) decreases total peripheral resistance and systemic arterial pressure in the rat (Weeks and Wingerson, 1964), cat (Holmes, Horton and Main, 1963), rabbit

42          *Jiro Nakano*

(Bergström and von Euler, 1963), mouse (Weeks *et al.*, 1969), chicken (Horton and Main, 1967), dog (Bergström *et al.*, 1964; Berti, Borroni, Fumagalli, Marchi and Zocche, 1964; Carlson and Orö, 1966; Glaviano and Masters, 1971; Maxwell, 1967; Nakano, 1972b; Nakano and McCurdy, 1967a, 1967b) and man (Bergström, Carlson, Ekelund and Orö, 1965a, Bergström, Carlson, Ekelund and Orö, 1965b; Bergström *et al.*, 1959b; Carlson *et al.*, 1969). $PGE_1$ usually increases the pulse pressure since it decreases the diastolic more than the systolic pressure. The cardiovascular effects of $PGE_1$ are markedly affected by the route of its administration. Bergström *et al.* (1964) showed that the depressor effect of the intravenously injected $PGE_1$ is markedly smaller than that of the intraarterially injected $PGE_1$ in anaesthetized dogs. Similar observations have been made by a number of investigators (Carlson and Orö, 1966, McGiff *et al.*, 1969b; Nakano, 1972b) in rats and dogs. These studies indicate that $PGE_1$ is effectively inactivated by a single circulation through the lungs. Many investigators (Weeks and Wingerson, 1964; Nakano and McCurdy, 1967a, 1967b; Lee, Covino, Takman and Smith, 1965; Weeks *et al.*, 1969; Carlson *et al.*, 1969; Maxwell, 1967) found that the intravenous injection of $PGE_1$ significantly increases the stroke volume and cardiac output in dogs and in rats (Fig. 6). The increase in stroke volume has been ascribed to the increase in systemic venous return by $PGE_1$ (Carlson *et al.*, 1969; Emerson, Kelks, Daugherty and Hodgman, 1971) since heart rate usually increases significantly.

The haemodynamic effects of the intravenous injections of $PGE_2$ appear to be qualitatively and quantitatively similar to those of $PGE_1$ in dogs and man. In dogs, the intravenous injection of $PGE_2$ (0.25-4.0 $\mu$g/kg) decreases systemic arterial pressure and increases heart rate and myocardial contractile force essentially in proportion to the

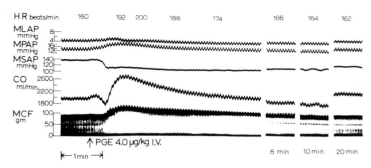

Fig. 6. Effects of the intavenous injection of $PGE_1$ on heart rate (HR), mean left atrial pressure (MLAP), mean pulmonary arterial pressure (MPAP), mean systemic arterial pressure (MSAP), cardiac output (CO) and myocardial contractile force (MCF) in a dog. Reproduced from Nakano and McCurdy (1967a) with permission of the publisher.

dose (Nakano, 1969). $PGE_2$ and $PGE_3$ decreases systemic arterial pressure in rats, rabbits and cats (Horton and Main, 1963) and in dogs (Weeks *et al.*, 1969). In general, $PGE_2$ is either equipotent to or slightly more active than $PGE_1$ (Weeks *et al.*, 1969), whereas $PGE_3$ is less active than $PGE_1$ in the three species of animals (Horton and Main, 1963).

### $PGA_1$ and $PGA_2$

The haemodynamic actions of the A compounds are qualitatively similar to those of $PGE_1$ and $PGE_2$ in dogs and rats (Bergström *et al.*, 1964; Lee *et al.*, 1965; Lee, McGiff, Kannegiesser, Aykent, Mudd and Frawley, 1971; Nakano and McCurdy, 1967a, 1967b, 1968; Nakano, 1968a, 1968b, 1969; Weeks *et al.*, 1969). The intravenous injection of $PGA_1$ or $PGA_2$ decreases systemic arterial pressure and total peripheral resistance markedly in rats (Weeks *et al.*, 1969; Pike *et al.*, 1967), dogs (Lee *et al.*, 1965; Nakano and McCurdy, 1967a, 1967b; Nakano, 1968a; Horton and Jones, 1969; Weeks *et al.*, 1969; Higgins, Vatner, Franklin and Braunwald, 1970), cats and rabbits (Horton and Jones, 1969). $PGA_1$ and $PGA_2$ have equipotent hypotensive action in both rats and dogs (Weeks *et al.*, 1969) or $PGA_2$ is about four times more potent than $PGA_1$ in cats (Horton and Jones, 1969). Several groups of investigators found greater hypotensive action of intravenously injected $PGA_1$ and $PGA_2$ than that of either $PGE_1$ or $PGE_2$ in dogs (Bergström, Carlson and Orö, 1967; Horton and Jones, 1969; Lee, 1968; Weeks, *et al.*, 1969), in rats (Weeks *et al.*, 1969), in rabbits (von Euler, 1936), cats (Horton and Jones, 1969), guinea-pigs (Änggård, 1966) and man (Christlieb, Dobrinsky, Lyons and Hickler, 1969; Carr, 1970a). It can be considered that the lungs inactivate $PGE_1$ and $PGE_2$ more readily than $PGA_1$ and $PGA_2$, since $PGE_1$ and $PGE_2$ have more favourable substrate specificity for PGDH purified from swine lungs than $PGA_1$ and $PGA_2$ *in vitro* (Nakano *et al.*, 1969). This observation is substantiated by the *in vivo* or the isolated lung circulation preparations (Ferreira and Vane, 1967; Biron and Boileau, 1969; McGiff *et al.*, 1969b; Nakano, 1970a). As seen in Fig. 7, the intravenous injection of $PGA_1$ or $PGA_2$ also increases heart rate, cardiac output, stroke volume and myocardial contractile force in dogs (Lee *et al.*, 1965; Nakano and McCurdy, 1967b; Nakano, 1968a; Weeks *et al.*, 1969; Higgins *et al.*, 1970) and rats (Weeks *et al.*, 1969). In patients with mild essential hypertension, the intravenous infusion of $PGA_1$ (0.3-1.32 $\mu g/kg/min$) increases heart rate, stroke volume and cardiac output as systemic arterial pressure falls (Christlieb *et al.*, 1969; Carr, 1970a). There is considerable individual difference in response to $PGA_1$, and no persistent hypotensive effect is observed. Post-infusion rebounding of systemic arterial pressure is common and is marked at times.

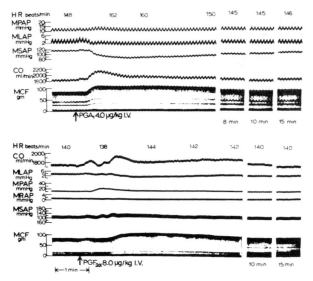

Fig. 7. Upper Tracing: The effects of the intravenous injection of PGA$_1$ on heart rate (HR), mean pulmonary arterial pressure (MPAP), mean left atrial pressure (MLAP), mean systemic arterial pressure (MSAP), cardiac output (CO) and myocardial contractile force (MCF) in a dog.

Lower Tracing: The effects of the intravenous injection of PGF$_{2\alpha}$ on heart rate (HR), cardiac output (CO), mean left atrial pressure (MLAP), mean pulmonary arterial pressure (MPAP), mean right atrial pressure (MRAP), mean systemic arterial pressure (MSAP) and myocardial contractile force (MCF) in a dog. Reproduced from Nakano and McCurdy (1967b) with permission of the publisher.

### *19-hydroxy-PGA$_1$, 19-hydroxy-PGB$_1$, dihydro-PGE$_1$, 15-keto-PGE$_1$, 15-R-PGA$_2$ and 15-R-PGE$_1$*

Horton and Jones (1969) observed that the intravenous injection of 19-hydroxy-PGA$_1$ decreases systemic arterial pressure in dogs, cats and rabbits. 19-hydroxy-PGA$_1$ is slightly less active than PGE$_1$ and 19-hydroxy-PGB$_1$ has negligible depressor activity in cats. Recently, Nakano (1971) observed that the cardiovascular effects of the intravenous injection of dihydro-PGE$_1$ and 15-keto-PGE$_1$ are qualitatively similar to those of PGE$_1$. The magnitude of the haemodynamic effects of dihydro-PGE$_1$ is slightly smaller than those of PGE$_1$ but markedly greater than those of 15-keto-PGE$_1$. Nakano (1969) also showed that the intravenous injection of up to 250 μg/kg of 15-epimer-PGA$_2$ (15-R-PGA$_2$) isolated from a Gorgonian, Plexaura homomala, and of 15-epimer-PGE$_1$ (15-R-PGE$_1$) causes no significant effect in heart rate, systemic arterial pressure or myocardial contractile force in anaesthetized dogs.

As originally postulated by von Euler (1935) the hypotensive action of E and A compounds is most likely due to the decrease in total peripheral resistance through their direct vasodilator action of almost all resistance vessels in different species of animals. During a hypotensive period, both $PGE_1$ and $PGA_1$ increase cardiac output considerably in dogs (Nakano and McCurdy, 1967a, 1967b). The hypotensive action of $PGE_1$ or $PGA_1$ persists after vagotomy (Horton and Jones, 1969), denervation of the carotid sinuses and bodies (Horton and Jones, 1969), and the administration of different anesthetics (Giles, Quiroz and Burch, 1969), atropine (von Euler, 1934a; Bergström *et al.*, 1959b), antihistamines (Berström *et al.*, 1959b), ganglionic blocking agents (Lee *et al.*, 1965; Carlson and Orö, 1966) beta-adrenoceptor blocking agents (Carlson and Orö, 1966; Nakano and McCurdy, 1967b) or the pretreatment with reserpine (Nakano, 1972b). It was demonstrated that the simultaneous administration of $PGE_1$ with catecholamines reduces the pressor effect of catecholamines in dogs (Bergström *et al.*, 1964; Steinberg *et al.*, 1964; Carlson and Orö, 1966). However, $PGE_1$ diminishes not only the pressor action of catecholamines but also that of vasopressin or angiotensin in cats (Holmes *et al.*, 1963), rats (Weeks and Wingerson, 1964) and in dogs (Carlson and Orö, 1966). Furthermore, the infusion of a ganglionic stimulating agent, DMPP, or the electrical stimulation of the central ends of the cut vagi increases systemic arterial pressure in dogs receiving continuous infusion of $PGE_1$ (Carlson and Orö, 1966). Hence, it is reasonable to conclude that an apparent antagonism between $PGE_1$ and catecholamines is neither specific nor pharmacologically competitive but most likely results from the summation of the two counteracting effects. The haemodynamic mechanisms responsible for the increase in cardiac output by E and A compounds may involve in three factors, i.e., (a) the decrease in total peripheral resistance, (b) the increase in myocardial contractile force and (c) the increase in systemic venous return.

### $PGF_{1\alpha}$ and $PGF_{2\alpha}$

$PGF_{1\alpha}$ and $PGF_{2\alpha}$ exert mild to moderate depressor action in cats and rabbits (Änggård and Bergström, 1963; Horton and Main, 1963) and pressor action in rats and dogs (DuCharme *et al.*, 1968; Nakano and McCurdy, 1968; Nakano and Cole, 1969) and in spiral chicks (Horton and Main, 1963, 1967). In chicks the effect may be pressor, depressor or biphasic (Horton and Main, 1967). The pressor action of $PGF_{2\alpha}$ is five times more potent than $PGF_{1\alpha}$ in dogs and rats, but is not so potent as angiotensin or noradrenaline. The dose of $PGF_{2\alpha}$ which stimulates nonvascular smooth muscle, usually causes no significant change on systemic arterial pressure in healthy males and in non-pregnant females (Karim, Trussell, Hillier and Patel, 1969). Hence, a simultaneous administration of both $PGF_{2\alpha}$ (2 $\mu g/kg/min$) and $PGE_2$ (0.2 $\mu g/kg/min$) decreases markedly systemic arterial pressure and increases heart rate in man (Karim *et al.*, 1969; Karim, Hillier, Trussell, Patel and Tamusauge, 1970). DuCharme *et al.* (1968) showed that in dogs the intravenous injection of $PGF_{2\alpha}$ (10 $\mu g/kg$) increases systemic arterial pressure, cardiac output and right atrial pressure whereas total peripheral resistance remains essentially unchanged. In contrast, Nakano and Cole (1969) showed that $PGF_{2\alpha}$ (8 $\mu g/kg$) increases systemic arterial pressure, cardiac output, myocardial contractile force and total peripheral resistance in dogs (Fig. 7). DuCharme *et al.* (1968) postulated that $PGF_{2\alpha}$ causes venoconstriction, increases systemic venous return and cardiac output, and hence increases systemic arterial pressure since total peripheral resistance remains unchanged. On the other hand, Nakano and McCurdy (1967b) and Nakano and Cole (1969) concluded that $PGF_{2\alpha}$ causes vasoconstriction in the regional arteries, and increases total peripheral resistance and systemic arterial pressure. In addition, the increased myocardial contractility and cardiac output produced by $PGF_{2\alpha}$ may contribute to increase systemic arterial pressure. In the dog heart-lung preparation, $PGF_{1\alpha}$ increases myocardial contractile force and cardiac output without producing any significant change in systemic arterial pressure (Katori, Takeda and Imai, 1970).

Carlson and Orö (1966) observed that the infusion of $PGE_1$ (0.4 $\mu g/kg/min$) into the common carotid artery raises systemic arterial pressure slightly. This pressor effect of $PGE_1$ is reversed after ganglionic blockade, suggesting reflex sympathetic vasoconstriction. However, Kaplan, Grega, Sherman and Buckley *et al.* (1969) postulated that extremely large amounts (5 $\mu g/kg$ or 0.4 $\mu g/kg/min$) of $PGE_1$ stimulate the central vasomotor centre to raise the systemic pressure when injected intraarterially into the vascularly isolated neurally intact head, perfused by a donor dog when the carotid sinus and body areas of the recipient have been denervated. On the other hand, a smaller but still fairly large dose (0.1 $\mu g/kg$) of $PGE_1$ has no effect on systemic arterial pressure (Nakano and McCurdy, 1968). Lavery, Lowe and Scroop (1970) found that the injection of $PGF_{2\alpha}$ (4-64 $ng/kg/min$) into the vertebral artery increases both systemic arterial pressure and cardiac output in anaesthetized dogs, while total peripheral resistance remains essentially unchanged and central venous pressure decreases. The infusion of $PGF_{2\alpha}$ into the internal carotid artery and intravenously has no significant cardiovascular effects, indicating that the cardiovascular effects of intravertebral injection of $PGF_{2\alpha}$ are due to activation of cardiovascular centres within the area of distribution of the vertebral artery. $PGF_{1\alpha}$ (9-60 $\mu g/min$) causes similar but less potent cardiovascular effects as compared to $PGF_{2\alpha}$. In contrast, the intravertebral injection of $PGE_1$ (4-360 ng/kg/min) causes tachycardia which is greater than that obtained with the intracarotid or intravenous infusions, but there is no significant effect on systemic arterial pressure.

### Vascular Smooth Muscle and Microcirculation

$PGA_2$ (0.1-0.3 µg/ml) causes neither contraction nor relaxation in the isolated rabbit aortic strips (Lee *et al.*, 1965). $PGE_1$, $PGE_2$, $PGA_1$ and $PGF_{1\alpha}$ cause contraction of the vascular smooth muscle from the isolated rabbit aortic strips or from the isolated dog coronary arterial strip (Strong and Bohr, 1967). In contrast, as seen in Fig. 8 these four prostaglandins cause a biphasic response to the small arterial strips from canine skeletal, mesenteric, and renal arteries, relaxing in response to low concentrations and contracting to high concentrations (Strong and Bohr, 1967). In the isolated mesenteric artery and vein strip, $PGE_1$ inhibits spontaneous contractions whereas $PGF_{1\alpha}$ and $PGF_{2\alpha}$ (10-200 ng/ml) stimulate them essentially in proportion to the concentration (Kadar and Sunahara, 1969). In the rat mesocaecum, the topical administration of $PGE_1$ (1-10 µg/ml) or the intravenous infusion of $PGE_1$ (2-4 µg/kg/min) produces a diffuse dilatation of metarterioles, precapillary sphincters and

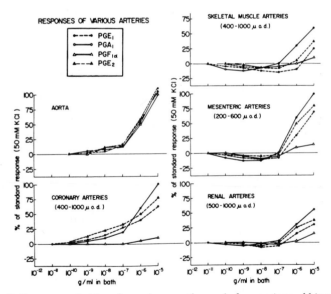

Fig. 8. Responses of strips of vascular smooth muscle from various rabbit arteries to geometrically increasing concentrations of four prostaglandins. Responses are expressed as per cent of the contractile response to 50 mM KC1. Reproduced from Strong and Bohr (1967) with permission of the authors and publisher.

muscular venules concomitant with a temporary augmentation of blood flow in the capillary network (Weiner and Kaley, 1969). On the other hand, the intravenous infusion of $PGF_{2\alpha}$ (10 μg/kg/min) increases systemic arterial pressure with a concomitant constriction of the metarterioles in both the mesocaecum and the cremaster muscle (Viguera and Sunahara, 1969).

Several workers (Lee *et al.*, 1965; Nakano and McCurdy, 1967b; Nakano, 1968b; Smith, McMorrow, Covino and Lee, 1968; Greenberg and Sparks, 1969; Fredholm, Oberg and Rosell, 1970a) showed in dogs that the intraarterial injection of $PGE_1$, $PGE_2$, $PGA_1$ or $PGA_2$ markedly decreases the small arterial perfusion pressure and the peripheral vascular resistance indicating the direct vasodilator action of the prostaglandins (Fig. 9 and 10). Furthermore, Greenberg and Sparks (1969) found that the intravenous administration of $PGE_1$ (0.01 to 10 μg/min) increases blood flow and limb volume, indicating an increase in vascular capacitance in the area studied. $PGE_1$ also increases capillary filtration coefficient, indicating either an increase in capillary permeability or increased capillary surface area due to decreased precapillary sphincter tone (Fig. 10). Generally, $PGE_1$ is a less potent vasodilator than bradykinin and eledoisin in the dog femoral or brachial artery. However, on a molar basis, $PGE_1$ is more potent than nitroglycerin, acetylcholine,

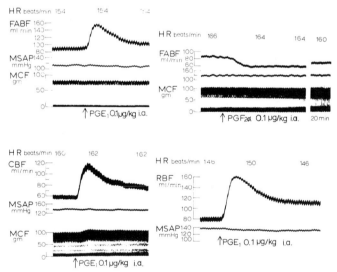

Fig. 9. Effects of the intraarterial injection of $PGE_1$ and $PGF_{2\alpha}$ on femoral arterial blood flow (FABF), coronary arterial blood flow (CBF) and renal arterial blood flow (RBF) in dogs. HR, MSAP and MCF denote heart rate, mean systemic arterial pressure and myocardial contractile force, respectively. Reproduced from Nakano (1968b) with permission of the publisher.

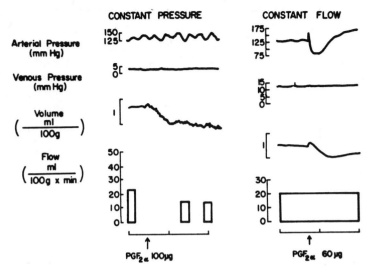

Fig. 10. Effect of $PGF_{2\alpha}$ on resistance and capacitance vessels during constant pressure and constant flow in a dog hind limb. Reproduced from Greenberg and Sparks (1969) with permission of the authors and publisher.

isoprenaline or histamine (Nakano and McCurdy, 1967b; Smith *et al.,* 1968; Nakano, 1968a, 1968b; Fredholm *et al.,* 1970a). It seems that E and A prostaglandins relax the resistance vessels, especially arterioles. In contrast, the effect of $PGF_{2\alpha}$ on the microcirculation in dogs remains controversial. $PGF_{2\alpha}$ causes little effect on the perfusion pressure in the dog hind limb, but considerable increase in small vein pressure, indicating that $PGF_{2\alpha}$ constricts predominantly the venous segments of the microcirculation (DuCharme *et al.,* 1968; Kadowitz, Sweet and Brody, 1971). In contrast, others (Nakano and Cole, 1969; Greenberg and Sparks, 1969) showed that $PGF_{2\alpha}$ also increases the perfusion pressure in the dog hind limb. Nakano (1968b) found that the intraarterial injection of $PGF_{2\alpha}$ (0.1 µg/kg) directly decreases the femoral and brachial arterial blood flows and increases the peripheral resistance in dogs.

There are variable results concerning the interaction between the prostaglandins and catecholamines and other vasoactive agents. Several workers observed that $PGE_1$, $PGE_2$ or $PGA_1$ reduces the vasoconstrictor action of noradrenaline, adrenaline and tyramine in the isolated small arterial strips (Strong and Bohr, 1967; Kadar and Sunahara, 1969; Viguera and Sunahara, 1969) and in the isolated dog limbs (Holmes *et al.,* 1963; Mayer, Abboud, Schmid and Mark, 1970; Weiner and Kaley, 1969; Kadowitz *et al.,* 1971). In contrast, others showed that $PGE_1$ or $PGA_1$ does not change the vascular response to noradrenaline or adrenaline in the isolated aortic strip (Lee *et al.,* 1965; Khairallah, Page and Türker, 1967) and in the dog hind limb (Daugherty, Schwinghamer, Swindall and Haddy, 1968) or increases the vasoconstrictor action of noradrenaline in the isolated hind limb (Kayaalp and Türker, 1968) and in the isolated mesenteric artery (Tobian and Viets, 1970). The effects of $PGE_1$ or $PGA_1$ on the vascular actions of other vasoactive agents are also variable. $PGE_1$ reduces the vasoconstrictor responses to angiotensin and serotonin, and the vasodilator action of nitroglycerin (Abdel-Sayed, Abboud, Hedwall and Schmid, 1970; Weiner and Kaley, 1969; Kadowitz *et al.*, 1971). In contrast, $PGE_1$ is found to increase the vasoconstrictor action of angiotensin, serotonin and vasopressin in the isolated aortic strip (Khairallah *et al.*, 1967) or causes no change in the responses to angiotensin in the aortic strip (Lee *et al.*, 1965) and to serotonin, histamine and bradykinin in small vessels (Weiner and Kaley, 1969).

### Heart Rate

$PGE_1$ does not change heart rate or has variable effects in the isolated rat, rabbit and cat hearts but it significantly increases in the isolated guinea-pig and frog heart (Berti *et al.*, 1965; Mantegazza, 1965; Lee *et al.*, 1965; Vergroesen, De Boer and Gottenbos, 1967). The positive chronotropic action of $PGE_1$ is not blocked by pretreatment with reserpine or by propranolol in the isolated guinea-pig heart (Berti *et al.*, 1965). Both $PGF_{1\alpha}$ and $PGF_{1\beta}$ cause no effect on heart rate (Vergroesen *et al.*, 1967), while neither $PGF_{2\alpha}$ nor $PGA_2$ alters heart rate in the isolated chicken and rabbit heart, respectively (Horton and Main, 1967; Lee *et al.*, 1965). In the dog heart-lung preparation, neither $PGE_1$ nor $PGF_{1\alpha}$ influences heart rate (Katori *et al.*, 1970).

In dogs, the intra-coronary injection of $PGE_1$ causes no change in heart rate (Nakano and McCurdy, 1967b). The intravenous injection of $PGE_1$ or $PGE_2$ increases heart rate significantly in human subjects (Bergström *et al.*, 1959a, 1965a; Steinberg *et al.*, 1964; Carlson *et al.*, 1969) and in dogs (Lee *et al.*, 1965; Carlson and Orö, 1966; Maxwell, 1967; Nakano, 1972b; Nakano and McCurdy, 1967a, 1968). Since the heart rate increasing effect of $PGE_1$ is completely abolished by propranolol (1 mg/kg), it is concluded that the increase in heart rate produced by $PGE_1$ in animals with intact circulation results from reflex sympathetic stimulation (Nakano and McCurdy, 1967a). The intravenous injection of either $PGA_1$ or $PGA_2$ more markedly increases heart rate than $PGE_1$ in dogs and in human subjects (Lee *et al.*, 1965; Nakano and McCurdy, 1968; Nakano, 1972b; Weeks *et al.*, 1969; Higgins *et al.*, 1970). The intravenous or intra-left atrial injection of $PGF_{2\alpha}$ slightly or moderately increases heart rate in anaesthetized dogs, although it increases systemic arterial pressure slightly (DuCharme *et al.*, 1968; Nakano and McCurdy, 1968; Nakano and Cole, 1969; Emerson, Kelks,

Daugherty and Hodgman, 1971). The tachycardiac effect of the intra-left atrial injection of $PGF_{2\alpha}$ is significantly greater than that of the intravenously injected $PGF_{2\alpha}$ in anaesthetized dogs (Nakano and Cole, 1969). Lavery *et al.* (1970) showed that, in anaesthetized dogs, the injection of either $PGF_{1\alpha}$ (9-50 $\mu$g/min) or $PGF_{2\alpha}$ (4-64 ng/kg/min) in the vertebral artery causes tachycardia which is unaffected by propranolol but abolished by vagotomy, whereas the intravenous or intracarotid infusion of the same dose of $PGF_{1\alpha}$ of $PGF_{2\alpha}$ has no effect. In contrast, the intravertebral, intravenous or intracarotid infusion of $PGE_1$ (4-360 ng/kg/min) causes tachycardia without any significant change in systemic arterial pressure. The magnitude of tachycardia produced by the intravertebral injection is greater than that by the intravenous or intracarotid infusion. From the above studies, it can be concluded that generally, prostaglandins cause little or no direct effect on heart rate, but affect heart rate indirectly through a reflex stimulation or inhibition on the sympathetic and vagal nerves plus its direct effect on the cardioaccelerator and inhibitor centres in the medulla.

## Myocardial Contractility and Cardiodynamics

$PGE_1$ (0.01-1 $\mu$g/ml or $10^{-5}$ M) or $PGF_{2\alpha}$ (1 $\mu$g/ml) exerts a positive inotropic action on the isolated, electrically driven rabbit atria (Tuttle and Skelly, 1968), the isolated guinea-pig atria (Sabatini-Smith, 1970) and the isolated dog papillary muscle preparations (Antonaccio and Lucchesi, 1970). $PGE_1$ produces no significant effect on the cardiac contractile force in the isolated cat and rabbit hearts (von Euler, 1935; Berti *et al.*, 1965; Mantegazza, 1965) or increased both heart rate and contractile force in the isolated rabbit heart (Wennmålm and Hedqvist, 1970). As seen in Fig. 11 and 12, $PGE_1$ increases myocardial contractile force in the isolated frog heart (Berti *et al.*, 1965; Klaus and Piccinini, 1967; Vergroesen and DeBoer, 1968), guinea-pig heart (Berti *et al.*, 1965; Mantegazza, 1965; Sobel and Robinson, 1969), rat heart (Berti *et al.*, 1965; Mantegazza, 1965; Vergroesen *et al.*, 1967), chicken heart (Horton and Main, 1967) and in the dog heart-lung preparation (Katori *et al.*, 1970). The positive inotropic action of $PGE_1$ is equivalent to that of adrenaline on a weight basis in the isolated guinea-pig heart (Berti *et al.*, 1965). Vergroesen *et al.* (1967) also found that $PGF_{1\alpha}$ or $PGF_{1\beta}$ (50 ng/ml) influences neither heart rate nor coronary blood flow, but exerts a pronounced positive inotropic action in the isolated rat and guinea-pig heart (Vergroesen *et al.*, 1967; Sobel and Robinson, 1969). $PGF_{1\beta}$ is much less active than the same concentration of $PGF_{1\alpha}$. On the other hand, Horton and Main (1967) and Lee *et al.* (1965) reported that $PGF_{2\alpha}$ (more than 5 $\mu$g) and $PGA_2$ (0.1-0.3 $\mu$g/ml) have no action on the force or rate of contraction in the isolated chicken and rabbit hearts,

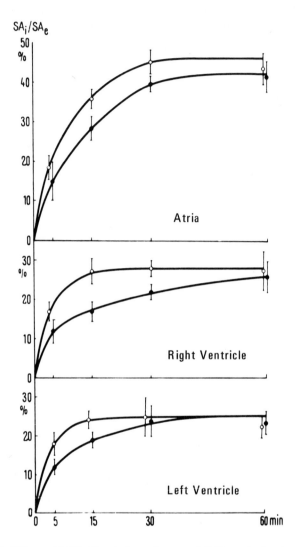

Fig. 11. Effects of PGE$_1$ (1 μg/ml) on the rate of Ca$^{++}$ uptake by the guinea-pig atria (upper), right ventricle (middle) and left ventricle (lower). Closed and open circles denote respectively, control and PGE$_1$. Reproduced from Klaus and Piccinini (1967) with permission of the authors and publisher.

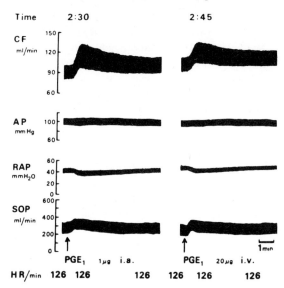

Fig. 12. Effects of the injection of PGE₁ into the left atrium (i.a.) and of that into the right vein (i.v.) on the coronary flow (CF), aortic pressure (AP), the right atrial pressure (RAP), systemic output (SOP) and heart rate (HR) in the dog heart lung preparation. Reproduced from Katori *et al.* (1970) with permission of the authors and publisher.

respectively. In the dog heart-lung preparation however, Katori *et al.* (1970) showed that $PGF_{1\alpha}$ increases myocardial contractile force without producing any change in heart rate (Fig. 12).

In anaesthetized dogs the intravenous injection of $PGE_1$ (0.25-4.0 $\mu$g/kg or 12.3 $\mu$g/min for 5 min) decreases systemic arterial pressure and increases myocardial contractile force markedly (Nakano and McCurdy, 1967a, 1968; Nakano and Cole, 1969; Emerson *et al.*, 1971). Maxwell (1967) and Nakano and Cole (1969) also showed that $PGE_1$ decreases left ventricular end-diastolic pressure, and increases both right and left ventricular work, dp/dt values of the left ventricular isometric tension and the peak tension and the df/dt value of myocardial contraction in anaesthetized dogs. A qualitatively similar effect on myocardial contractility in dogs is observed with an intravenous injection of $PGE_2$, $PGA_1$ and $PGA_2$ (Nakano and McCurdy, 1968; Nakano, 1969).

The intravenous injection of $PGF_{2\alpha}$ (1-10 $\mu$g/kg or 58.2 $\mu$g/min for 5 min) increases myocardial contractile force slightly (Nakano and McCurdy, 1968; Nakano and Cole, 1969; Emerson *et al.*, 1971) or produces no change in dogs (DuCharme *et al.*, 1968). Furthermore, the intracoronary injection of $PGE_1$ (0.1 $\mu$g/kg or 2-8 $\mu$g/min) increases both coronary arterial blood flow and myocardial contractile force in the area perfused (Nakano and McCurdy, 1967a; Nakano, 1968b; Hollenberg, Walker and McCormick, 1968; Nutter and Crumly, 1970) (Fig. 9). During this period, heart rate and systemic arterial pressure remain essentially unchanged. Since the supernormal increase in coronary blood flow does not result in an increase in myocardial contractile force in dogs (Nakano, 1966), the increased myocardial contractile force by the intracoronary arterial injection of $PGE_1$ is due to its direct positive inotropic action on the myocardium. On the other hand, the intracoronary injection of either $PGF_{1\alpha}$ or $PGF_{2\alpha}$ causes little or no effect on myocardial contractile force (Hollenberg *et al.*, 1968).

While in dogs $PGE_2$, $PGA_1$ and $PGA_2$ markedly increase myocardial contractile force (Nakano, 1970a; Nutter and Crumly, 1970), an epimer of $PGA_2$, $15$-R-$PGA_2$, produces no effect on myocardial contractile force (Nakano, 1969). Nutter and Crumly (1970) showed that the intracoronary injection of $PGE_1$ or $PGA_1$ increases myocardial contractile force and decreases the internal diameter of the left ventricle without producing any significant change in heart rate in anaesthetized dogs.

The underlying mechanism responsible for the positive inotropic action of prostaglandins remains unknown. Since the positive inotropic action of $PGE_1$ is frequently not associated with an increase in heart rate, it is most likely that this action may not be secondary to the change in heart rate (Berti *et al.*, 1965; Katori *et al.*, 1970). The positive inotropic action does not appear to be mediated through beta adrenergic stimulation by either direct or reflexly increased catecholamine release. As seen in Fig. 13, the positive inotropic action of $PGE_1$ is not blocked

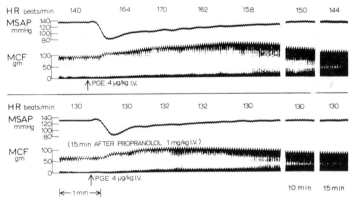

Fig. 13. Effects of $PGE_1$ on heart rate (HR), mean systemic arterial pressure (MSAP) and myocardial contractile force (MCF) in an anaesthetized dog before and after the administration of propranolol. Reproduced from Nakano and McCurdy (1967a) with permission of the publisher.

by propranolol (1 mg/kg) or by pretreatment with reserpine in the isolated guinea-pig heart (Berti *et al.,* 1965; Mantegazza, 1965) and in anaesthetized dogs (Nakano and McCurdy, 1967a). The positive inotropic action of $PGE_1$ and $PGF_{1\alpha}$ is associated with the increased myocardial adenylcyclase activity in the isolated guinea-pig heart (Sobel and Robison, 1969) and with the increased intracellular cyclic AMP concentration in the rat heart (Curnow and Nuttall, 1971). Furthermore, Piccinini, Pomarelli and Chiarra (1969) and Curnow and Nuttall (1971) found that $PGE_1$ activates phosphorylase and inhibits glycogen synthetase in the myocardium *in vitro* and *in vivo* respectively.

The positive inotropic action of $PGE_1$ in EDTA-treated dogs is significantly smaller than that in control dogs, suggesting the participation of $Ca^{++}$ in this effect of $PGE_1$ on myocardial contractility in dogs (Nakano, Cole and Ishii, 1968a). Klaus and Piccinini (1967) showed that the positive inotropic action of $PGE_1$ in the isolated guinea-pig or frog heart is coupled with an increase in the rate of $^{45}Ca$ uptake from the perfusion medium (Fig. 11). The total myocardial $Ca^{++}$ content and the amount of exchangeable cellular $Ca^{++}$ are not affected. They concluded that the positive inotropic action of $PGE_1$ is related to myocardial $Ca^{++}$ metabolism, and can be most probably explained by an increase in the membrane permeability to $Ca^{++}$ similar to the action of adrenaline. Likewise, $PGE_1$ or $PGF_{2\alpha}$ (1 $\mu$g/ml) enhances the uptake of $Ca^{++}$ by fragments of cardiac sarcoplasmic reticulum in the isolated guinea-pig atria (Sabatini-Smith, 1970). Mantegazza (1965) found that, with normal $Ca^{++}$ concentrations, $PGE_1$ causes little change in myocardial contractile force, but in the presence of half the usual $Ca^{++}$ concentrations, $PGE_1$ consistently increases myocardial contractile force. Tuttle and Skelly (1968) showed that $PGE_1$ significantly increases the sensitivity of atrial muscle to ouabain in the isolated, electrically driven rabbit atrium. $PGE_1$ produces effects on intracellular $K^+$ which are similar to those produced by high concentrations of ouabain. Vergroesen and DeBoer (1968) showed that $PGE_1$ exerts a marked positive inotropic action in the potassium-intoxicated frog heart, and restores normal function in the potassium arrested heart. Furthermore, they concluded that $PGE_1$ antagonized the effect of $K^+$ rather than enhancing the effect of $Ca^{++}$. Nakano and McCurdy (1967a) and Hollenberg *et al.* (1968) showed that $PGE_1$ does not block the positive inotropic action of noradrenaline in dogs. Wennmålm and Hedqvist (1970) and Hedqvist (1970) showed that in the rabbit the infusion of $PGE_1$ markedly diminishes the noradrenaline release from the heart by cardiac sympathetic nerve stimulation, markedly reduces myocardial contractile force and slightly decreases the positive chronotropic action of nerve stimulation. They concluded that $PGE_1$ in low concentrations ($8 \times 10^{-8} - 3 \times 10^{-7}$ M) interferes with the function of the sympathetic neuro-effector system of the rabbit heart. This interference seems to be based mainly on a prejunctional action leading to decreased release of noradrenaline from the nerve terminals and subsequently to a decrease of the mechanical response to sympathetic nerve stimulation.

## Systemic Venous Return

In dogs in which cardiac input was kept constant by means of a Sigmamotor pump, the intravenous injection of $PGE_1$ (4 µg/kg) increases heart rate, decreases systemic and pulmonary arterial pressures, and right and left atrial pressures (Nakano and McCurdy, 1968; Nakano and Cole, 1969; Nakano and Kessinger, 1970). On the other hand, $PGE_1$ and $PGA_1$ cause a biphasic change in systemic venous return, an initial marked increase being followed by slight decrease before return to control values. Emerson *et al.* (1971) confirmed the observations made by Nakano and Cole on the effect of $PGE_1$ on the systemic venous return.

DuCharme *et al.* (1968) showed that the intravenous injection of 10 µg/kg of $PGF_{2\alpha}$ decreases total venous capacitance in anaesthetized dogs, in which cardiac output is kept constant by pumping blood from the right atrium to the pulmonary artery. $PGF_{2\alpha}$ increases the right atrial pressure, whereas systemic arterial pressure increases slightly. When a pressure stabilizer reservoir is inserted on the venous side, $PGF_{2\alpha}$ causes a shift of blood into the stabilizer reservoir. Hexamethonium, phenoxybenzamine or denervation abolishes the effect of $PGF_{2\alpha}$ on the cutaneous veins of the perfused paw, but neither of these drugs prevents the reduction of venous capacitance by $PGF_{2\alpha}$ in the whole animal. As discussed before, DuCharme *et al.* (1968) postulated that the hypertensive action of $PGF_{2\alpha}$ in dogs is due to the increase in cardiac output, which is caused by an increase in central venous pressure resulting from peripheral venoconstriction and subsequent increase in systemic venous return. Their postulate has recently been refuted by Lavery *et al.* (1970), who demonstrated that $PGF_{2\alpha}$ decreases central venous pressure in dogs as cardiac output increases. Nakano and Cole (1969) found that the intravenous injection of $PGF_{2\alpha}$ (8 µg/kg) increases systemic and pulmonary arterial pressure, and decreases systemic venous return in anaesthetized dogs. Recently Emerson *et al.* (1971) found that $PGF_{2\alpha}$, causes a decrease or biphasic change in systemic venous return in anaesthetized dogs, an initial short increase being followed by a sustained decrease. However, they also observed that $PGF_{2\alpha}$ not infrequently reduces systemic venous return without an initial phase of increase. It seems that $PGF_{2\alpha}$ may produce different degrees of circulatory changes dependent upon the cardiovascular or sympathetic state prior to its administration.

## Pulmonary Circulation

The intravenous administration of $PGE_1$ or $PGE_2$ increases pulmonary arterial pressure but reduces pulmonary vascular resistance in anaesthetized dogs (Nakano and McCurdy, 1967b, 1968; Maxwell, 1967; Giles *et al.*, 1969; Said, 1968). In the isolated rabbit lung preparation, Hauge, Lunde and Waaler (1967) showed that $PGE_1$ dilates pulmonary vascular beds and and decreases pulmonary vascular resistance in control dogs as well as in dogs treated with propranolol and phentolamine. The intravenous or intrapulmonary arterial injection of $PGE_1$ decreases pulmonary arterial perfusion pressure in dogs in which either cardiac input or pulmonary arterial blood flow is kept constant by means of a Sigmamotor pump (Nakano and Cole, 1969; Nakano and Kessinger, 1970) (Fig. 14). Hyman (1969) showed that the infusion of $PGE_1$ (0.8-1.3 $\mu$g/kg/min for 10 min) into the pulmonary lobar artery decreases mean pulmonary arterial pressure, lobar arterial perfusion pressure and small pulmonary lobar vein pressure as systemic arterial pressure decreases in dogs while the left atrial pressure remains unchanged. In anaesthetized dogs, Giles *et al.* (1969) found that the intravenous or intracoronary infusion of $PGE_1$ (0.33-0.67 $\mu$g/kg/min) not only decreases pulmonary vein pressure but also pulmonary blood volume in anaesthetized dogs. In contrast, Said (1968) and Anderson, Tsagaris and Kuida (1971) found that $PGE_2$ increases both pulmonary arterial and venous pressures without producing any significant change in the left atrial and pulmonary wedge pressures in dogs and calves respectively.

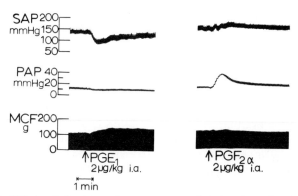

Fig. 14. Effects of the intrapulmonary artery administration of a single dose (2 $\mu$g/kg) of $PGE_1$ and $PGF_{2\alpha}$ on the systemic arterial pressure (MSAP) and the perfusion pressure in the left pulmonary artery (MPAP) of a dog in which left pulmonary arterial blood flow was kept constant by a Sigmamotor pump through the period of the experiment. Reproduced from Nakano and Kessinger (1970) with permission of the publisher.

Änggård and Bergström (1963) observed that the intravenous administration of $PGF_{2\alpha}$ decreases systemic arterial pressure and increases heart rate and right ventricular systolic pressure (hence pulmonary arterial systolic pressure) in cats. In contrast, the intravenous administration of 8-10 $\mu$g/kg of $PGF_{2\alpha}$ markedly increases pulmonary arterial pressure in dogs (DuCharme *et al.*, 1968; Nakano and McCurdy, 1968; Hyman, 1969) and calves (Anderson *et al.*, 1971). As seen in Fig. 14, the intraarterial injection of $PGF_{2\alpha}$ increases the pulmonary arterial pressure even when pulmonary blood flow is kept constant, indicating the direct vasoconstrictor action of $PGF_{2\alpha}$. $PGF_{2\alpha}$ also directly constricts pulmonary veins and/or venules, and increases pulmonary venous pressure in dogs (DuCharme *et al.*, 1968; Said, 1968; Hyman, 1969). Therefore, it is concluded that the increased pulmonary arterial pressure is secondary to the increased pulmonary venous pressure by $PGF_{2\alpha}$.

## Coronary Circulation and Myocardial Metabolism

Berti *et al.* (1965) found that $PGE_1$ (10 $\mu$g) does not change coronary blood flow, whereas others (Mantegazza, 1965; Vergroesen *et al.*, 1967; Willebrands and Tasseron, 1968) showed that $PGE_1$, $PGE_2$ or $PGA_1$ increases coronary blood flow in the isolated rat heart. The magnitude of the coronary dilator action of $PGA_1$ is significantly smaller than that of $PGE_1$. Although Vergroesen *et al.* (1967) showed that neither $PGF_{1\alpha}$ nor $PGF_{1\beta}$ influences coronary blood flow, others (Wildebrands and Tasseron, 1968) found that $PGF_{1\alpha}$ (0.5 $\mu$g/ml) increases both coronary blood flow and myocardial contractile force in the isolated rat heart. Several workers (Berti *et al.*, 1965; Mantegazza, 1965; Wennmålm and Hedqvist, 1970) found that $PGE_1$ (1-5 $\mu$g) increases coronary blood flow in the isolated guinea-pig, rabbit and cat heart. The effects of $PGE_1$ are more prolonged than those of the same dose of adrenaline, and are not blocked by pronethalol, propranolol or by the pretreatment with reserpine (Berti *et al.*, 1965).

In the dog heart-lung preparation, Katori *et al.* (1970) found that the injection of $PGE_1$ (3 $\mu$g) into the left atrium or the intravenous injection of $PGE_1$ (20 $\mu$g) markedly increases coronary blood flow, cardiac output and myocardial contractile force, although both heart rate and systolic arterial pressure remain essentially unchanged. In addition, $PGE_1$ decreases coronary A-V oxygen difference and changes very little the myocardial oxygen consumption and oxygen extraction coefficient. Hence, they concluded that the increase in coronary arterial blood flow produced by $PGE_1$ is due not to the enhanced myocardial contractility but to a direct coronary vasodilator action of this compound. The coronary vasodilator action and other haemodynamic actions of $PGF_{1\alpha}$

are qualitatively similar to those of $PGE_1$ but the magnitude of the effects of $PGF_{1\alpha}$ is considerably smaller than those of $PGE_1$. The magnitude of the coronary vasodilator action of $PGE_1$ is, however, approximately 1/50 that of nitroglycerin in heart-lung preparations.

In anaesthetized dogs, several workers (Nakano and McCurdy, 1967a, 1967b, 1968; Nakano, 1968b; Hollenberg *et al.,* 1968; Nutter and Crumly, 1970) showed that the injection of $PGE_1$ or $PGA_1$ (0.1 µg/kg or 0.1-12.5 µg/min) into the coronary artery increases coronary arterial blood flow and decreases the coronary vascular resistance markedly without producing any significant change in heart rate and mean systemic arterial pressure (Fig. 9). Nakano and McCurdy (1967a, 1967b, 1968) observed that the increase in the coronary blood flow is associated with an increase in myocardial contractile force in the area perfused by the artery. Propranolol blocks neither the positive inotropic action of $PGE_1$, nor its coronary vasodilator action. They also found that the intracoronary arterial injection of $PGE_1$ counteracts the coronary vasoconstrictor action of the intracoronary injection of lysine[8]-vasopressin, and increases coronary blood flow and myocardial contractile force to levels markedly above control (Nakano, 1968a, 1972b) (Fig. 15). The duration and magnitude of the coronary

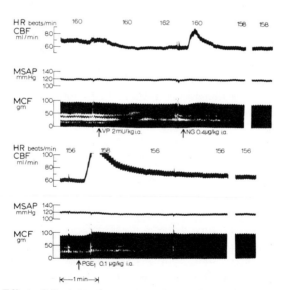

Fig. 15. Effect of the intracoronary arterial injection of lysine-vasopressin (VP), nitroglycerin (NG) and $PGE_1$ on heart rate (HR), coronary arterial blood flow (CBF), mean systemic arterial pressure (MSAP) and myocardial contractile force (MCF) in the dog. Reproduced from Nakano (1972b) with permission of the publisher.

vasodilator action of $PGE_1$ (0.1 $\mu$g/kg) are considerably longer and greater than those of nitroglycerin (0.4 $\mu$g/kg). The intracoronary arterial injection of $PGF_{2\alpha}$ (0.1 $\mu$g/kg) neither influences coronary arterial blood flow nor myocardial contractile force in dogs. $PGF_{1\alpha}$ and $PGF_{2\alpha}$ (4-12 $\mu$g/min) have no effect or only slightly increase myocardial blood flow while contractile force remains unchanged (Hollenberg *et al.*, 1968). None of these three prostaglandins has an effect on ECG.

In dogs, several workers (Maxwell, 1967; Higgins *et al.*, 1970; Bloor and Sobel, 1970) observed that the intravenous infusion of $PGE_1$ (0.3-3 $\mu$g/kg/min) increases heart rate, coronary arterial blood flow and cardiac output whereas it decreases systemic arterial pressure, and total and coronary peripheral resistance. Furthermore, $PGE_1$ decreases coronary sinus oxygen content and increases coronary A-V oxygen difference and myocardial oxygen consumption. Because of the greater increase in myocardial oxygen consumption than in cardiac work, cardiac 'efficiency' decreases. When heart rate is maintained constant by atrial drive (180/min), $PGA_1$ still markedly decreases the coronary peripheral vascular resistance (Higgins *et al.*, 1970). $PGE_1$ and $PGA_1$ also decrease the coronary vascular resistance after beta adrenoceptor blockade with propranolol and cholinergic blockade with atropine (Hedwall, Abbdel-Sayed, Schmid and Abboud, 1970). Since $PGA_1$ increases coronary sinus oxygen tension with unaltered myocardial oxygen extraction, they concluded that $PGA_1$ increases coronary arterial blood flow by its direct coronary vasodilator effect in dogs. Bloor and Sobel (1970) found that the intravenous injection of $PGF_{2\alpha}$ does not affect the coronary vascular bed in their dogs.

Maxwell (1967) found that $PGE_1$ infused intravenously decreases glucose and free fatty acid concentrations and increases lactate concentrations in the coronary sinus blood, indicating the increased uptake of glucose and free fatty acids and decreased uptake of release of lactate by the myocardium. On the other hand, $PGE_1$ does not affect pyruvate concentrations in the coronary sinus blood. Wildebrands and Tasseron (1968) also showed that, as both coronary blood flow and myocardial contractile force increase, both $PGE_1$ (0.5 $\mu$g/ml) and $PGF_{1\alpha}$ (0.5 $\mu$g/ml) not only increase myocardial oxygen consumption but also increase $C^{14}O_2$ production from $C^{14}$-glucose and $C^{14}$-palmitate, indicating an enhancement of the substrate oxidation in the myocardium by $PGE_1$ and $PGF_{1\alpha}$. Glaviano and Masters (1971) found that $PGE_1$ depresses coronary blood flow and myocardial uptake of free fatty acids, and increases myocardial content of triglycerides although myocardial glucose uptake increases. They concluded that $PGE_1$ inhibits basal lipolysis in the myocardium. As discussed previously, $PGE_1$ was found to enhance the activity of adenyl cyclase in the guinea pig heart (Sobel and Robison, 1969) and to increase the intracellular cyclic AMP concentrations in the rat heart (Curnow and Nuttall, 1971). Furthermore, $PGE_1$ activates phosphorylase activity in the guinea pig heart (Piccinini *et al.,* 1969) and in the rat heart (Curnow and Nuttall, 1971), and decreases the activity of glycogen synthetase in the rat heart (Curnow and Nuttall, 1971).

## Splanchnic, Hepatic, Portal and Splenic Circulations

Von Euler (1935) showed that crude prostaglandin (probably mostly $PGE_1$) increases portal venous pressure and blanching of the liver and produces the pooling of blood in the portal circulation in anaesthetized cats. The intraarterial injection of 0.6-1.2 $\mu$g of $PGE_1$, $PGE_2$, $PGA_1$ and $PGA_2$ or the intraarterial or intravenous infusion of 50 ng/kg/min of $PGE_1$ decreases the peripheral resistance and increases markedly the blood flow in the superior mesenteric artery in dogs (Lee, 1968; Shehadeh, Price and Jacobson, 1969; Higgins *et al.,* 1970). The increase in cardiac output was proportional to that in the arterial blood flow (Higgins *et al.,* 1970). Nakano and Cole (1969) observed that the injection of $PGE_1$ (4 $\mu$g/kg) into a femoral vein decreases significantly the systemic arterial pressure and causes a biphasic change in the portal venous pressure, an initial increase being followed by a decrease. In contrast, they found that the injection of the same dose of $PGE_1$ into the portal vein does not change the systemic arterial pressure, but again produces a biphasic change in the venous pressure. However, the speed and duration of the initial increase and secondary decrease are slower and more prolonged with the intraportal administration than with the intrafemoral vein administration. The rapid metabolism of $PGE_1$ in the lungs by PGDH (Änggård and Samuelsson, 1964, 1966; Nakano *et al.,* 1969; Nakano, 1970a; Nakano and Prancan, 1971) and also in the liver by non-specific beta- and omega-oxidation (Hamberg, 1968; Samuelsson, 1970) may largely account for the absence of the hypotensive action of $PGE_1$ injected into the portal vein.

Lee (1968) and Shedadeh *et al.* (1969) demonstrated that the intraarterial injection of $PGF_{2\alpha}$ (0.6-1.2 $\mu$g/ml) or the continuous intraarterial infusion of $PGF_{2\alpha}$ (0.1-1.0 $\mu$g/kg/min) increases the peripheral resistance and decreases blood flow in the superior mesenteric artery in anaesthetized dogs, indicating a vasoconstrictor action of $PGF_{2\alpha}$ in the peripheral vascular beds. Nakano and Cole (1969) also found that the injection of $PGF_{2\alpha}$ (8 $\mu$g/kg) into a femoral vein increases systemic and pulmonary arterial pressure, portal venous pressure and myocardial contractility and decreases systemic venous return significantly. In contrast, the intra-portal injection of the same dose of $PGF_{2\alpha}$ decreases systemic and pulmonary arterial pressure, right atrial pressure and myocardial contractile force. The duration and magnitude of the increase in the portal venous pressure is more prolonged and greater with the injection of $PGF_{2\alpha}$ into the portal vein than that into a femoral vein.

In the isolated perfused dog spleen, the intraarterial infusion of $PGE_1$ or $PGE_2$ (2 $\mu g/min$) increases splenic arterial blood flow and volume as splenic vascular resistance decreases (Davies and Withrington, 1968). $PGE_1$ is slightly less potent in reducing splenic vascular resistance than acetylcholine, and $PGE_2$ is considerably less effective than either. The splenic vasodilator action of $PGE_1$ or $PGE_2$ is not blocked by either phenoxybenzamine or propranolol. The splenic vascular responses to adrenaline, noradrenaline, angiotensin and sympathetic nerve stimulation are not modified by the simultaneous intraarterial infusion of $PGE_1$ or $PGE_2$ (Davies and Withrington, 1968, 1969). The intraarterial infusion of low concentrations (less than 0.1 $\mu g/ml$) of $PGF_{2\alpha}$ increases splenic arterial blood flow and produces a marked reduction in splenic vascular resistance while higher concentrations (more than 0.1 $\mu g/ml$) of $PGF_{2\alpha}$ increases splenic vascular resistance (Davies and Withrington, 1971). Little action on splenic volume is observed by any arterial concentration of $PGF_{2\alpha}$. The reductions in splenic vascular resistance caused by low arterial concentrations of $PGF_{2\alpha}$ are reversed by phenoxybenzamine (Davies and Withrington, 1971). On the other hand, the infusion of $PGF_{1\alpha}$, $PGA_1$ or $PGA_2$ slightly increases splenic volume and splenic arterial blood flow (Davies and Withrington, 1968, 1969). Hedqvist and Brundin (1969) and Hedqvist (1970, 1971) observed that $PGE_1$ or $PGE_2$ inhibits the pressor response to injected noradrenaline as well as to noradrenaline locally released by electrical stimulation of the splenic nerve in the isolated cat spleen perfused at a constant rate. On the other hand, Davies and Withrington (1971) have been unable to observe any appreciable interaction between $PGF_{2\alpha}$ and the splenic responses to sympathetic nerve stimulation, adrenaline and noradrenaline.

**Gastric Circulation**

$PGE_1$ and $PGA_1$ inhibit histamine-induced gastric secretion as gastric mucosal blood flow decreases significantly in dogs (Wilson and Levine, 1969; Jacobson, 1970). Recently, Nakano, Prancan and Kessinger (1971) showed that the intravenous injection of $PGE_1$ and $PGA_1$ (0.25-4.0 $\mu g/kg$) decreases mean systemic arterial pressure, mean gastric arterial perfusion pressure and gastric peripheral vascular resistance in dogs, in which the entire stomach is perfused constantly with arterial blood by a Sigmamotor pump. The magnitude of the haemodynamic changes by the intravenously injected $PGA_1$ is significantly greater than that by the intravenously injected $PGE_1$. The intraarterial injection of $PGE_1$ or $PGA_1$ (0.6-10 ng/kg) also decreases gastric arterial perfusion pressure and peripheral vascular resistance without producing any significant change in mean systemic arterial pressure and heart rate in similar dog preparations. The magnitude of the haemodynamic effects of the intraarterially injected $PGE_1$ is significantly greater than that of the intraarterially injected $PGA_1$. This study indicates that in dogs both $PGE_1$ and $PGA_1$ are potent vasodilators in the gastric peripheral vascular beds and increase the gastric blood flow, although a local redistribution of blood flow may occur indirectly, secondary to its antacid action.

### Renal Circulation

Barger and Herd (1967) demonstrated that in dogs the intraarterial injection of $PGA_2$ increases the renal cortical blood flow and decreases the outer medullary blood flow, suggesting that $PGA_2$ causes a redistribution of the renal blood flow from the outer medulla to the cortex. Several investigators (Johnston, Herzog and Lauler, 1967; Nakano and McCurdy, 1967a, 1968; Nakano, 1968a; McGiff *et al.*, 1969b) found that the intraarterial injection of $PGE_1$, $PGE_2$, $PGA_1$ or $PGA_2$ increases the renal arterial blood flow markedly and decreases the renal peripheral vascular resistance in anaesthetized dogs (Fig. 9). The intraarterial injection of $PGE_1$ (1 µg), $PGE_2$ (0.6-1.2 µg) or $PGA_2$ (0.6-1.2 µg) may initially decrease and then increases total renal blood flow in dogs (Lee, 1968). On the other hand, the intraarterial injection of $PGF_{2\alpha}$ (0.1 µg/kg) increases the renal peripheral vascular resistance and decreases the renal arterial blood flow (Nakano and McCurdy, 1967a, 1968). The magnitude of the haemodynamic effects of the intraarterial injection of $PGE_1$ is significantly greater than that of $PGA_1$. McGiff *et al.* (1969b) and Higgins *et al.* (1970) observed that intravenous injection of $PGA_1$ or $PGA_2$ (5 ng/kg/min or 0.01-1 µg/kg) also increases renal arterial blood flow whereas the intravenous injection of the same dose of $PGE_1$ has no effect in dogs. In contrast, Murphy, Hesse, Evers, Hobika, Mostert, Szolnoky, Schooners, Abramczyk and Grace (1970) showed that in normotensive dogs the intravenous injection of $PGE_1$ (1 µg/kg) or $PGA_1$ (0.48-1.32 µg/kg/min) decreases transiently renal arterial blood flow. On the other hand, the same dose of $PGE_1$ or $PGA_1$ increases the renal arterial blood flow markedly in hypertensive dogs (Murphy *et al.*, 1970) and in patients with essential hypertension (Carr, 1970a). $PGA_1$ causes a greater increase in renal blood flow than cardiac output (Carr, 1970a).

### Ovarian, Uterine and Placental Circulations

Von Euler (1938) first showed that crude prostaglandin (mostly $PGE_1$) increases the resistance of human placental vessels. Hillier and Karim (1968) demonstrated that $PGE_1$ (0.2-1.4 µg/ml) decreases the isometric contraction of a longitudinal or circular strip of the human umbilical and placental arteries obtained from women who had a Caesarian section at 34-42 weeks gestation in a full term delivery. On the other hand, $PGE_2$ (0.04-0.8 $\mu$g/ml), $PGF_{1\alpha}$ (0.8-4 $\mu$g/ml) and $PGF_{2\alpha}$ (0.04-0.8 $\mu$g/ml) produce contractions of the umbilical and placental blood vessels. $PGE_2$ and $PGF_{2\alpha}$ are essentially equipotent in their action on these vascular smooth muscles. In contrast, $PGE_1$, $PGE_2$ and $PGF_{2\alpha}$ have no effect on the umbilical cord and placental blood vessels from women who aborted spontaneously at 19-20 weeks of pregnancy. Pharriss *et al.* (1970) concluded that the intravenous injection of $PGF_{2\alpha}$ (0.1-1 mg) constricts the utero-ovarian veins and decreases its blood flow for one hour or more in rats, rabbits and dogs (Fig. 5). Pharriss *et al.* (1970) postulated, therefore, that the luteolytic action of $PGF_{2\alpha}$ is due to the congestion of the ovaries by its direct vasoconstrictor action on the ovarian-uterine veins. However, the results of the studies made by Behrman *et al.* (1971) and McCracken (1971) are not in agreement with the hypothesis postulated by Pharriss *et al.* (1970) since they found that $PGF_{2\alpha}$ significantly inhibited steroidogenesis without producing significant change in the ovarian blood flow in rats and sheep. Recently, Nakano and Prancan (unpublished data) found that in pregnant dogs near term, the intravenous injection of $PGE_2$ (1 $\mu$g/kg/min for 15 min) decreases systemic arterial pressure whereas the same amount of $PGF_{2\alpha}$ increases it. However, both $PGE_2$ and $PGF_{2\alpha}$ increases the uterine arterial perfusion pressure, uterine venous pressure and the peripheral resistance in the uterine vascular beds in pregnant dogs at near term. The increase in the peripheral resistance is due either to the vasoconstrictor action of $PGE_2$ and $PGF_{2\alpha}$ or to the increased extra-vascular support by uterine contraction.

## Carotid and Cerebral Circulations

The intraarterial injection of $PGE_1$ (0.1 $\mu$g/kg or 1 $\mu$g), $PGA_1$ (0.1 $\mu$g/kg) or $PGA_2$ (0.6-1.2 $\mu$g) decreases the peripheral vascular resistance and increases the blood flow markedly in a common carotid artery in dogs (Nakano and McCurdy, 1967a; Nakano, 1968b; Lee, 1968). During this period, no significant change occurs in mean systemic arterial pressure, heart rate and myocardial contractile force, hence indicating the direct vasodilator effect of $PGE_1$, $PGA_1$ and $PGA_2$ in the carotid arteries. Lavery *et al.* (1970) found both $PGF_{2\alpha}$ and $PGF_{1\alpha}$ (4-64 $\mu$g/kg/min) increase the vertebral arterial blood flow as mean systemic arterial pressure increases.

Katsuki, Onomae, Ino and Ito (1969) reported that in dogs the intravenous injection of $PGE_1$ (3 $\mu$g/kg) markedly decreases systemic arterial blood flow and markedly increases blood flows in the internal carotid artery and cerebral cortex, whereas $PGE_1$ slightly increases the external carotid arterial blood flow. On the other hand, the intravenous injection of $PGF_{1\alpha}$ (3 µg/kg) changes neither systemic arterial pressure nor cerebral and carotid circulations. However, the larger dose (20 µg/kg) of $PGF_{1\alpha}$ slightly increases systemic arterial pressure and slightly decreases blood flow in the common carotid artery, whereas the internal carotid arterial flow remains essentially unchanged. Recently, White, Denton and Robertson (1971) showed that, in dogs and rhesus monkeys, the intra-carotid infusion of $PGE_1$ (0.1-10 µg/kg/min) dilates the cerebral blood vessels whereas $PGF_{2\alpha}$ constricts the same vessels. On the other hand, $PGA_1$ has no effect on the cerebral blood vessels.

## Extremity Circulation

Von Euler (1939) first reported that crude prostaglandin (probably mostly $PGE_1$) dilates the blood vessels and increases the blood flow in the isolated, perfused rabbit hind leg. Many investigators have shown that the intraarterial injection of $PGE_1$, $PGE_2$, $PGA_1$ or $PGA_2$ increases the blood flows and decreases the peripheral vascular resistance in both brachial, femoral and iliac arteries in dogs (Lee *et al.*, 1965; Lee, 1968; Nakano and McCurdy, 1967a; Nakano, 1968b, 1972a; Smith *et al.*, 1968; Horton and Jones, 1969; Abdel-Sayed *et al.*, 1970; Higgins *et al.*, 1970; Kadowitz *et al.*, 1971), cats (Holmes *et al.*, 1963), rabbits (Holmes *et al.*, 1963), frogs (von Euler, 1936) and man (Bevegård and Orö, 1969). These studies indicate that $PGE_1$ exerts directly a potent vasodilator action in the brachial and femoral arteries in different species of animals and in man, since the vasodilator effect occurs without any significant change in the remainder of the cardiovascular system. Daugherty *et al.* (1968) showed that the intravenous infusion of $PGE_1$ (0.97 µg/min) increases both skin and muscle blood flows by the same degree with little effect in the systemic arterial pressure.

DuCharme *et al.* (1968) and Mark, Schmid, Eckstein and Wendling (1971) showed that the intraarterial infusion or intravenous injection of $PGF_{2\alpha}$ produces little change in the femoral arterial perfusion pressure but increases considerably the small vein pressure in the isolated dog hind limb in which arterial blood flow is kept constant. Hodgman, Jelke, Swindall and Daugherty (1970) showed that the intraarterial infusion of $PGF_{2\alpha}$ decreases the skin blood flow but does not influence the skeletal muscle blood flow in the isolated dog forelimb. Total limb vascular resistance rises progressively due to a large increase in skin artery, small vessel and venous resistance. These workers concluded that $PGF_{2\alpha}$ increases the venous vascular resistance alone or more than the arteriolar resistance in dogs. On the other hand, Greenberg and Sparks (1969) and Nakano (1968b) showed that the intraarterial injection of $PGF_{2\alpha}$

decreases blood flow and increases peripheral resistance in both brachial and femoral arteries in dogs (Fig. 9 and 10) indicating that $PGF_{2\alpha}$ significantly constricts the resistance vessels. Generally, the vasoconstrictor action of $PGF_{2\alpha}$ is considerably smaller than that of noradrenaline or angiotensin in dogs (Nakano, 1968b, 1972b). DuCharme *et al.* (1968) showed that the vasoconstrictor effect of $PGF_{2\alpha}$ on the small limb veins is abolished by denervation or the administration of hexamethonium or phenoxybenzamine, and is restored by electrical stimulation of the lumbar sympathetic trunk. This may indicate that the venoconstrictor effect of $PGF_{2\alpha}$ is influenced by sympathetic stimulation. On the other hand, Nakano *et al.* (1968a, 1968b) showed that the vasoconstrictor effect of $PGF_{2\alpha}$ is not blocked by phenoxybenzamine (0.5 mg/kg) or methysergide (1 $\mu$g/kg), indicating that $PGF_{2\alpha}$ constricts directly the regional blood vessels.

## Nasal Circulation

Stovall and Jackson (1967) showed that the injection of $PGE_1$, $PGE_2$, $PGF_{1\alpha}$ or $PGA_1$ into a common carotid artery constricts the small vessels in the nasal mucosa, resulting in a dose-related decrease in the airway resistance in the nasal cavity in anaesthetized dogs (Fig. 16). $PGE_1$ and $PGE_2$ are the most potent vasoconstrictors of the nasal blood vessels, the threshold dose ranging from 1 to 50 ng. The potency of $PGA_1$ and $PGF_{1\alpha}$ is about 1/100 that of $PGE_1$ or $PGE_2$. The maximum effect produced by $PGE_1$ or $PGE_2$ is about equivalent to that produced by an equal dose of adrenaline. However, the duration of the action of prostaglandins is approximately seven times longer than that of adrenaline. Likewise, Änggård (1969) and Jackson (1970) observed that the topical application of $PGE_1$ (10-100 $\mu$g) increases nasal patency through nasal vasoconstriction for 3-12 hours in approximately 40-60%

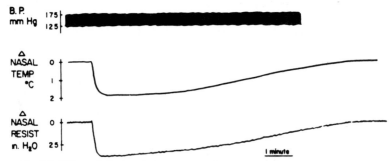

Fig. 16. Effect of the intracarotid arterial injection of $PGE_2$ on systemic arterial pressure (BP), nasal temperature and nasal airway resistance in the dog. Reproduced from Stovall and Jackson (1967) with permission of the authors and publisher.

of the subjects studied. It remains uncertain whether the prostaglandins exist in the nasal mucosa or how prostaglandins constrict the blood vessels in this particular area.

## Nervous System

Prostaglandins ($PGE_1$, $PGE_2$, $PGF_{1\alpha}$ and $PGF_{2\alpha}$) and prostaglandin-like substances occur in the brain (Ambache, 1966; Samuelsson, 1964; Coceani and Wolfe, 1965; Coceani, Pace-Asciak and Wolfe, 1968; Horton and Main, 1966, 1967; Holmes and Horton, 1967) cerebellum (Coceani and Wolfe, 1965; Ramwell and Shaw, 1966) spinal cord (Ramwell, Shaw and Jessup, 1966b; Coceani *et al.*, 1968) and spinal fluid (Feldberg and Myers, 1966). Furthermore, these prostaglandins are found to be released spontaneously in small quantities (Coceani and Wolfe, 1965; Ramwell and Shaw, 1966) or in larger quantities by electrical stimulation or by central nervous stimulation with picrotoxin, penetylenetetrazol and strychnine (Coceani and Wolfe, 1965; Ramwell and Shaw, 1966). In addition, prostaglandins are released from the peripheral nerve endings either spontaneously or by electrical stimulation or by acetylcholine, serotonin, dopa, tranylcypromine or ACTH. The tissues studied include diaphragm (Ramwell, Shaw and Kucharski, 1965; Ramwell and Shaw, 1967), hindlimb (Ramwell *et al.*, 1966b), spleen (Davies, Horton and Withrington, 1966; Bennett, Friedmann and Vane, 1967), stomach (Bennett *et al.*, 1967; Coceani, Pace-Asciak, Volta and Wolfe, 1967), epididymal adipose tissue (Shaw, 1966; Ramwell and Shaw, 1967) and adrenal gland (Ramwell, Shaw, Douglas and Poisner, 1966a). Catecholamines do not appear to evoke prostaglandin release (Ramwell *et al.*, 1966a) or vice versa (Horton, 1969). The administration of phentolamine, phenoxybenzamine, hyosine, hexamethonium or tetra-doxin blocks partially or completely prostaglandin release evoked by the peripheral nerve stimulation (Davies *et al.*, 1966; Ramwell *et al.*, 1966b; Bennett *et al.*, 1967; Coceani *et al.*, 1967).

Horton (1964) and Horton and Main (1965, 1966) studied the pharmacological actions of prostaglandins on the central nervous system in cats and chicken (Tables 2 and 3). In conscious cats, the intraventricular injection of $PGE_1$, $PGE_2$ or $PGE_3$ (7-20 µg/kg) causes transient sedation, and prolonged stupor and catatonia, but no ataxia (Horton, 1964). In contrast, the intraventricular injection of $PGF_{2\alpha}$ or the prostaglandin precursors, di-homo-linolenic acid and arachidonic acid, cause no detectable changes in the behaviours of cats. In mice, the subcutaneous injection of $PGE_1$ causes decreased spontaneous activity, and ptosis which is prevented by pretreatment with imipramine. In addition, $PGE_1$ prolongs hexobarbitone sleeping time and antagonizes electrical and penetylenetetrazol-induced convulsions in mice (Holmes

Table 2

Actions of prostaglandins on the central nervous system in the cat

| Anesthetic | State of CNS | Route of injection | Prostaglandin | Response |
|---|---|---|---|---|
| None | Intact | Lateral ventricle | $E_1$, $E_2$, $E_3$, $F_{2\alpha}$ | Sedation, stupor, catatonia<br>No effect |
| | | Intravenous | $E_1$ | Slight sedation |
| | | Intravenous | $E_1$, $F_{2\alpha}$ | (1) Potentiation of decerebrate rigidity<br>(2) Contraction of gastrocnemius muscle |
| None | Midcollicular decerebration | Iontophoretic | $E_1$, $E_2$, $F_{2\alpha}$ | Excitation or inhibition of medullary neurones |
| None | Spinal section at $C_2$, brain destroyed | Intravenous | $E_1$ | (1) Contraction of gastrocnemius muscle, not abolished by acute, dorsal root section<br>(2) Potentiation of crossed extensor reflex<br>(3) No effect on patellar reflex |
| Pentobarbitone | Intact | Intravenous | $E_1$ | (1) Abolition of tremor<br>(2) Reduction in gastrocnemius muscle tension |
| | | Lateral ventricle | $E_1$ | No effect on tremor |
| | | Direct application to cerebral cortex | $E_1$ | No effect on tremor |
| Chloralose | Intact | Intraaortic | $E_1$<br>$F_{1\alpha}$, $F_{2\alpha}$ | Inhibition of spinal monosynaptic reflexes<br>Potentiation and/or inhibition of spinal monosynaptic reflexes |
| | | Iontophoretic | $E_1$ | No effect on cortical neurones |

Reproduced from Horton (1969) with permission of the author and publisher.

Table 3

Actions of prostaglandins on the central nervous system in the chick

| Anaesthetic | State of CNS | Route of injection | Prostaglandin | Response |
|---|---|---|---|---|
| None | Intact | Intravenous | $E_1$, $E_2$, $E_3$ $F_{1\alpha}$, $F_{2\alpha}$ | Sedation, loss of righting reflex |
| None | Spinal section at $C_4$ | Intravenous | $F_{2\alpha}$ | Contraction of extensor muscles (1) Contraction of gastrocnemius muscle |
| | Decapitated | | $E_2$ | (2) Potentiation of crossed extensor reflex Potentiation of crossed extensor reflex |
| Chloralose | Intact | Intravenous | $F_{2\alpha}$ | (1) Contraction of gastrocnemius muscle (2) Potentiation of crossed extensor reflex |
| | | | $E_1$ | Inhibition of crossed extensor reflex |
| Urethane | Intact | Intravenous | $F_{2\alpha}$ | (1) Contraction of gastrocnemius muscle (2) Abolition of tremor |
| | | | $E_1$ | Abolition of tremor |
| | | Cerebral cortex | $E_1$ | Abolition of tremor |

Reproduced from Horton (1969) with permission of the author and publisher.

and Horton, 1967). Milton and Wendlandt (1970) observed that in conscious cats the injection of small doses (28 nmoles to 28 $\mu$moles) of $PGE_1$ into the third ventricle rapidly increases the rectal temperature by as much as $3°C$. The temperature rise is accompanied by violent shivering and piloerection. The cats appear to be sedated without any evidence of catatonia when large doses (28-280 $\mu$moles) are injected into the lateral ventricle. $PGA_1$ and $PGF_{1\alpha}$ also exert lesser pyretic action whereas $PGF_{2\alpha}$ has no effect. The intraperitoneal administration of 4-acetamidophenol (4-Ac) (0.3 mmoles/kg) 30 min before the prosta-glandins prevents the temperature rise due to $PGA_1$ and $PGF_{1\alpha}$. When 4-Ac is given after the injection of these prostaglandins, it reduces the established fever. In contrast, 4-Ac is unable to prevent the onset of fever, or to reduce a fever already induced by $PGE_1$. Milton and Wendlandt (1970) postulated that $PGE_1$ may be acting as a modulator in temperature regulation in the hypothalamus and that the action of antipyretics may interfere with the release of $PGE_1$ by 5-hydroxytryp-tamine (5-HT) or pyrogen. Furthermore, they suggested that this mecha-nism would explain why 5-HT fever and not $PGE_1$ is affected by 4-AC in cats. Very recently, Vane and his colleagues (Vane, 1971; Ferreira, Moncada and Vane, 1971; Smith and Willis, 1971) reported that indomethacin, aspirin and sodium salicylate (in descending order of potency) block the synthesis of $PGE_2$ and $PGF_{2\alpha}$ from arachidonic acid in the guinea-pig lung homogenate, and the production of the prostaglandins in the isolated dog spleen induced by adrenaline, and in a suspension of the human platelets induced by thrombin. It can be speculated that both pyrogens and 5-HT induce fever by triggering the production and release of prostaglandins in the temperature regulating centre in the hypothalamus, and the antipyretics may act by inhibiting the prostaglandin synthesis there (Collier, 1971).

In rats, microelectrophoresis of noradrenaline, cyclic AMP and gamma-aminobutyric acid (GABA) markedly reduces the spontaneous discharge of Purkinje cells in the cerebellum (Hoffer, Siggins and Bloom, 1969; Siggins, Hoffer and Bloom, 1971). A phosphodiesterase inhibitor, aminophylline, has not only similar effect, but also potentiates the effect by noradrenaline and cyclic AMP. Both $PGE_1$ and $PGE_2$ effectively antagonize the response to noradrenaline and aminophylline, but not that to cyclic AMP and GABA (Figs. 17 and 18). $PGF_{1\alpha}$, $PGF_{2\alpha}$, linoleic acid and linolenic acid have negligible effects (Siggins *et al.*, 1971). $PGE_1$ produces similar antagonistic action on the spontaneous activity of single neurones and their response to noradrenaline in the rat cortex and rabbit cerebellar Purkinje cells, but has no effect in the rat reticular formation and hippocampus areas (Siggins *et al.*, 1971). These observations suggest that the endogenous prostaglandins may physio-logically function to modulate adrenergic functions in some areas of CNS.

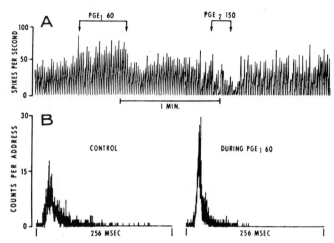

Fig. 17. Effects of microelectrophoretic application of $PGE_1$ and $PGE_2$ on spontaneous Purkinje cell discharge. (A) Effects of drug application on mean discharge frequency. Duration of drug application indicated by arrows, numbers after each drug indicate ejection current in nanoamperes. (B) Interspike interval histograms of the same cell during the control period and during application of $PGE_1$: 1000 spikes and 0.25 msec address interval used for each histogram. The peak of the histogram represents the most probable interspike interval of single spike discharge. Note that the increase in mean discharge produced by $PGE_1$ is accompanied by a decrease in the population of long pauses (tail of the histogram) but little change in the most probable interspike interval (22 msec). Reproduced from Hoffer *et al.* (1969) with permission of the authors and publisher. Copyright 1969 by the American Association for the Advancement of Science.

In chicks, $PGE_1$, $PGE_2$ or $PGE_3$ (25 µg/kg) injected intravenously induces a marked sedation with cessation of spontaneous movements, closure of the eyes and loss of righting reflexes (Horton, 1964). In contrast, $PGF_{2\alpha}$ produces no sedation, but extension and abduction of the legs and dorsiflexion of the neck (Horton and Main, 1965). The effect on the legs appears to be due to an action of $PGF_{2\alpha}$ directly on the spinal cord, since it can be abolished by cutting the sciatic nerve and elicited in the chick after mid-cervical cord transection (Horton and Main, 1967). Furthermore, in spinal or decerebrate cats, gastrocnemius muscle tension is increased by either $PGE_1$ or $PGF_{2\alpha}$ given intravenously but not intraarterially to the muscle. The response in spinal cats is abolished by sciatic nerve section but not by dorsal root section (Horton and Main, 1965; Horton and Main, 1967). The action of $PGE_1$ or $PGF_{2\alpha}$ presumably is a direct facilitation of excitatory pathways rather than an inhibition of inhibitory pathways, since $PGE_1$ does not inhibit the crossed extensor reflex brought about by stretching of the ipsilateral

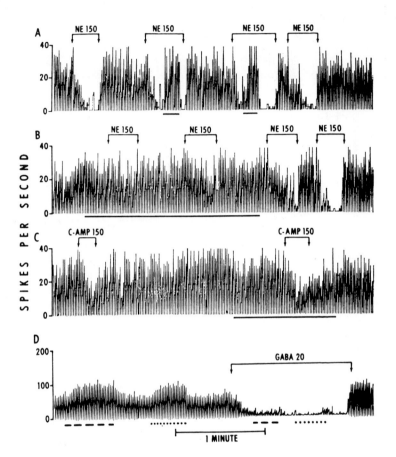

Fig. 18. Selective antagonism by prostaglandins of Purkinje cell responses to noradrenaline (NE). A, B and C represent consecutive records from the same cell. D illustrates another cell from a different preparation. Duration of NE, cyclic AMP, and γ-aminobutyric acid microelectrophoresis indicated by arrows. Numbers after each drug indicate ejection current A. nanoamperes. Black lines beneath the records in A, B and C represent microelectrophoresis of $PGE_1$, 80 na. The dashed and dotted lines beneath the record in D represents microelectrophoresis of $PGE_1$, 125 na and $PGE_2$, 125 na, respectively. Concentrations of prostaglandin which have no direct effect on mean discharge rate (B) antagonize the depressant effects of NE (A, B) but not cyclic AMP (C). Even doses of prostaglandin which directly increase mean discharge rates have no effect on the depressant effects of γ-aminobutyric acid (D). Reproduced from Hoffer *et al.* (1969) with permission of the authors and publisher. Copyright 1969 by the American Association for the Advancement of Science.

hamstring muscle or by electrical stimulation of the peroneal nerve. The crossed extensor reflex in the spinal chick and cat is potentiated by both $PGF_{2\alpha}$ and $PGE_1$, but no significant changes have been observed on the mono-synaptic patellar reflex in the cat with $PGE_1$ (Horton and Main, 1966). In the anaesthetized cat, both $PGF_{1\alpha}$ and $PGE_1$ usually inhibit mono-synaptic spinal reflexes for a considerably long period (Duda, Horton and McPherson, 1968).

In the lightly anaesthetized chick or cat, tremor which is frequently observed during recovery from anaesthesia, is abolished by the intravenous injection of $PGE_1$ or its direct application to the cerebral hemispheres (Horton and Main, 1967). From these observations, it seems evident that prostaglandins exert a direct effect on the spinal cord. However, the upper motor neurones would modulate the effects of prostaglandins on the spinal cord in cats and chicks. Although Krnjevic (1965) did not observe any significant effects of $PGE_1$ on cortical neurones in cats, Avanzino, Bradley and Wolstencroft *et al.* (1966) showed that $PGE_1$, $PGE_2$ and $PGE_3$ administered into the medulla (medial reticular formation) exert a marked stimulating action on the brain-stem neurones in unanaesthetized, decerebrate cats. About 20-30% of neurones are stimulated and a smaller proportion are inhibited, whereas the remainder (60%) show no response. Short-lasting tachyphylaxis to E prostaglandins frequently occurs but there is no cross tachyphylaxis between the three E prostaglandins. Acetylcholine also produces either excitation or inhibition, but the direction of its effect on the same neurone is not related to that of the prostaglandins. Coceani, Dreifuss, Puglisi and Wolfe (1969) found that local superfusion of $PGF_{2\alpha}$ (10 $\mu$g/ml) over the surface of the medulla oblongata reduces markedly synaptic transmission.

In the anaesthetized chick with intact brain, the eye-opening and the depressor responses to $PGF_{2\alpha}$ are not abolished by spinal transection. Contractions of the cat nictitating membrane elicited by pre-ganglionic cervical nerve stimulation are unaffected by $PGE_1$ injected either intravenously or into the common carotid artery. However, relaxations of the nictitating membrane after cessation of stimulation are more rapid in the period immediately following $PGE_1$ administration (Holmes *et al.*, 1963).

$PGE_1$ does not appear to be a pain-producing substance since $PGE_1$ (0.1 to 50 $\mu$g/ml) applied to exposed blister bases on the human forearm does not give rise to any sensation of pain or itch (Horton, 1969). In contrast, bradykinin (0.1 $\mu$g/ml) and serotonin (0.01$\mu$g/ml) are effective in producing pain on these preparations (Horton, 1969). $PGE_1$ in a large concentration (100 $\mu$g/ml) produces a barely detectable sensation of pain, but it is about half as potent as its precursor, di-homo-$\gamma$-linoleic acid, and arachidonic acid (Horton and Main, 1966).

**Renal System**

It has been found that crude lipid extracts of the renal medulla of the dog, pig (Hickler, Lauler, Saravis, Vagnucci, Steiner and Thorn, 1964; Muirhead, Daniels, Booth, Freyburger and Hinman, 1965), Rabbit (Lee *et al.,* 1965; Hickler *et al.,* 1964; Strong, Boucher, Nowaczynski and Genest, 1966), rat (Hickler *et al.,* 1964) and man (Lee *et al.,* 1965; Hickler *et al.,* 1964; Strong *et al.,* 1966) exert a transient but potent vasodepressor action in rats and dogs. The circulatory actions of some of these lipids are similar to those of E and A prostaglandins. Lee *et al.* (1965) and Daniels, Hinman, Leach and Muirhead (1967) found that the major depressor lipids of the rabbit kidney are prostaglandins, especially $PGE_2$ and $PGA_2$. $PGE_1$ and $PGF_{2\alpha}$ also appear to be present in the renal medulla. The renal prostaglandins are also biosynthesized from the precursor fatty acids, linoleic acid and arachidonic acid (Hamberg, 1969; van Dorp, 1971), and released by nerve stimulation (Dunham and Zimmerman, 1970) and by factors which decrease the renal blood flow (McGiff, Crowshaw, Terragno, Lonigro, Strand, Williamson, Ng and Lee, 1969a). The released prostaglandins are metabolized very rapidly by PGDH in the renal cortex and medulla (Nakano, 1970b; Änggård, 1971; Nakano and Prancan, 1971), and hence appear in the renal vein. However, recently, Edwards, Strong and Hunt (1969) and McGiff *et al.* (1969a) found that prostaglandin-like substances increase in the renal venous blood in animals with renal ischemia and in patients with essential and renal hypertension.

As discussed in the previous section on the cardiovascular actions of prostaglandins,both E and A compounds increase markedly renal blood flow, and may redistribute the blood flow from the medulla to the cortex. Although the mechanism involved remains unknown, prosta-glandins significantly modify the renal function in animals with or without renal hypertension. In anaesthetized dogs, Johnston *et al.* (1967) and Vander (1968) showed that the injection of subhypotensive doses (0.1-2 $\mu$g/min) of $PGE_1$ or $PGE_2$ into one renal artery significantly increase total renal plasma flow, urinary flow, sodium excretion and free water clearance in the ipsilateral kidney. On the other hand, glomerular filtration rate (GFR) remains unchanged, and p-amino-hippurate (PAH) extraction ratio decreases in the ipsilateral kidney. These renal effects of $PGE_1$ must be due to its direct action on the kidney, and is not mediated by the extrarenal neurohumoral regulatory mechanism since there are no effects on the contralateral kidney. On the other hand, Murphy *et al.* (1970) showed that the intravenous injection of $PGE_1$ (1 $\mu$g/kg for 3 min) markedly reduces renal blood flow, urinary flow and sodium excretion, and causes little changes in inulin, creatinine and PAH clearance in normotensive dogs. In contrast, the same dose of $PGE_1$

increases renal blood flow but decreases all other parameters measured in hypertensive dogs. $PGA_1$ also decreases all parameters measured in normotensive dogs, but increases inulin, creatinine and PAH clearances and urinary flow and decreases markedly renal blood flow and urinary sodium excretion in hypertensive dogs. These data are not in accord with the observations made by the previous workers (Johnston *et al.*, 1967; Vander, 1968).

Recently, in patients with essential hypertension, Lee *et al.* (1971) found that the intravenous infusion of $PGA_1$ (0.1-2.1 µg/kg/min) significantly increases effective renal plasma flow (ERPF), GFR, urinary flow and sodium and potassium excretion without producing any significant change in systemic arterial pressure (Figs. 19 and 20). Higher doses (2.1-11.2 µg/kg/min) of $PGA_1$ decrease systemic arterial pressure markedly and reduce previously elevated ERPF, GFR, urinary flow and sodium and potassium excretion to or toward preinfusion levels. Thus, decreased renal perfusion due to reduction in systemic arterial pressure offsets the direct renal vasodilating and natriuretic action of $PGA_1$. Conseqently, normotension induced by $PGA_1$ in hypertensive patients is associated with a normal renal blood flow and a normal renal sodium excretion. Carr (1970a) also showed that the intravenous infusion of $PGA_1$ (1.3 µg/kg/min) significantly increases GRF and ERPF as systemic arterial pressure decreases and cardiac output increases markedly in patients with essential hypertension. During the infusion of $PGA_1$, urinary flow, sodium and potassium excretion, and free water clearance

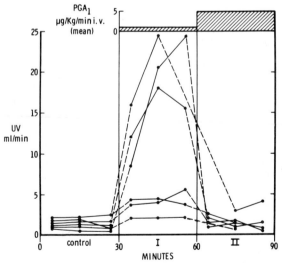

Fig. 19. Effect of $PGA_1$ on urine flow (UV) in essential hypertension. Reproduced from Lee *et al.* (1971) with permission of the authors and publisher.

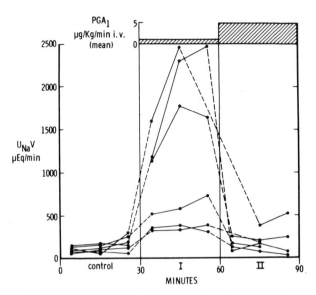

Fig. 20. Effect of $PGA_1$ on sodium excretion ($U_{Na}V$) in essential hypertension. Reproduced from Lee *et al.* (1971) with permission of the authors and publishers.

($C_{H_2O}$) increase markedly whereas solute free water clearance ($T^CH_2O$) decreases.

The basic mechanism responsible for the effect of prostaglandins on the renal function remains uncertain. It is reasonable to assume that the redistribution of the renal blood flow may influence the tubular transport mechanism by offsetting the countercurrent multiplier system as seen with ethacrynic acid and furosemide (Barger and Herd, 1967). Furthermore, the direct effect of prostaglandins on the water reabsorption and Na transport mechanism in the renal tubules should be taken into consideration. Recently, attempts have been made to elucidate the subcellular mechanism responsible for natriuresis and water diuresis induced by prostaglandins. It was found that $PGE_1$ inhibits water permeability induced by vasopressin and theophylline in the isolated toad bladder (Orloff, Handler and Bergström, 1965) and in the isolated perfused collecting tubules of the rabbit kidney (Orloff and Grantham, 1967). However, $PGE_1$ alone has no effect on water permeability (Orloff *et al.*, 1965). Since the anti-diuretic action of vasopressin is closely associated with the adenyl cyclase activity and the intracellular concentrations of cyclic AMP, Orloff *et al.* (1965) and Grantham and Orloff (1968) suggested that $PGE_1$ may inhibit competitively adenyl cyclase activity with vasopressin in the site of water permeability in the toad bladder and in the isolated rat collecting tubules. Very recently, Lipson and Sharp (1971) showed that in the toad bladder, $PGE_1$ inhibits the osmotic water flow response induced by vasopressin and theophylline but not by cyclic AMP by itself (Fig. 21). The inhibition of the vasopressin response may be by competitive interaction with adenyl cyclase. In contrast to the effects on water flow, $PGE_1$ by itself stimulates sodium transport across the bladder. This stimulation of transport can be potentiated by theophylline, suggesting an action of $PGE_1$ on adenyl cyclase and consequent stimulation of

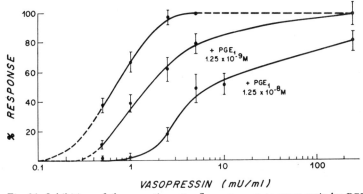

Fig. 21. Inhibition of the osmotic water flow response to vasopressin by $PGE_1$. Reproduced from Lipson and Sharp (1971) with permission of the authors and publisher.

sodium transport by cyclic AMP. $PGE_1$ was not shown to interact with the same receptor sites that vasopressin occupies for its stimulation of sodium transport. The action of $PGE_1$ on adenyl cyclase to stimulate sodium transport and inhibit water flow, provides confirmation that two distinct adenyl cyclases exist in the toad bladder, one responsible for sodium transport and the other for water flow and that the cyclic AMP released must be compartmentalized (Peterson and Edelman, 1964; Orloff and Handler, 1967: Lipson, Hynie and Sharp, 1971).

Lee (1968) has postulated that renal prostaglandins may be responsible for some form of essential hypertension and also may counteract the renin elaborating mechanism by enhancing the renal cortical blood flow as a consequence of the renal blood flow redistribution. Presently, it remains uncertain, however, whether renal prostaglandin may play a role in a homeostatic mechanism in patients with renal hypertension. Vander (1968) and Carr (1970b) showed that $PGE_1$ or $PGE_2$ infused into the renal artery or $PGA_1$ (0.48-1.32 $\mu g/kg/min$) infused intravenously has no detectable effect on renin release in normotensive dogs and in patients with essential hypertension, respectively. Muirhead, Brooks, Kosinski, Daniels and Hinman (1966) and Muirhead, Leach, Brown, Daniels and Hinman (1967) showed that large doses of $PGE_2$ (15-29 $\mu$g/kg/day), $PGA_1$ (5-100 $\mu$g/kg/min) and $PGF_{1\alpha}$ (15-30 $\mu$g/kg/day) decreased systemic arterial pressure in dogs with renoprival hypertension. However, further testing of the antihypertensive action of extremely large doses of prostaglandins failed to confirm the early reports (Bergström *et al.,* 1968).

## Metabolism

### *Lipid Metabolism*

Lipolysis *in vitro* (adipose tissue or isolated fat cells): Steinberg, Vaughan, Nestel and Bergström (1963) and Steinberg *et al.* (1964) first observed that $PGE_1$ reduces the release of glycerol or free fatty acid (FFA) from the rat epididymal adipose tissue, indicating the direct antilipolytic action of $PGE_1$. Subsequently, many investigators (Bergström and Carlson, 1965; Bergström *et al.,* 1967; Berti, Lentati and Grafnetta, 1967; Böhle, Ditschuneit, Ammon and Dobert, 1966a; Böhle, Rettberg, Ditschuniet and Dobert, 1967; Carlson *et al.,* 1968a, 1969; Carlson, Ekelund and Orö, 1970a, 1970b; Stock and Westermann, 1966; Mandel and Kuehl, 1967; Paoletti, Lentati and Karolkiewicz, 1967; Steinberg and Vaughan, 1967; Stock, Böhle and Westermann, 1967; Vaughan, 1967) confirmed the inhibition by $PGE_1$ of basal glycerol and FFA releases from adipose tissue or from isolated fat cells of fed rats. $PGE_1$ is one of the most potent antilipolytic substances known. As little as 1 ng/ml of $PGE_1$ reduces basal glycerol and FFA release and 100 ng/ml inhibits it maximally (Steinberg *et al.,* 1964; Carlson, 1967; Fain, 1967). Several workers (Bergström and Carlson, 1965; Stock and Westermann, 1966; Carlson, 1967; Stock *et al.,* 1967; Micheli, 1969, 1970) showed that $PGE_1$ does not inhibit lipolysis in adipose tissue from fasted rats, rabbits and dogs. Occasionally, $PGE_1$ increases lipolysis in the fasted dogs. However, other workers (Fain, 1967; Kupiecki, 1967; Bizzi, Veneroni, Garattini, Puglisi and Paoletti, 1967) found that $PGE_1$ does inhibit lipolysis in the adipose tissue and isolated fat cells from fasted rats. Kupiecki (1967) also found that the essential fatty acid (FFA) concentration is decreased in tissue taken from fasted rats pretreated with $PGE_1$. $PGE_1$ also inhibits the lipolytic effect of noradrenaline on EFA deficient fat cells (Bergström and Carlson, 1965; Bizzi *et al.,* 1967). Haessler and Crawford (1966, 1967) observed that in the adipose tissue from fasted rats the inhibition of $PGE_1$ of both basal and adrenaline-stimulated lipolysis is dependent upon the presence of glucose in the incubation medium. In contrast, Bergström and Carlson (1965) showed that $PGE_1$ exerts no antilipolytic action in a glucose-containing medium.

$PGE_1$ reduces lipolysis in rat adipose tissue and isolated fat cells treated with various lipolytic agents, such as adrenaline and noradrenaline (Steinberg *et al.*, 1963, 1964; Stock and Westermann, 1966; Böhle *et al.*, 1966a, 1967; Carlson, 1967; Bizzi *et al.*, 1967; Fain, 1967), ACTH and TSH (Fain, 1967; Stock and Westermann, 1966; Boberg, Micheli and Rammer, 1970), tri-iodothyronine (Mandel and Kuell, 1967), glucagon (Steinberg *et al.*, 1963), vasopressin (Vaughan, 1964), growth hormone (Böhle *et al.*, 1966a, 1967; Fain, 1967) and theophylline (Mühlbachova, Solyom and Puglisi, 1967; Solyom, Puglisi and Mühlbachova, 1967; Fain, 1968a, 1968b; Stock, Aulich and Westermann, 1968) (Fig. 22). Very low concentrations of $PGE_1$ significantly inhibit the lipolytic effect of adrenaline. Excessive amounts of $PGE_1$ only partially (41%) inhibit the lipolytic effect of submaximal concentrations of adrenaline, glucagon and ACTH in either rat adipose tissue (Weeks and Walk, 1967) or in the isolated rat fat cells (Blecher, Merlino, Ro'Ane and Flynn, 1969). The antagonism of $PGE_1$ and catecholamines, ACTH, glucagon or theophylline has been found to be competitive (Fain, 1967; Stock *et al.*, 1968) (Fig. 23), noncompetitive (Mühlbachova *et al.*, 1967) and mixed, the noncompetitive component

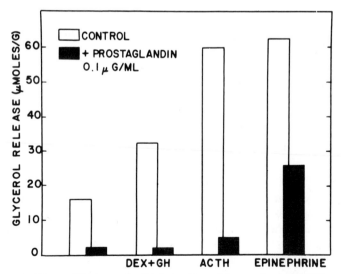

Fig. 22. Effect of $PGE_1$ on the lipolytic effect of dexamethasone (DEX), growth hormone (GH), ACTH and epinephrine (adrenaline) in isolated rat fat cells. Reproduced from Fain (1967) with permission of the author and publisher.

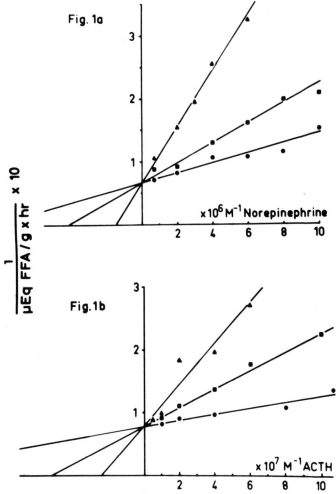

Fig. 23. Competitive inhibition of norepinephrine (noradrenaline)-induced lipolysis by $PGE_1$. Reproduced from Stock *et al.* (1968) with permission of the author and publisher.

being more prominent in a medium with half the usual calcium (Fassina and Contessa, 1967). Furthermore, Fassina and Contessa (1967) found that the inhibitory effect of $PGE_1$ on noradrenaline-induced lipolysis is enhanced in low $Ca^{++}$ and/or low $K^+$ medium, while Fain (1968a) found that this effect is not dependent upon $K^+$ concentrations in the fat cells.

$PGE_1$ (1 ng/ml) also inhibits glycerol and FFA release evoked by electrical stimulation of the sympathetic nerves to the rat epididymal fat pad *in vitro* (Berti and Usardi, 1964) and in canine subcutaneous adipose tissue *in situ* (Fredholm and Rosell, 1970). Since prostaglandin released from the fat pad can also be evoked by nerve stimulation in comparable concentrations (Ramwell and Shaw, 1967; Fredholm, Rosell and Strandberg, 1970b), it has been postulated that $PGE_1$ may play a physiological role as feedback regulation of hormone-stimulated lipolysis in the adipose tissue.

The basal and noradrenaline-stimulated lipolysis of the isolated human subcutaneous adipose tissue are reduced respectively by 10 ng/ml and 1 µg/ml of $PGE_1$ (Carlson, 1967; Bergström and Carlson, 1965; Micheli, Carlson and Hallberg, 1968). $PGE_1$ (1 µg/ml) depresses noradrenaline-stimulated glycerol release in human subcutaneous and omental adipose tissue (Carlson and Hallberg, 1968). In rabbit omental and perirenal adipose tissue, $PGE_1$ has no effect on basal glycerol release but reduces slightly lipolysis stimulated by noradrenaline or ACTH (Micheli, 1969, 1970). In dog omental adipose tissue or subcutaneous adipose tissue, low doses of $PGE_1$ inhibits noradrenaline-induced lipolysis (Micheli, 1970; Fredholm and Rosell, 1970), whereas high concentrations of $PGE_1$ stimulates it (Micheli, 1970).

The antilipolytic potencies of several other prostaglandins have been determined on rat adipose tissue or isolated fat cells. $PGF_{1\alpha}$ and $PGF_{2\alpha}$ are much weaker than $PGE_1$ or $PGE_2$ (Butcher and Baird, 1968, 1969; Steinberg *et al.*, 1964) and $PGF_{1\beta}$ is completely inactive (Butcher and Baird, 1969; Butcher, Pike and Sutherland, 1967; Steinberg *et al.*, 1964). $PGE_2$ is almost three times more potent than $PGE_1$ in adipose tissue and isolated fat cells (Steinberg *et al.*, 1964; Christ and Nugteren, 1970). Among several other prostaglandin analogues, $\omega$-homo-$PGE_1$ (21 : 3 $\omega$7) and dihomo-$PGE_1$ (the C-22 analogue) have activity roughly equal to that of $PGE_1$ (Bergström *et al.*, 1968; Christ and Nugteren, 1970), whereas nor-$PGE_1$, nor-$PGE_2$ and dinor-$PGE_2$ have very feeble or no antilipolytic action (Böhle and May, 1968). $PGA_1$ exerts little or no antilipolytic action (Bergström *et al.*, 1967; Nakano *et al.*, 1968a).

Lipolysis *in vivo:* Bergström *et al.* (1964, 1965a, 1965b) showed that in dogs $PGE_1$ injected intravenously lowers elevated plasma FFA and glycerol levels which have been increased by noradrenaline, suggesting an inhibitory effect of $PGE_1$ on the hormone-induced lipolysis in adipose tissue (Bergström *et al.*, 1964, 1965a, 1965b). $PGE_1$ inhibits not only the efflux of labelled palmitate into the plasma, but also the effect on FFA mobilization by either adrenaline or the sympathetic ganglion stimulant, DMPP (Bergström, Carlson and Orö, 1966; Steinberg *et al.*, 1964). In rats, as seen in adipose tissue *in vitro,* the intravenous infusion of $PGE_1$ reduces the elevated FFA induced by noradrenaline, ACTH, and exposure to cold (Berti *et al.*, 1967). A relatively large parenteral dose or the intravenous or intra-aortic infusion of $PGE_1$ reduces plasma FFA levels in rabbits (Böhle *et al.*, 1966a, 1966b, 1967), guinea pigs

(Berti *et al.*, 1967) and rats (Berti *et al.*, 1967; Kupiecki, 1967). However, the intravenous infusion of the relatively small dose (0.2 $\mu$g/kg/min) into man or the dog increases plasma glycerol and FFA levels (Bergström *et al.*, 1965a, 1965b, 1966). In man, this dose of $PGE_1$ only slightly reduces the elevation in glycerol and plasma FFA induced by simultaneous noradrenaline infusion (Bergström *et al.*, 1965a, 1965b; Carlson *et al.*, 1970a). However, in dogs, larger doses (0.4 to 1.6 $\mu$g/kg/min) of $PGE_1$ decrease plasma glycerol and FFA levels (Bergström *et al.*, 1966). Ganglion blocking agents prevent the increase in plasma FFA induced by low doses of $PGE_1$ (Bergström *et al.*, 1966; Carlson, 1967). This suggests that the increase of plasma FFA is due to the reflexly increased sympathetic activity by hypotension. Nitroglycerine and other hypotensive drugs also increase plasma FFA in the dog (Bergström *et al.*, 1968; Steinberg and Pittman, 1966). In unanaesthetized dogs, $PGE_1$ lowers, but $PGA_1$ raises plasma FFA (Steinberg and Pittman, 1966) since $PGA_1$ exerts no or very little antilipolytic effect but is a greater depressor agent than $PGE_1$. In fasted rats, intravenous injection of $PGE_1$ has a biphasic effect on plasma FFA, an initial fall being followed by a rise, before returning to control (Kupiecki, 1967). Carlson *et al.* (1968a, 1970a, 1970b) showed that, in man $PGE_1$ and $PGA_1$ (0.056-0.56 $\mu$g/kg/min) infused intravenously increases plasma FFA levels slightly. On the other hand, the intravenous infusion of $PGF_{1\alpha}$, $PGF_{1\beta}$ and $PGF_{2\alpha}$ (0.32 or 0.56 $\mu$g/kg/min) causes no effect on plasma FFA levels. The intravenous injection of $PGE_2$ or $PGE_3$ also lowers noradrenaline-induced elevation of plasma FFA in dogs, whereas $PGF_{1\alpha}$ has no effect (Bergström *et al.*, 1964). $PGA_1$ either raises or does not change plasma FFA (Bergström *et al.*, 1967; Steinberg and Pittman, 1966).

## Mode of the antilipolytic action of prostaglandins

The mechanisms responsible for a hormone-stimulated hypothesis for the lipolysis and the biochemical site of the antilipolytic action of prostaglandins have been proposed by several investigators (Steinberg, 1967; Bergström *et al.*, 1968; Horton, 1969; Butcher and Baird, 1969; Stock *et al.*, 1968). Several hormones activate adenyl cyclase to form cyclic AMP which is converted to $5'$ AMP by phosphodiesterase in the adipose tissue. Hormone-sensitive lipase, which hydrolyzes triglyceride in the adipose tissue, is activated by cyclic AMP-dependent-proteinkinase (Kuo and Greengard, 1969) and appears to be rate-limiting (Steinberg and Vaughan, 1967). Hence, a second messenger, cyclic $3'$, $5'$ AMP seems to play a key role in mediating the lipolytic actions of catecholamines and other hormones by activating this lipase (Butcher and Sutherland, 1967; Robison, Butcher and Sutherland, 1967). In addition, lipolysis is greatly influenced by availability of glucose in the adipose tissue. Glucose metabolism is closely related to re-esterification of FFA by providing $\alpha$-glycerophosphate, which cannot be formed from glycerol in adipose tissue.

$PGE_1$ opposes the catecholamine-induced elevations of both plasma FFA and glycerol *pari passu* in intact dogs (Bergström *et al.,* 1964). $PGE_1$ mainly acts on the lipolytic process in the adipose tissues. $PGE_1$ decreases the adrenaline-induced activation of hormone sensitive lipase in the rat adipose tissue (Steinberg *et al.,* 1964), through the decreased concentrations of cyclic AMP in the fat cells (Butcher and Baird, 1969). Adrenaline, glucagon and ACTH increase the intracellular levels of cyclic AMP, thus enhancing hormone sensitive lipase in adipose tissue *in vitro* (Steinberg and Vaughan, 1967; Rizack, 1961; Butcher *et al.,* 1967). $PGE_1$ decreases cyclic AMP and thus inhibits the hormone-induced lipolysis (Butcher *et al.,* 1967; Butcher and Sutherland, 1967). It remains to be clarified whether $PGE_1$ decreases the intracellular concentration of cyclic AMP by inhibition of the adenyl cyclase (Steinberg, 1967; Fain, 1967) or enhances its destruction by stimulating the phosphodiesterase in the fat cell (Mühlbachova *et al.,* 1967). Since $PGE_1$ does not inhibit stimulation of lipolysis by exogenous cyclic AMP or dibutyryl cyclic AMP, it appears to act before activation of the hormone sensitive lipase system by cyclic AMP (Steinberg and Vaughan, 1967; Peterson, Patterson and Ashmore, 1968). Stock *et al.* (1967) postulated that $PGE_1$ inhibits the availability of ATP (the substrate) for adenyl cyclase in the cell membrane. Recently, however, Butcher and Baird (1969) found that $PGE_1$ affects neither adenyl cyclase nor phosphodiesterase, but does decrease in cyclic AMP in fat cells through an unknown mechanism. Belcher *et al.* (1969) showed that the lipolytic effect of noradrenaline, ACTH and glucagon is never completely inhibited by $PGE_1$, even at excessive concentrations, although complete inhibition is obtained by appropriate concentrations of propranolol. This observation suggests that the isolated fat cells may have at least two different types of activation receptor sites for hormones, and that $PGE_1$ binds to only one type of site.

Theophylline stimulates lipolysis by inhibiting phosphodiesterase (Butcher and Sutherland, 1967; Butcher *et al.,* 1967). $PGE_1$ inhibits competitively theophylline-induced lipolysis in rat adipose tissue (Mühlbachova *et al.,* 1967; Solyom *et al.,* 1967; Steinberg and Vaughan, 1967; Stock *et al.,* 1967) and in rat fat cells (Fain, 1968a; 1968b). At high concentrations of theophylline, $PGE_1$ is relatively ineffective, either because of the competitive inhibition or because in the presence of virtually complete inhibition of phosphodiesterase the rate of formation of cyclic AMP is no longer rate-limiting (Steinberg, 1967; Steinberg and Vaughan, 1967). At given concentrations, $PGE_1$ inhibits theophylline-induced lipolysis to a greater degree than noradrenaline and also the maximum inhibition is greater (Mühlbachova *et al.*, 1967).

In rat epididymal fat tissue, $PGE_1$ inhibits the increases in lipolysis and in cyclic AMP induced by adrenaline (Butcher and Baird, 1969) but paradoxically, $PGE_1$ *per se* increases cyclic AMP to levels without inducing lipolysis (Butcher *et al.*, 1967; Butcher and Baird, 1969). In contrast, in isolated fat cells, $PGE_1$ *per se* has no effect on cyclic AMP levels but, inhibits the adrenaline-induced increase in cyclic AMP as well as FFA release (Butcher and Baird, 1969). This result indicates that tissues other than fat cells in the adipose tissue are responsbile for the increased cyclic AMP by $PGE_1$. The results of the effects of prostaglandins appear to be variable among investigators. This variability can be in part explained by such factors as age and species differences of the animals used, tissue difference, and nutritional and hormonal states of the adipose tissues.

*Lipoprotein lipase and cholesterol*

Böhle *et al.* (1967) found that in rabbits $PGE_1$ given intravenously decreases the increased FFA and ketone bodies levels induced by heparin whereas the heparin-induced increase in plasma glycerol is not affected. Although Solyom *et al.* (1970) showed that $PGE_1$ does not affect incorporation of $^3$H-palmitate (re-esterification) in the isolated rat adipose tissue, Böhle *et al.* (1967) and Haessler and Crawford (1966) found that $PGE_1$ enhances the uptake and re-esterification of FFA in the rabbits *in vivo* and in the adipose tissues. $PGE_1$ does not influence the heparin-induced release or activation of human lipoprotein lipase. In contrast, Berti *et al.* (1967) found that $PGE_1$ increases the activity of cardiac lipoprotein lipase in rats and pigs. Recently, Schweppe and Jungmann (1970) found that, in the rat liver *in vitro,* both $PGE_1$ and $PGF_{1\alpha}$ produce a concentration-dependent inhibition of the biosynthesis of cholesteryl palmitate, oleate and linoleate as well as that of fatty acids.

**Carbohydrate Metabolism**

Relatively few studies have been made of the effect of prostaglandins on carbohydrate metabolism. Most workers have found that the intravenous injection of $PGE_1$ causes significant hyperglycemia in dogs (Bergström *et al.*, 1966), rabbits (Böhle *et al.*, 1966b), rats (Paoletti *et al.*, 1967; Böhle and May, 1968), (Fig. 24) and guinea pigs (Berti *et al.*, 1967). Böhle and May observed that incubation of rat liver slices with various concentrations of $PGE_1$ *in vitro* induces a dose-dependent decrease in glycogen content of the tissue. On the other hand, $PGE_1$ fails

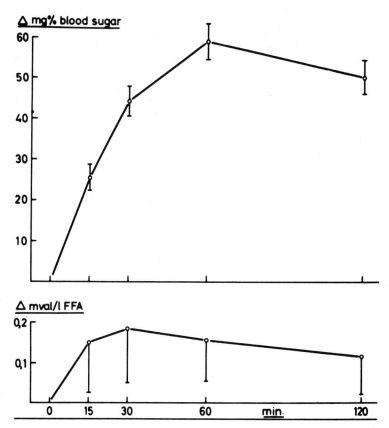

Fig. 24. Effect of the intraperitoneal injection of PGE$_1$ (1 mg/kg) on blood glucose and free fatty acid levels in rats. Reproduced from Böhle and May (1968) with permission of the authors and publisher.

to increase blood glucose in adrenalectomized rats (Bergström *et al.,* 1968). Furthermore, many unrelated hypotensive agents can induce hyperglycemia in dogs (Bergström *et al.,* 1968). These observations indicate that two separate mechanisms may be responsible for the genesis of PGE$_1$-induced hyperglycemia, i.e., (a) direct glycogenolytic action of PGE$_1$ in the liver and (b) reflexly increased secretion of catecholamines secondary to the hypotensive action of PGE$_1$ (Bergström *et al.,* 1968; Böhle and May, 1968). From the *in vivo* experiments, it appears that the direct glycogenolytic effect of PGE$_1$ is rather feeble as compared to the latter mechanism for the production of hyperglycemia. In dogs, PGE$_1$ blocks the increase in plasma FFA levels induced by noradrenaline or DMPP, but has no effect upon the simultaneous hyperglycemia

P—4

(Bergström *et al.*, 1964, 1966; Steinberg and Pittman, 1966). $PGE_1$ further increases theophylline-induced hyperglycemia in the rabbit (Paoletti *et al.*, 1967). Carlson *et al.* (1970b) showed that in healthy males, the intravenous infusion of $PGE_2$, $PGA_1$, $PGF_{1\alpha}$, $PGF_{1\beta}$ and $PGF_{2\alpha}$ causes no effect or non-consistent changes in blood glucose levels.

$PGE_1$ not only inhibits basal and hormone-induced lipolysis but also influences some aspects of glucose metabolism in adipose tissue in a manner similar to insulin. $PGE_1$ $(0.1\text{-}1.0\,\mu g/ml)$ stimulates glucose uptake, glucose oxidation, $^{14}CO_2$ production and triglyceride synthesis from both $^{14}C$-glucose and $^{14}C$-acetate in the isolated rat adipose tissue (Böhle *et al.*, 1966a, 1966b, 1967; Haessler and Crawford, 1967; Vaughan, 1967). $PGE_1$ $(10\,\mu g/kg)$ given intraperitoneally to intact rats increases ·the incorporation of $^{14}C$-glucose into the glycogen in the diaphragm and adipose tissue essentially in proportion to the dose (Böhle *et al.*, 1966a, 1966b; Böhle and May, 1968) although it does not affect glucose uptake by the diaphragm. In contrast, *in vitro*, $PGE_1$ stimulates glycogen synthesis in the adipose tissue. $PGA_1$ has neither of these effects (Vaughan, 1967).

*Protein Metabolism*

Holmes (1965) observed that $PGE_1$ (up to 1 mg/ml) does not have any effect on the growth of several micro-organisms *in vitro*, although several unsaturated fatty acids (lauric, undecenoic and ricinoic acids) inhibited the growth. Rudden and Johnson (1967) also found that both $PGE_1$ and $PGF_{1\alpha}$ have only slight effects on the synthesis of protein and nucleic acid in a cell-free system from E. Coli (Strain B).

**Endocrine System**

Very recently, considerable attention has been focused on the biological actions of the prostaglandins on the endocrine system *in vivo* and *in vitro*. Presently, it is rather premature to make a general statement, but it appears that prostaglandins not only participate in the synthesis and release of the different hormones in the hypothalamus and pituitary gland, but also play a role on the stimulation of the trophic hormones on the target glands and on the modulation of the actions of different hormones. One can predict, with reasonable certainty, that more exciting observations will be made in the very near future to elucidate these complex interactions between hormones and prostaglandins on the endocrine target tissues and the physiological roles of prostaglandins on the endocrine functions. Since it has been described in detail in a previous section, the effects of prostaglandins on the ovary will not be discussed here.

## Pituitary Gland

Peng, Six and Munson (1970) showed that the intravenous injection of $PGE_1$ (0.5-2 $\mu$g/rat) increases plasma and adrenal corticosterone levels in rats, as the cholesterol and ascorbic acid levels in the adrenal cortex decreases markedly. Although Zor, Kaneko, Lowe, Bloom and Field (1969b) found that these changes are not observed in hypophysecto-mized rats, Flack, Jessup and Ramwell (1969) showed that $PGE_2$ stimulates steroidogenesis in hypophysectomized rats. However, the effective dose (1 mg/kg, i.p.) was far beyond the physiological range. $PGE_1$ is relatively specific since neither $PGA_1$ nor $PGF_{2\alpha}$ depletes adrenal ascorbic acid at a dose 10 times that of $PGE_1$. $PGE_1$ does not affect adrenal ascorbic acid in cortisol-treated rats or in hypophysecto-mized rats. These observations indicate that $PGE_1$ has no ACTH-like action on the adrenal cortex, but acts by stimulating ACTH release (Peng *et al.,* 1970). Morphine markedly inhibits the adrenal ascorbic acid response to $PGE_1$ in intact rats, suggesting that $PGE_1$ does not directly act on the anterior pituitary gland but on some part of the central nervous system, possibly the hypothalamus to release ACTH. However, the inhibition of morphine on the action of prostaglandins at receptor sites cannot be excluded (Sanner, 1971). Peng *et al.* (1970) concluded that the prostaglandins function as a hypothalamic hormone, (corticotrophin-releasing factor, CRF), mediating ACTH release in stress. MacLeod and Lehmeyer (1970) found that, in the isolated rat anterior pituitary gland, $PGE_1$ and $PGE_2$ ($10^{-6}$M) markedly increased the incorporation of $^3$H-leucine into growth hormone and its release. $PGE_1$ ($10^{-8}$M) and $PGA_1$ ($10^{-6}$M) increased growth hormone synthesis but not release, whereas $PGF_{2\alpha}$ ($10^{-6}$M) was without effect on either synthesis or release of growth hormone. In contrast, Schofield (1970) observed that, in heifer pituitary slices, $PGE_1$ ($5 \times 10^{-8} - 5 \times 10^{-6}$M) increases growth hormone release. Vale, Rivier and Guillemin (1971) also found that $PGE_1$ ($2.8 \times 10^{-5} - 10^{-6}$M) stimulated secretion of TSH as well as ACTH in the rat pituitary gland *in vitro*. A prostaglandin antagonist, 7-oxa-13-prostynoic acid, decreases $PGE_1$-stimulated TSH and ACTH secretion. Vilhardt and Hedqvist (1970) found that the intracarotid injection of $PGE_2$ (1-20 $\mu$g) increases urine osmolarity and markedly decreases the urine flow volume in rats, indicating its stimulatory effect on vasopressin secretion (Fig. 25). The synthesis and release of prolactin are not affected by $PGE_1$ (MacLeod, Lehmeyer and Frontham, 1971). Likewise, $PGE_1$, $PGA_1$, $PGB_1$ and $PGF_{1\alpha}$ (2-200 $\mu$g/ml) do not appear to stimulate the release of the lutenizing hormone *in vitro* (Zor, Kaneko, Schneider, McCann and Field, 1970).

The mode of the action of the prostaglandins on the pituitary gland remains uncertain. However, there appears to be a close relationship

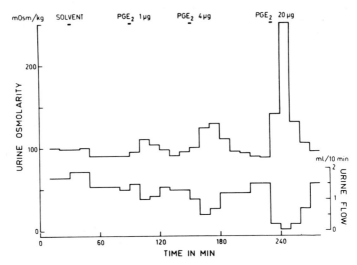

Fig. 25. Effects of the injection of $PGE_2$ into the carotid artery on urine osmolarity and release of a water-loaded rat. Reproduced from Vilhardt and Hedqvist (1970) with permission of the authors and publisher.

between the action of the prostaglandins and the cyclic AMP system in the hypothalamus and pituitary gland for the synthesis and release of the pituitary hormones.

Zor *et al.* (1969b) showed that, in the isolated rat anterior pituitary gland, $PGE_1$, $PGA_1$, $PGB_1$ and $PGF_{1\alpha}$ (2-200 μg/ml) increase formation of cyclic AMP, but there is a marked variation in their potency. $PGE_1$ is the most effective and $PGF_{1\alpha}$ the least. $PGE_1$ also stimulates [3]H-adenine incorporation into [3]H-labelled cyclic AMP in intact pituitary *in vitro*, although it markedly increases adenyl cyclase activity in the pituitary homogenates. $PGE_1$ (10 μg/ml) added *in vitro* has no effect on cyclic AMP concentrations in hypothalamic fragments. Vilhardt and Hedqvist (1970) postulated that the vasopressin-releasing action of $PGE_2$ is mediated through its action on the hypothalamic nuclei or on ganglia at higher levels of the brain.

### Adrenal Gland

Flack *et al.* (1969) reported that small doses (1.4 to 2.4 × 10$^{-6}$ M) of $PGE_1$, $PGE_2$ or $PGF_{1\alpha}$ increases steroidogenesis in the superfused adrenal glands obtained from hypophysectomized rats. This effect is mimicked in part by both ACTH and cyclic AMP. All three responses are inhibited by cyclohexamide. Saruta and Kaplan (1971) showed that in beef adrenal slices, both $PGE_1$ and $PGE_2$ (100 μg/g) stimulate adrenal steroidogenesis whereas $PGA_1$, $PGF_{1\alpha}$ and $PGF_{2\alpha}$ have no detectable effect. $PGE_1$ and $PGE_2$ have a greater stimulatory effect upon aldosterone and corticosterone biosynthesis than upon cortisol. Inhibitors of protein synthesis, puromycin and actinomycin D, inhibit the adrenal steroidogenesis induced by $PGE_1$ and $PGE_2$. $PGE_1$ has an additive effect to that of angiotensin, even at doses of angiotensin that appear to be maximal for its effect, suggesting that $PGE_1$ may act in a manner different from angiotensin.

*Thyroid Gland*

Several investigators showed that both TSH (5 mU/ml) and $PGE_1$ or $PGE_2$ (1-10 $\mu$g/ml or $10^{-7}$ to $5 \times 10^{-5}$ M) increase adenyl cyclase activity, cyclic AMP concentration, glucose oxidation and colloid droplet formation (endocytosis) in canine thyroid slices (Kaneko, Zor and Field, 1969; Onaya and Solomon, 1969; Zor, Bloom, Lowe and Field, 1969a; Zor *et al.*, 1969b; Dekker and Field, 1970; Ahn and Rosenberg, 1970; Field *et al.*, 1971), canine thyroid homogenates (Zor *et al.*, 1969b), bovine thyroid slices (Burke, 1970a; Burke, Kowalski and Babiarz, 1971), sheep thyroid mitochondria (Burke, 1970a) and sheep thyroid slices (Burke, 1970b) (Table 4). In addition both TSH and $PGE_1$ increase iodide trapping in the bovine thyroid slices (Burke *et al.*, 1971), and also stimulate organic binding of iodine, thyroxine synthesis and proteolysis of $^{131}$I-labelled iodoprotein in canine thyroid slices even in the presence of perchlorate (Ahn and Rosenberg, 1970). However, $PGE_1$ does not reproduce the action of TSH on incorporation of $^{32}$P into phospholipids in either sheep thyroid slices (Burke, 1970b) or canine thyroid slices (Zor *et al.*, 1970; Dekker and Field, 1970). Zor *et al.* (1969a) and Ahn and Rosenberg (1970) reported that $PGE_1$ neither potentiated nor

Table 4

Comparative effects of different prostaglandins and TSH on various parameters of thyroid metabolism

| Parameter | $PGA_1$ | $PGB_1$ | $PGE_1$ | $PGF_{1\alpha}$ | TSH |
|---|---|---|---|---|---|
| Adenyl cyclase | ↑ 0.2 | ↑ 0.2 | ↑ 0.2 | ↑ 0.2 | ↑ |
| Cyclic AMP | ↑ 100 | ∘ 100 | ↑ 1 | ∘ 100 | ↑ |
| $^{14}CO_2$ | ↑ 100 | ↑ 100 | ↑ 1 | ↑ 10 | ↑ |
| $^{32}$Phospholipid | ↓ 100 | ∘ 100 | ↑ 100 | ↑ 100 | ↑ |
| Coloid droplets | ↑ 100 | ↑ 100 | ↑ 1 | ↑ 100 | ↑ |

Dose in $\mu$g
Reproduced from Field *et al.* (1971) with permission of the authors and publisher.

inhibited the effects of TSH in canine thyroid slices. In contrast, Onaya and Solomon (1970) and Burke (1970a) found that the effects of $PGE_1$ and $PGE_2$ on adenyl cyclase, glucose oxidation and endocytosis are additive with TSH. The stimulatory effects of TSH and $PGE_1$ on adenyl cyclase and glucose utilization are inhibited by excessive iodide, but the effect on the thyroid endocytosis is unaffected (Burke, 1970a). Furthermore, the effects of TSH and $PGE_1$ on adenyl cyclase and iodide trapping in the thyroid slices are inhibited by a prostaglandin antagonist, 7-oxa-prostynoic acid. On the other hand, the stimulatory effects of $PGE_1$ on the endocytosis, glucose utilization and $^{131}I$ release are inhibited by a lysosomal stabilizer, chlorpromazine (Onaya and Solomon, 1970).

Burke (1970a) also found that $PGF_{1\alpha}$ and $PGF_{1\beta}$ ($2.5 \times 10^{-6}$ to $5 \times 10^{-5}$ M) increase adenyl cyclase activity and endocytosis in sheep thyroid mitochondria and ovine thyroid slices, but do not increase glucose utilization. On the other hand, Zor *et al.* (1969b) and Dekker and Field (1970) showed that $PGF_{1\alpha}$ (10 $\mu$g/ml) increases glucose oxidation but has little or no effect on cyclic AMP and endocytosis, although these effects are observed with higher doses (100 $\mu$g/ml) of $PGF_{1\alpha}$. Both $PGF_{1\alpha}$ and $PGF_{1\beta}$ abolish submaximal TSH effects on thyroid glucose oxidation (Burke, 1970a). Similarly, high doses (100 $\mu$g/ml) of $PGA_1$ and $PGB_1$ increase glucose utilization and endocytosis but only $PGA_1$ increases cyclic AMP concentrations (Zor *et al.*, 1969b; Dekker and Field, 1970). In the dog (Onaya and Solomon, 1970) and in the mouse (Burke, 1970a), $PGE_1$, $PGE_2$, $PGF_{1\alpha}$ or $PGF_{1\beta}$ (50-200 $\mu$g) increases the release of $^{131}I$ from the thyroid (Table 5). However, Burke (1970a) showed that when added to submaximal dose of TSH or long-acting thyroid stimulator (LATS) it leads to a significant reduction in hormonal effect. He concluded that the various phases of thyroid hormone synthesis such as adenyl cyclase activation, endocytosis and glucose utilization, are not enhanced in concert, and TSH and perhaps LATS and prostaglandins compete for a common adenyl cyclase receptor site(s) in thyroid.

*Testicle*

In the hypophysectomized rats, Kuehl, Patanelli, Tarnoff and Humes (1970b) observed that neither $PGE_1$ nor $PGE_2$ increases adenyl cyclase activity and cyclic AMP concentrations in the testicle. Furthermore, both prostaglandins have no effect on the LH- or FSH-stimulated adenyl cyclase activity. Ellis and Batista (1969) showed that $PGE_1$ participates in regulating testicular function. $PGE_1$ acts to modulate androgen synthesis as well as overall prostaglandin synthesis and testicular contraction in rabbits. Hargrove, Johnson and Ellis (1971) also observed

Table 5

Effect of prostaglandins on mouse thyroid $^{131}$I release

| Substance[a] | Response index (% of 0-h Blood $^{131}$I) | | |
|---|---|---|---|
| | 3 h | 8 h | 24 h |
| 6% BSA[b] | 103 ± 14 | 138 ± 22 | 156 ± 27 |
| TSH, 0.2 mU | 329 ± 51 | 206 ± 32 | 171 ± 30 |
| PGE$_1$, 50 μg | 155 ± 16 | 141 ± 23 | 153 ± 25 |
| PGE$_2$, 50 μg | 193 ± 22 | 152 ± 19 | 149 ± 21 |
| PGE$_{1α}$, 50 μg | 147 ± 13 | 143 ± 15 | 157 ± 18 |
| PGF$_{1β}$, 50 μg | 134 ± 15 | 141 ± 16 | 137 ± 22 |
| PGE$_1$, 100 μg | 232 ± 28 | 176 ± 24 | 165 ± 27 |
| PGE$_2$, 100 μg | 331 ± 42 | 256 ± 27 | 182 ± 33 |
| PGF$_{1α}$, 100 μg | 207 ± 22 | 161 ± 26 | 173 ± 28 |
| PGF$_{1β}$, 100 μg | 193 ± 26 | 157 ± 27 | 169 ± 29 |
| PGE$_1$, 200 μg | 231 ± 34 | 169 ± 25 | 153 ± 25 |
| PGE$_2$, 200 μg | 322 ± 43 | 261 ± 24 | 174 ± 30 |
| PGF$_{1α}$, 200 μg | 219 ± 25 | 167 ± 29 | 152 ± 26 |
| PGF$_{1β}$, 200 μg | 198 ± 23 | 152 ± 27 | 147 ± 28 |

Values are means ± S.E.M. a: 0.5 ml per mouse. b: 6% Bovine serum albumin prepared in ethanol-Na$_2$CO$_3$ solution used for prostaglandins.

Reproduced from Burke (1970a) with permission of the author and publisher.

that in rabbits PGE$_1$ (more than $3.6 \times 10^{-8}$ M) decreases the testicular tone and blocks completely its contraction.

## Parathyroid

In calvaria isolated from foetal rats at term, Chase and Auerbach (1970) showed that both parathyroid hormone and PGE$_1$ and PGE$_2$ increase the concentrations of cyclic AMP in the skeletal tissue, whereas PGF$_{1α}$ and PGF$_{2α}$ have no effect. Neither propranolol nor phentolamine blocks PGE$_1$- or parathyroid hormone-stimulated effect on cyclic AMP in the skeletal tissue. When PGE$_2$ and parathyroid hormone are added together at suboptimal concentrations, the effects are additive. None of the prostaglandins tested influence adenyl cyclase and phosphodiesterase activities in the rat calvaria, whereas parathyroid hormone causes significant stimulation of adenyl cyclase. The activation of adenyl cyclase by parathyroid hormone is not affected by PGE$_1$.

Klein and Raisz (1970) observed that prostaglandins stimulate resorption of foetal rat bone in 48-96 hr tissue culture. Both $PGE_1$ and $PGE_2$ cause increased release of previously incorporated $^{45}Ca$ into the medium, losses of stable and labelled calcium from the bone and morphological changes of osteoclastic resorption. The effects of E prostaglandins are similar to those of parathyroid hormone $(10^{-7} - 10^{-8} M)$. As seen with parathyroid hormone, the effects of $PGE_1$ is inhibited by thyrocalcitonin and cortisol. $PGA_1$ and $PGF_{1\alpha}$ also stimulate bone reabsorption but only at higher doses $(10^{-6} M)$. Furthermore, *in vivo* an injection of $PGE_1$ in parathyroidectomized rats does not increase serum calcium concentrations, while parathyroid hormone (4-40 U/rat) is effective (Klein and Raisz, 1970).

*Pancreas*

Many pharmacological agents and hormones are known to influence the secretion of insulin. Recently, several investigators (Turtle, Littleton and Kipnis, 1968; Sussman and Vaughan, 1967) found that insulin release from the beta cells is closely related to the intracellular concentrations of cyclic AMP and/or the activities of adenyl cyclase and phosphodiesterase. While studying the stimulatory effect of tranylcypromine on insulin release, Bressler, Vargas-Cordon and Lebovitz (1968) found that $PGE_1$ produces a dose-dependent increase in plasma insulin and also hyperglycaemia in mice. The hyperglycaemia detected following $PGE_1$ administration is insufficient to account for this increased secretion of insulin, and thus the effect of $PGE_1$ may well be mediated via intracellular cyclic AMP. It is of interest that a beta adrenergic blocking agent, MJ 1999, blocks the increased insulin secretion induced by $PGE_1$. In dogs, Maxwell (1967) showed that $PGE_1$ decreases both blood glucose and FFA levels, but does not change the insulin-like activity in the blood. All of the other investigators found that $PGE_1$ increases blood glucose in many species of animals *in vivo*. If $PGE_1$ does increase insulin release, it must not be offset by the hyperglycaemic factors induced by $PGE_1$ (Bergström *et al.*, 1968; Böhle and May, 1968).

### Haematological System

Kloeze (1967) first reported that *in vitro* in low concentrations (0.05-5 µg/ml) of $PGE_1$ markedly inhibits ADP-induced aggregation of rat, pig and human platelets using a turbinometrical method (Fig. 26). $PGE_1$ was also found to reduce ADP-induced glass adhesiveness of rat platelets. In contrast, the same concentrations of $PGE_2$ stimulate ADP-induced aggregation and adhesiveness of pig and rat platelets. Emmons, Hampton, Harrison, Honour and Mitchell (1967) demonstrated

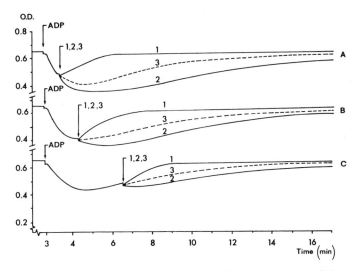

Fig. 26. Platelet aggregation in diluted, citrated platelet-rich plasma of the pig at 37° after addition of: (1) $PGE_1$ $(1.4 \times 10^{-6}M)$; (2) $PGE_2$ $(1.4 \times 10^{-6}M)$; (3) saline (control). ADP concentration $(10^{-6}M)$. Reproduced from Kloeze (1967) with permission of the author and publisher.

that $PGE_1$ also inhibits the aggregation and adhesiveness of human platelets induced by ADP, ATP, noradrenaline, serotonin, thrombin or connective tissue extract. It also inhibits the changes in platelet electrophoretic mobility produced by ADP and noradrenaline. The inhibitory effects of $PGE_1$ on platelet aggregation and adhesiveness are effectively counteracted by the addition of $Ca^{++}$ (Emmons *et al.*, 1967). Subsequently, many investigators have confirmed this phenomenon except for the action of $PGE_2$. Chandrasekhar (1967), Wolfe and Shulman (1969) and Weeks *et al.* (1969) found that $PGE_2$, iso-$PGE_1$ and dinor-$PGE_1$ also exert weaker but qualitatively similar inhibitory effects on the human, rabbit and rat platelets. The discrepancy of the results remains unsolved. The other prostaglandins, $PGA_1$, $PGA_2$, $PGF_{1\alpha}$, $PGF_{1\beta}$, $PGF_{2\alpha}$ and $PGF_{2\beta}$ are without effect even with high concentrations (up to 100 $\mu$g/ml) (Kloeze, 1967; von Euler and Eliasson, 1967; Weeks *et al.*, 1969; Sekhar, 1970; Kloeze, 1970b). Recently, Shio *et al.* (1970) also found that $PGE_1$ inhibits ADP-induced sphericalization as well as aggregation of rat platelets, whereas $PGE_2$ has no effect. Mürer (1971) found that clot retraction is also inhibited by $PGE_1$. This action is effectively counteracted by the addition of $Ca^{++}$.

Emmons *et al.* (1967) observed that a single intravenous injection of $PGE_1$ (5-30 $\mu$g/kg) or intravenous infusion of $PGE_1$ (0.4-1.6 $\mu$g/kg/min) suppresses platelet thrombus formation in injured cerebral arteries in rabbits. In contrast, Carlson, Irion and Orö (1968b) found that the intravenous infusion of $PGE_1$ (0.05-0.1 $\mu$g/kg/min for 30 min) has no apparent effect on platelet aggregation in three healthy human subjects. Recently, Kloeze (1970a) also found that neither $PGE_1$ nor $PGE_2$ injected intravenously interferes with the coagulation process (prothrombin time) in rats *in vitro*. However, Kloeze (1970b) found that $PGE_1$ and $\omega$-homo-$PGE_1$ inhibit ADP-aggregation of rat platelets *in vivo*. Both E compounds inhibit transient thrombocytopenia induced by the intravenous injection of ADP in rats. $PGE_1$ also increases the $LD_{50}$ of ADP injected in large amounts into young rats which die of respiratory arrest and coma. This phenomenon is attributed to the $PGE_1$-induced inhibition of platelet aggregation. Kloeze (1970c) also reported that $PGE_1$ (0.1-4 $\mu$g/min) applied topically inhibits the formation and growth of platelet thrombi in rats, induced by an electric stimulus in cortical veins. In contrast, $PGF_{1\alpha}$ appeared to be ineffective. Sekhar (1970) also showed that $PGE_1$ exerts a very potent thrombolytic effect against ADP-induced platelet thrombi *in vitro*. A single intravenous injection of $PGE_1$ (3 mg/kg) inhibits platelet aggregation in blood samples withdrawn from rats 30 min following the injection. Platelet aggregation is also inhibited significantly in rats given by an intravenous infusion of $PGE_1$ (1.8 mg/kg/day).

The underlying mechanisms responsible for the inhibitory actions of prostaglandins on the platelet aggregation and adhesiveness induced by ADP and other agonists remain uncertain. However, there appears to be a close relationship between prostaglandins and cyclic AMP system on this phenomenon. In contrast to other systems, catecholamines reduce and $PGE_1$ enhances adenyl cyclase activity and cyclic AMP concentrations in the human and animal platelets as well as leucocytes (Wolfe and Shulman, 1969, 1970; Zieve and Greenough, 1969; Marquis, Vigdahl and Tavormina, 1969; Marquis *et al.*, 1970; Vigdahl, Marquis and Tavormina, 1969; Vigdahl and Marquis, 1970; Robison, Arnold and Hartmann, 1969; Robison, Cole, Arnold and Hartmann, 1971; Cole, Robison and Hartmann, 1970; Scott, 1970; Moskowitz, Harwood, Reid and Krishna, 1971; Mills and Smith, 1971). These observations strongly suggest that the platelet aggregation is closely linked to the activation of adenyl cyclase and the concentration of cyclic AMP. Either the inhibitors of adenyl cyclase (adrenaline, noradrenaline, phenylephrine and $Ca^{++}$) or the stimulators of cyclic AMP phosphodiesterase (imidazole) stimulate platelet aggregation (Marquis *et al.*, 1970; Wolfe and Shulman, 1970). On the other hand, dibutyryl cyclic AMP, and the stimulators of adenyl cyclase (prostaglandins) and the inhibitors of phosphodiesterase (caffeine, theophylline, papaverine, ethaverine, dioxyline, dipyramidole and compounds RA 233) which increase cyclic AMP concentrations in the platelets, inhibit the platelet aggregation (Vigdahl and Marquis, 1970;

Cole *et al.,* 1970; Robison *et al.,* 1971). Hence, the effect of $PGE_1$ on the platelet aggregation is markedly influenced by the concentrations of $Ca^{++}$ (Vigdahl *et al.,* 1969; Wolfe and Shulman, 1970) or by the addition of imidazole or the phosphodiesterase inhibitors listed above (Fig. 27). Wolfe and Shulman (1970) showed that thrombin induces a rapid simultaneous release from platelets of ADP and $Ca^{++}$ in a constant ratio.

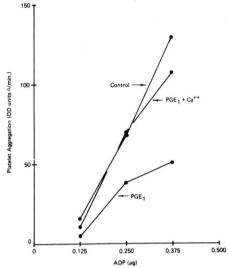

Fig. 27. Decrease in $PGE_1$-inhibition of ADP-induced platelet aggregation by $Ca^{++}$. Concentrations utilized: $PGE_1$, $2 \times 10^{-8}$ M; $CaCl^2$, $5 \times 10^{-4}$M. Reproduced from Vigdahl *et al.* (1969) with permission of the authors and publisher.

$PGE_1$, theophylline and dibutyryl cyclic AMP inhibit this release reaction as well as lactate production and the subsequent aggregation of platelets. Usually, the prostaglandins ($PGF_{1\alpha}$, $PGF_{1\beta}$ and $PGF_{2\alpha}$) which do not inhibit platelet aggregation produce little or no effect on adenyl cyclase activity and cyclic AMP concentrations (Wolfe and Shulman, 1969; Scott, 1970). It is known that $Ca^{++}$ is important in overall clotting mechanism as well as the action of $PGE_1$ on platelet aggregation. However, Ferri, Galatylas and Piccinini (1965) observed that $PGE_1$ can restore coagulation time to normal in a calcium deficient system. Emmons *et al.* (1967) reported that $PGE_1$ does not affect recalcification time in whole rabbit blood. The physiological significance of these two observations remain uncertain.

*Eye*

Many investigators (Waitzman and King, 1967; Beitch and Eakins, 1969; Eakins, 1971; Waitzman, 1970) demonstrated that introduction of very small doses (0.1-0.5 $\mu$g) of $PGE_1$ or $PGE_2$ into the anterior chamber of the rabbit eye results in a dose-dependent sustained elevation of intraocular pressure (IOP), sometimes associated with meiosis (Fig. 28). $PGE_1$ is equipotent to $PGE_2$ on these actions. $PGA_1$, $PGF_{1\alpha}$ and $PGF_{2\alpha}$ also exert qualitatively similar effects in the rabbit and cat eyes but the magnitude of their actions is markedly smaller than those of $PGE_1$.

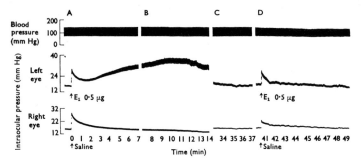

Fig. 28. Effect of $PGE_1$ on the intraocular pressure (IOP) of the rabbit. A. Intracameral injection of $PGE_1$ (0.5 $\mu$g) in 10 $\mu$l 0.9% NaCl solution in the left eye, 10 $\mu$l 0.9% NaCl solution injected into the control right eye. B. Peak response in the test eye. C. Return of IOP in the test eye to normal. D. Intracameral injections repeated as in A. Note the failure of the second injection of $PGE_1$ to produce a sustained rise in IOP. Reproduced from Beitch and Eakins (1969) with permission of the authors and publisher.

$PGF_{1\alpha}$ has the least action or none in the rabbit eye (Waitzman and King, 1967; Beitch and Eakins, 1969). In contrast to their actions in the rabbit eye, Waitzman and King (1967) showed that intraocular administration of $PGE_1$ (2.5 $\mu$g) $PGE_2$ (2.5 $\mu$g) or $PGF_{1\alpha}$ (125 $\mu$g) causes no effect on the IOP of cats and monkeys. On the other hand, Eakins (1971) observed that in the cat $PGE_1$ and $PGE_2$ (1 $\mu$g) produce a variable increase in IOP accompanied by ocular vasodilatation and meiosis. Usually much larger doses are required to elevate IOP in the cat than in the rabbit. Both E compounds also increase the protein content of aqueous humour, which is related to the magnitude of the sustained increase in IOP in both cats and rabbits (Beitch and Eakins, 1969; Eakins, 1971). On the other hand, Waitzman and King (1967) found that $PGE_1$ increases IOP without producing any significant change in the protein content of the aqueous humour. Since $PGE_1$ increases IOP without producing meiosis in cats and monkeys, Waitzman (1970) concluded that the meiotic action of $PGE_1$ does not result from the elevation of IOP. Stabilization of the blood-aqueous barrier with polyphloretin (PPP) markedly reduced both the IOP responses and the effect of $PGE_2$ on the protein content of the aqueous humour (Beitch and Eakins, 1969). From their observations, it was concluded that the production of local ocular vasodilatation and increased permeability of the blood aqueous barrier play an important role in the effect of prostaglandins on the IOP in cats and rabbits.

Waitzman and King (1967) studied the interaction between prostaglandins and catecholamines (noradrenaline, isoprenaline and phenylephrine) on the IOP and meiosis. In the rabbit and cat, both noradrenaline and isoprenaline antagonize the actions of $PGE_1$ on meiosis and IOP (Waitzman, 1970). These effects are observed even in the presence of retrobulbar anaesthesia. In the rabbit and cat the magnitude of the antagonistic action of noradrenaline on $PGE_1$-induced meiosis was markedly greater than that of isoprenaline. On the contrary, the magnitude of the antagonistic action of isoprenaline on the increasing action of $PGE_1$ on the IOP is markedly greater than that of noradrenaline. Phenoxybenzamine blocks completely the antagonistic action of noradrenaline, and blocks partially that of isoprenaline on the meiosis and the increased IOP induced by $PGE_1$ (Waitzman, 1970). In contrast, propranolol is ineffective in antagonising the effect of either isoprenaline or noradrenaline on the ocular actions of $PGE_1$. Waitzman (1970) also found that $PGE_1$ or $PGE_2$ antagonizes both catecholamine- and atropine-induced mydriasis in the rabbit.

*Skin*

*Man, guinea pig, rabbit and rat :* Carlson *et al.* (1969) observed that the intravenous infusion of $PGE_1$ (0.032-0.58 μg/kg/min) causes a flushing of the face, arms and hands in healthy human subjects, the degree and extent of this action being essentially in proportion to the dose. In some of the subjects, however, the flushing diminishes and changes to pallor with higher doses of $PGE_1$. Horton and Main (1963, 1967) found that both $PGE_1$ and $PGE_2$ (0.4 μg) increase the gastrocnemius venous outflow and cutaneous venous outflow in anaesthetized cats. On the other hand, both $PGE_3$ and $PGF_{1\alpha}$ (0.8 μg) were less effective on the cutaneous and skeletal muscle blood flows.

Several investigators (Ambache, 1961; Horton and Main, 1963; Solomon, Juhlin and Kirschenbaum, 1968; Weiner and Kaley, 1969; Kaley and Weiner, 1971; Juhlin and Michaelsson, 1969; Crunkhorn and Willis, 1971) found that the intradermal injection of $PGE_1$ or $PGE_2$ (5-10 μg) produces a small wheal, and an area of redness lasting for 2-10 hours, and an increased vascular permeability of the skin of the guinea pig, rats and man, as evidenced by extravasation of protamine blue (Table 6). However, a large dose (100 μg) of $PGE_1$ has little effect, while an extremely large dose (250 μg) of $PGE_1$ produces erythema for one hour in the rabbit skin (Solomon *et al.,* 1968). Erythema and redness

Table 6

Effect of prostaglandins on vascular permeability
in rat skin

| Agent tested | Dose | Relative* potency % |
|---|---|---|
| 0.9 % saline | .05 ml | 15 |
| PG vehicle | .05 ml | 15 |
| $PGE_1$ | .05 $\mu$g | 76 |
| $PGE_1$ | .50 $\mu$g | 100 |
| $PGA_1$ | .05 $\mu$g | 25 |
| $PGA_1$ | .50 $\mu$g | 35 |
| $PGF_{2\alpha}$ | .05 $\mu$g | 10 |
| $PGF_{2\alpha}$ | .50 $\mu$g | 10 |
| Bradykinin | .50 $\mu$g | 80 |
| Histamine | .05 $\mu$g | 64 |
| Serotonin | .05 $\mu$g | 72 |

* Relative to 0.5 $\mu$g of $PGE_1$ (100%).
Reproduced from Kaley and Weiner (1971) with
permission of the authors and publisher.

induced by $PGE_1$ are not associated with pruritus but with tenderness
(Solomon *et al.,* 1968). In contrast, Horton and Main (1963) found that
$PGE_1$ has no effect on production of pain in the human blister base.
Continuous intravenous infusion of $PGE_1$ (3 mg/kg/day) to conscious
unrestained rats also results in a swelling of the hind feet after three
days. This swelling subsides a day or two after terminating the infusion.
In no instances have large doses of $PGA_1$, $PGF_{1\alpha}$ or $PGF_{2\alpha}$, given acutely
intradermally or chronically intravenously, had any significant effect on
the skin in guinea pig, rat, rabbit or man. Injection of adrenaline or
noradrenaline blanches the erythema and flattens the wheal, whereas
neither lignocaine nor diphenhydramine has any effect on the cutaneous
lesions induced by $PGE_1$ (Solomon *et al.,* 1968). In contrast, in the rat
skin, Horton and Main (1963), Crunkhorn and Willis (1971) and Kaley
and Weiner (1971) concluded that the increased permeability and oedema
formation induced by $PGE_1$ or $PGE_2$ are predominantly due to the
histamine release from the mast cells, since pretreatment with
mepyramine greatly reduces the response to $PGE_2$ and the addition of
methysergide gives complete inhibition. Previously it was shown that
$PGE_1$ induces a $Ca^{++}$-dependent degranulation and disruption of rat
peritoneal mast cells (Cabut and Vincenza, 1967). However, recently
Mannaioni (1970) reported that $PGE_1$ does not interfere either with the
release or with the uptake of histamine in murine neoplastic mast cells *in*

*vitro.* This may be due to the fact that murine neoplastic cells are resistant to the lytic substances or may inactivate $PGE_1$ rapidly. In essential fatty acid (EFA)-deficient rats, it is not certain whether the effect of $PGE_1$ on permeability is caused by the changes in skin permeability to water. All attempts to treat EFA deficiency in rats and mice by prostaglandins have been unsuccessful (Bergström *et al.*, 1968). Willoughby (1968) demonstrated that the intravenous injection of $PGF_{2\alpha}$ (10-50 $\mu g/kg$) antagonizes the increased venular permeability to plasma protein induced by the intradermal injection of histamine, serotonin, bradykinin or lymph node-permeability factor in conscious rats. Pretreatment with low doses of $PGF_{2\alpha}$ suppresses the increased permeability after thermal injury in anaesthetized rats. In contrast, $PGE_1$ is without effect on these mediators or the inflammatory response.

From the recent observations of the cutaneous effects of the prostaglandins, it appears obvious that the prostaglandins play a great role on the genesis of the inflammatory processes (Kaley and Weiner, 1971; Crunkhorn and Willis, 1971). It is of interest that the prostaglandins have been found in acutely inflamed tissues (Giroud and Willoughby, 1970; Willis, 1969). Very recently, indomethacin, aspirin, and sodium salicylate were found to inhibit the synthesis of prostaglandins in lungs, platelets and spleen (Vane, 1971; Ferreira *et al.*, 1971; Smith and Willis, 1971). Collier (1971) postulated that these non-steroidal anti-inflammatory drugs may act on the prostaglandin-mediated inflammatory processes in the skin or other tissues *in vivo.*

*Frog:* Fassina and Contessa (1967) first observed that $PGE_1$ ($10^{-7}$ to $2 \times 10^{-6} M$) increases the short circuit current (SCC) and $Na^+$ transport in the isolated surviving frog skin. Furthermore, $PGE_1$ has no effect on the Na-K dependent ATPase of human erythrocyte membranes and calf heart (Fassina and Contessa, 1967; Fassina *et al.*, 1969). Furthermore, Fassina *et al.* (1969) observed that the action of $PGE_1$ on the SCC is inhibited by an excess of $Ca^{++}$ of the removal of $Na^+$ in the medium, and also in the presence of ouabain or digitoxin. These observations indicate that the action of $PGE_1$ on frog skin is dependent on the normal rate of $Na^+$ transport which is involved in $Na^+$-$K^+$ dependent ATPase, Fassina *et al.* (1969) concluded that $PGE_1$ stimulates the process responsible for $Na^+$ transport indirectly by permitting delivery of more $Na^+$ to the site of the action. Furthermore, they implicated the possible role of $Ca^+$ on the action of $PGE_1$ on the frog skin since a competitive antagonism is found to exist between the $Na^+$ transport action of $PGE_1$ and the concentration of $Ca^{++}$ in the frog skin. Ramwell and Shaw (1970) not only confirmed the above observations made by Fassina *et al.* (1969), but also observed that $PGE_1$ decreases $Ca^{++}$ content of the skin due to its direct stimulating action on $Ca^{++}$ efflux across the outer membrane. They concluded that the $PGE_1$ may remove $Ca^{++}$ from the membrane, and thereby permit $Na^+$ entry, thus increasing adenyl cyclase activity in the frog skin (Ramwell and Shaw, 1970). It is not certain, however, whether this chain of biophysical and enzymatic reaction induced by $PGE_1$ in the frog skin is applicable to the mammalian skin as well as many heterogenous tissues in the body (Robison *et al.*, 1971).

*Chicken:* Kischer (1967) demonstrated that $PGE_1$ and $PGB_1$ (1-100 $\mu g/ml$), when applied in culture to back skin of the chick embryo, stimulated epidermal proliferation and keratinization, whereas development of the down feather organ is completely blocked by both compounds. The effect of $PGB_1$ on the skin is 10 times greater than that of $PGE_1$. $PGF_{1\alpha}$ has no such effects. Using the electron-microscope, Kischer (1969) also found that tonofilaments appear much sooner in $PGE_1$- or $PGB_1$-treated explants than in controls, and are distributed at all levels of the epidermis. Furthermore, the cristae of mitochondria in epidermal cells of treated skins are long, closely apposed, and oriented parallel to the longest axis of the organelle as contrasted with a transverse orientation for them in control epidermis. There is increased deposition of collagen in the mesenchyme of treated skins as contrasted to that observed in controls. Unusual structures (inclusion bodies) occur throughout the stratified and superficial epidermis of treated skin and these are composed of fine filaments and granules which are also associated with tonofilaments. In addition, numerous small vacuoles appear in the epidermal cells of treated skins and seem to develop from cisternae of the Golgi apparatus or endoplasmic reticulum. It was concluded that these observations are consistent with an accelerated maturation process, but may be correlated with a specific and irreversible change in a metabolic event necessary for feather development (Kischer, 1969).

## 4. PROSTAGLANDIN INHIBITORS

Recently, Fried *et al.* (1969) synthesized analogues of $PGE_1$ and $PGF_1$, 7-oxa-$PGE_1$, 7-oxa-$PGF_{1\alpha}$ and 7-oxa-13,14-prostynoic acid. It was found that these compounds antagonize competitively the smooth muscle stimulating effect of $PGE_1$ in the isolated gerbil colon (Fried *et al.*, 1969, 1971) and also the effect of $PGE_1$ on the stimulation of the pituitary gland (Vale *et al.*, 1971). The same inhibitor also competitively inhibits the effects of $PGE_1$ and $PGE_2$ on the adenylcyclase activity in the mouse ovary (Kuehl *et al.*, 1970a). Burke *et al.* (1971) showed that 7-oxa-prostynoic acid inhibits the stimulatory actions of both TSH and $PGE_1$ on adenylcyclase and iodide trapping in the bovine thyroid slices.

However, Nakano (1971b) found that one of these 7-oxa compounds, 7-oxa-13,14-prostynoic acid, does not inhibit the vasodilator effect of $PGE_1$ on the isolated dog hind limb preparation. $15$-R-$PGE_1$, $PGB_1$ and 7-oxa-prostynoic acid inhibit uncompetitively or competitively the enzymatic activity of prostaglandin dehydrogenase *in vitro* when $PGE_1$ is used as a substrate (Nakano *et al.,* 1969; Shio *et al.,* 1970; Marrazzi and Matschinsky, 1971). However, Nakano and Kessinger (1970a) showed that neither $PGB_1$ nor $15$-R-$PGE_1$ inhibits the direct vasodilator action of $PGE_1$ in the dog.

Recently, Eakins and Karim (1970) and Eakins, Karim and Miller (1970) demonstrated that a cell membrane stabilizer, polyphloretin phosphate (PPP) competitively antagonizes the effects of $PGE_2$ and $PGF_{2\alpha}$ on intestinal contraction (Table 9). Beitch and Eakins (1969) also found that PPP blocks the effects of $PGE_1$ on the eye (meiosis and increased intraocular pressure) in rabbits and cats. In rabbits, PPP also inhibits the hypotensive action of $PGF_{2\alpha}$ but does not have any effect on the hypotensive action of $PGE_2$ (Eakins and Karim, 1970; Eakins *et al.,* 1970; Eakins, 1971). Recently, Nakano and Prancan (unpublished data) also showed that PPP has no effect in the direct vasodilator action of $PGE_2$ in the isolated dog *in situ* hind limb preparations. Furthermore, these workers found that PPP does not affect the pulmonary vasoconstrictor action of $PGF_{2\alpha}$ in dogs in which the pulmonary arterial blood flow is kept constant by means of a Sigmamotor pump. Sanner

Table 7

Effect of polyphloretin phosphate (PPP) on some smooth muscle actions of prostaglandins *in vitro*

| *Preparation* | *Prostaglandins* | *Response* | *Antagonism by PPP* |
|---|---|---|---|
| Colon, Jird | $F_{2\alpha}$, $E_2$ | Contraction | + |
| Jejunum, Rabbit | $F_{2\alpha}$, $E_2$ | Contraction | + |
| Uterus, Rabbit (N.P.) | $F_{2\alpha}$, $E_2$ | Contraction | + |
| Uterus, G. pig (N.P. & P.) | $F_{2\alpha}$, $E_2$ | Contraction | + |
| Uterus, Rat (N.P. & P.) | $F_{2\alpha}$, $E_2$ | Contraction | + |
| Uterus, Monkey (N.P.) | $F_{2\alpha}$, $E_2$ | Contraction | + |
| Trachea, Rabbit | $E_2$ | Relaxation | − |
| Umbilical cord, Human | $E_1$ | Relaxation | − |
| | $E_2$, $F_{2\alpha}$ | Contraction | − |

N.P. = Nonpregnant

P. = Pregnant

Reproduced from Eakins (1971) with permission of the author and publisher.

(1969, 1971) found that both a dibenzoxazepine hydrazide derivative, Compound SC-19220, and morphine sulphate inhibit the smooth muscle stimulating effect of $PGE_1$ in the isolated guinea-pig ileum. However, Nakano and Prancan (unpublished data) found that the vasodilator effect of $PGE_2$ is not blocked by SC-19220 in the isolated dog hind limb preparations. Presently, it appears that no specific agent which antagonizes the circulatory actions of prostaglandins is available.

## 5. SUMMARY AND CONCLUSION

Numerous recent studies reveal that prostaglandins are present ubiquitously and exert potent pharmacological actions on different organs and tissues. Although the precise roles of prostaglandins in health and disease remain uncertain, it appears that prostaglandins may modulate local biochemical functions as well as regional circulations, and may influence the physiological functions of the hormones and neurotransmitters. For the past three or four years, progress in research on prostaglandins has been phenomenally rapid and extensive in many biomedical fields. With reasonable certainty, one can anticipate more exciting observations on the prostaglandins which may better our understanding of human physiology and pathophysiology, perhaps leading to therapeutic applications of these potent substances in the near future.

## ACKNOWLEDGMENTS

The author wishes to express his gratitude to Dr J. R. McCurdy, Mr A. V. Prancan, Mr J. M. Kessinger, Mrs N. Morsy, Mrs C. L. Kessinger and Mr Mike Distler for their excellent technical assistance and to Miss K. Hugos and Mrs L. Nakano for their aid in the preparation of this manuscrupt. He is also indebted to Drs J. I. Moore and M. Koss for their invaluable criticisms on the manuscript.

This work was supported in part by research grants from U.S. Public Health Service (HE 11848) and from the Oklahoma Heart Association.

# REFERENCES

Abdel-Sayed, W., Abboud, F. M., Hedwall, P. R. and Schmid, P. G. (1970). Vascular responses to prostaglandin $E_1$ ($PGE_1$) in muscular and cutaneous beds. *Circulation 42 Suppl. III,* 126.

Ahn, C. S. and Rosenberg, I. N. (1970). Iodine metabolism in thyroid slices: Effects of TSH, dibutyryl cyclic 3',5'-AMP, NaF and prostaglandin $E_1$. *Endocrinology,* 86, 396.

Ambache, N. (1961). Prolonged erythema produced by chromatographically purified irin. *Journal of Physiology (London),* 160, 3p.

Ambache, N. (1966). Biological characterization of, and structure-action studies on, smooth muscle contracting hydroxy-acids. *Memoirs Society for Endocrinology,* 14, 19.

Anderson, F. L., Tsagaris, T. J. and Kuida, H. (1971). Effect of prostaglandins on bovine pulmonary circulation. *Federation Proceedings,* 30, 380.

Änggård, A. (1969). The effect of prostaglandins on nasal airway resistance in man. *Annals of Otology, Rhinology & Laryngology,* 78, 657.

Änggård, E. (1966). The biological activities of three metabolites of prostaglandin $E_1$. *Acta Physiologica Scandinavica,* 66, 509. Karger, Basel/New York.

Änggård, E. (1970). Pharmacology of the prostaglandins. *Proceedings of the 4th International Congress of Pharmacology,* 4, 7.

Änggård, E. (1971). Studies on the analysis and metabolism of the prostaglandins. *Annals of the New York Academy of Sciences,* 180, 200.

Änggård, E. and Bergström, S. (1963). Biological effects on an unsaturated trihydroxy acid ($PGF_{2\alpha}$) from normal swine lung. *Acta Physiologica Scandinavica,* 58, 1.

Änggård, E. and Samuelsson, B. (1964). Metabolism of prostaglandin $E_1$ in guinea pig lung: the structure of two metabolites. *Journal of Biological Chemistry,* 239, 4097.

Änggård, E. and Samuelsson, B. (1966). Purification and properties of a 15-hydroxy-prostaglandin dehydrogenase from swine lung. *Arkiv för Kemi,* 25, 293.

Antonaccio, M. J. and Lucchesi, B. R. (1970). The interaction of glucagon with theophylline, $PGE_1$, isoproterenol, ouabain and $CaCl_2$ on the dog isolated papillary muscle. *Life Sciences,* 9, 1081.

Asplund, J. (1947). Some preliminary experiments in connection with the effect of prostaglandin on the uterus and tubae *in vivo. Acta Physiologica Scandinavica,* 13, 109.

Avanzino, G. L., Bradley, P. B. and Wolstencroft, J. H. (1966). Actions of prostaglandins $E_1$, $E_2$ and $F_{2\alpha}$ on brain stem neurones. *British Journal of Pharmacology,* 27, 157.

Barger, A. C. and Herd, J. A. (1967). Study of renal circulation in the unanesthetized dog with inert gases: external counting. *Proceedings of the 3rd International Congress of Nephrology,* Karger, Basel/New York, 1, 174

Bedwani, J. R. and Horton, E. W. (1968). The effects of prostaglandins $E_1$ and $E_2$ on ovarian steroidogenesis. *Life Sciences,* 7, 389.

Behrman, H., Yoshinaga, K. and Greep, R. (1971). Extraluteal effects of prostaglandins. *Annals of the New York Academy of Sciences,* 180, 426.

Beitch, B. R. and Eakins, K. E. (1969). The effects of prostaglandins on the intraocular pressure of the rabbit. *British Journal of Pharmacology*, 37, 158.

Blecher, M., Merlino, M. S., Ro'Ane, J. T. and Flynn, P. D. (1969). Independence of the effects of epinephrine, glucagon and adrenocorticotropin on glucose utilization from those on lipolysis in isolated rat adipose cells. *Journal of Biological Chemistry*, 244, 3423.

Bennett, A. and Fleshler, B. (1970). Prostaglandins and the gastrointestinal tract. *Gastroenterology*, 59, 790.

Bennett, A., Friedmann, C. A. and Vane, J. R. (1967). The release of prostaglandin $E_1$ from the rat stomach. *Nature* (London), 216, 873.

Bergström, S. and Carlson, L. A. (1965). Influence of the nutritional state on the inhibition of lipolysis in adipose tissue by prostaglandin $E_1$ and nicotinic acid. *Acta Physiologica Scandinavica*, 65, 383.

Bergström, S., Carlson, L. A., Ekelund, L. G. and Orö, L. (1965a). Cardiovascular and metabolic response to infusions of prostaglandin $E_1$ and to simultaneous infusions of noradrenaline and prostaglandin $E_1$ in man. *Acta Physiologica Scandinavica*, 64, 332.

Bergström, S., Carlson, L. A., Ekelund, L. G. and Orö, L. (1965b). Effect of prostaglandin $E_1$ on blood pressure, heart rate and concentration of free fatty acids of plasma in man. *Proceedings of the Society for Experimental Biology and Medicine*, 118, 110.

Bergström, S., Carlson, L. A. and Orö, L. (1964). Effects of prostaglandins on catecholamine induced changes in the free fatty acids of plasma and in blood pressure in the dog. *Acta. Physiologica Scandinavica*, 60, 170.

Bergström, S., Carlson, L. A. and Orö, L. (1966). Effect of different doses of prostaglandin $E_1$ on free fatty acids of plasma, blood glucose and heart rate in the non-anesthetized dog. *Acta Physiologica Scandinavica*, 67, 185.

Bergström, S., Carlson, L. A. and Orö, L. (1967). A note on the cardiovascular and metabolic effects of prostaglandin $A_1$. *Life Sciences*, 6, 449.

Bergström, S., Carlson, L. A. and Weeks, J. R. (1968). The prostaglandins: A family of biologically active lipids. *Pharmacological Reviews*, 20, 1.

Bergström, S., Duner, H., Euler, U. S. von, Pernow, B. and Sjövall, J. (1959a). Observations on the effects of infusion of prostaglandin E in man. *Acta Physiologica Scandinavica*, 45, 145.

Bergström, S., Eliasson, R., Euler, U. S. von and Sjövall, J. (1959b). Some biological effects of two crystalline prostaglandin factors. *Acta Physiologica Scandinavica*, 45, 133.

Bergström, S. and Euler, U. S. von (1963). The biological activity of prostaglandin $E_1$, $E_2$ and $E_3$. *Acta Physiologica Scandinavica*, 59, 493.

Bergström, S. and Sjövall, J. (1957). The isolation of prostaglandin. *Acta Physiologica Scandinavica*, 11, 1086.

Berti, F., Borroni, V., Fumagalli, R., Marchi, P. and Zocche, G. P. (1964). Sull attivita pressoria della prostaglandina. *Atti della Accademia lombarda*, 19, 397.

Berti, F., Lentati, R. and Usardi, M. M. (1965). The species specificity of prostaglandin $E_1$ effects on isolated heart. *Med. Pharmac. Exp.*, 13, 233.

Berti, F. and Usardi, M. N. (1964). Investigations on a new inhibitor of free fatty acid mobilization. *Giornale dell, Arteriosclerosi*, 2, 261.

Berti, F., Lentati, R. and Grafnetta, D. (1967). Effeti della sommistrazioni di prostaglandina $E_1$ sulla lipasi lipoproteica cardica. *Bolletino della Societa italiana di biologica sperimentale*, **43**, 515.

Bevegård, S. and Orö, L. (1969). Effect of prostaglandin $E_1$ on forearm blood flow. *Scandinavian Journal of Clinical and Laboratory Investigation*, **23**, 347.

Bickers, W. and Main, R. J. (1941). Patterns of uterine motility. In the normal ovulatory and anovulatory cycle, after castration, coitus and missed abortion. *Journal of Clinical Endocrinology*, **1**, 992.

Biron, P. and Boileau, J. C. (1969). Fate of vasopressin and oxytocin in the pulmonary circulation. *Canadian Journal of Physiology*, **47**, 713.

Bizzi, A. and Veneroni, E., Garattini, S., Puglisi, L. and Paoletti, R. (1967). Hypersensitivity to lipid mobilizing agents in essential fatty acid (EFA) deficient rats. *European Journal of Pharmacology*, **2**, 48.

Blatchley, F. R. and Donovan, B. T. (1969). Luteolytic effect of prostaglandins in the guinea pig. *Nature* (London), **221**, 1065.

Bloor, C. M. and Sobel, B. E. (1970). Enhanced coronary blood flow following prostaglandin infusion in the conscious dog. *Circulation 42: Suppl. III*, 111.

Böberg, J., Micheli, H. and Rammer, L. (1970). Effect of nicotinic acid on ACTH and noradrenaline stimulated lipolysis in the rabbit. II. *In vitro* studies including comparison with prostaglandin $E_1$. *Acta Physiologica Scandinavica*, **79**, 299.

Böhle, E., Ditschuneit, H., Ammon, J. und Döbert, R. (1966a). Über die Wirkung von Prostaglandin $E_1$ ($PGE_1$) auf den Fett- und Kohlenhydratstoffwechsel des isolierten Rattenfettgewebes. *Verhandlungen der Deutchen Gesellschaft für innere Medizin*, **72**, 465.

Böhle, E., Döbert, E., Ammon, J. und Ditschuneit, H. (1966b). Über Stoffwechselwirkungen von Prostaglandinen. I. Der Einfluss von Prostaglandin $E_1$ auf den Glucose-und Fettstoffwechsel des epididymalen Fettgewebes der Ratte. *Diabetologia*, **2**, 162.

Böhle, E., Döbert, R. und Merkl, I. M. (1967). Über die Wirkung von Prostaglandin $E_1$ und Insulin auf die heparininduzierte Triglycerihydrolyse. *A. Gesamte Exp. Med.*, **144**, 285.

Böhle, E. and May, B. (1968). Metabolic effects of prostaglandin $E_1$ upon lipid and carbohydrate metabolism. In: *Prostaglandin Symposium of the Worcester Foundation* (ed. P. W. Ramwell and J. E. Shaw), p. 115, Interscience, New York.

Böhle, E., Rettberg, H., Ditschuneit, H. H., Döbert, R. H. and Ditschuneit, H. (1967). Tierexperimentelle Untersuchungen über die Beeinflussung des Fettund Kohlenhydratstoffwechsels durch Prostaglandin $E_1$. *Verhandlungen der Deutchen Gesellschaft für innere Medizin*, **73**, 797.

Bressler, R., Vargas-Cordon, M. and Lebovitz, H. E. (1968). Tranylcypromine: A potent insulin secretagogue and hypoglycemic agent. *Diabetes*, **17**, 617.

Brundin, J. (1968). The effect of prostaglandin $E_1$ on the response of the rabbit oviduct to hypogastic nerve stimulation. *Acta Physiologica Scandinavica*, **73**, 54.

Bundy, G., Lincoln, F., Nelson, N., Pike, J. and Schneider, W. (1971). Novel prostaglandin syntheses. *Annals of the New York Academy of Sciences*, **180**, 76.

Burke, G. (1970a). Effects of iodide on thyroid stimulation. *Journal of Clinical Endocrinology and Metabolism*, **30**, 76.

Burke, G. (1970b). On the role of adenyl cyclase activation and endocytosis in thyroid slice metabolism. *Endocrinology*, **86**, 353.

Burke, G. (1970c). Effects of prostaglandins on basal and stimulated thyroid function. *American Journal of Physiology,* **218**, 1445.

Burke, G., Kowalski, K. and Babiarz, D. (1971). Effects of thyrotropin, prostaglandin $E_1$ and a prostaglandin antagonist on iodide trapping in isolated thyroid cells. *Life Sciences,* **10**, 513.

Butcher, R. W. and Baird, C. E. (1968). Effects of prostaglandins on adenosine 3', 5'-monophosphate levels in fat and other tissues. *Journal of Biological Chemistry,* **243**. 1713.

Butcher, R. W. and Baird, C. E. (1969). The regulation of cyclic AMP and lipolysis in adipose tissue by hormones and other agents. In: Drugs Affecting Lipid Metabolism (ed. N. L. Holmes, L. A. Carlson and R. Paoletti), p. 5, Plenum Press, New York.

Butcher, R. W., Pike, J. E. and Sutherland, E. W. (1967). The effects of prostaglandin $E_1$ on adenosine 3', 5',-monophosphate levels in adipose tissue. In: Prostaglandins (ed. S. Bergström and B. Samuelsson), p. 133, Almqvist and Wiksell, Stockholm.

Butcher, R. W. and Sutherland, E. W. (1967). The effects of the catecholamines, adrenergic blocking agents, prostaglandin $E_1$ and insulin on cyclic AMP levels in the rat epididymal fat pad in vitro. *Annals of the New York Academy of Sciences,* **139**, 849.

Bygdeman, M. (1964). The effect of different prostaglandins on the human myometrium in vitro. *Acta Physiologica Scandinavica,* **63**, (Suppl. 242), 1.

Bygdeman, M. (1967). Studies of the effects of prostaglandins in seminal plasma on human myometrium in vitro. In: Prostaglandins (ed. S. Bergström and B. Samuelsson), p. 71, Almqvist and Wiksell, Stockholm.

Bygdeman, M. and Eliasson, R. (1963a). The effect of prostaglandin from human seminal fluid on the motility of the non-pregnant human uterus in vitro. *Acta Physiologica Scandinavica,* **59**, 43.

Bygdeman, M. and Eliasson, R. (1963b). A comparative study on the effect of different prostaglandin compounds on the motility of the isolated human myometrium. *Medicina Experimentalia,* **9**, 409.

Bygdeman, M. and Hamberg, M. (1967). The effect of eight new prostaglandins on human myometrium. *Acta Physiologica Scandinavica,* **69**, 320.

Bygdeman, M., Kwon, S. and Wiqvist, N. (1967). The effect of prostaglandin $E_1$ on human pregnant myometrium *in vivo*. In: Prostaglandins (ed. S. Bergström and B. Samuelsson), p. 93, Almqvist and Wiksell, Stockholm.

Cabut, M. S. and Vincenzi, L. (1967). Preliminary investigations on the mast cell degranulation and histamine and heparin release induced by prostaglandin $E_1$. In: Prostaglandins (ed. S. Bergström and B. Samuelsson), p. 237, Almqvist and Wiksell, Stockholm.

Cahn, R. S., Ingold, C. K. and Prelog, V. (1956). The specification of asymmetric configuration in organic chemistry. *Experientia,* **12**, 81.

Carlson, L. A. (1967). Cardiovascular and metabolic effects of prostaglandins. *Progress in Biochemical Pharmacology,* **3**, 94.

Carlson, L. A., Ekelund, L. G. and Orö, L. (1968a). Clinical and metabolic effects of different doses of prostaglandin $E_1$ in man. *Acta Medica Scandinavica,* **183**, 423.

Carlson, L. A., Ekelund, L. G. and Orö, L. (1970a). Effect of intravenous prostaglandin $E_1$ on noradrenaline-stimulated mobilization of plasma free fatty acids in man. *Acta Medica Scandinavica,* **188**, 379.

Carlson, L. A., Ekelund, L. G. and Orö, L. (1969). Circulatory and respiratory effects of different doses of prostaglandin $E_1$ in man. *Acta Physiologica Scandinavica,* **75,** 161.

Carlson, L. A., Ekelund, L. G. and Orö, L. (1970b). Clinical, metabolic and cardiovascular effects of different prostaglandins in man. *Acta Medica Scandinavica,* **188,** 553.

Carlson, L. A. and Halleberg, D. (1968). Basal lipolysis and effects of noradrenaline and prostaglandin $E_1$ on lipolysis in human subcutaneous and omental adipose tissue. *Journal of Laboratory and Clinical Medicine,* **71,** 368.

Carlson, L. A., Irion, E. and Orö, L. (1968b). Effect of infusion of prostaglandin $E_1$ on the aggregation of blood platelets in man. *Life Sciences,* **7,** 85.

Carlson, L. A. and Orö, L. (1966). Effect of prostaglandin $E_1$ on blood pressure and heart rate in the dog. *Acta Physiologica Scandinavica,* **67,** 89.

Carr, A. A. (1970a). Hemodynamic and renal effects of a prostaglandin, $PGA_1$, in subjects with essential hypertension. *American Journal of Medical Sciences,* **259,** 21.

Carr, A. A. (1970b). Effects of $PGA_1$ on plasma renin activity in man. *Clinical Research,* **18,** 60.

Chandrasekhar, N. (1967). Inhibition of platelet aggregation by prostaglandins. *Blood,* **30,** 554.

Chase, L. R. and Auerbach, G. D. (1970). The effect of parathyroid hormone on the concentration of adenosine $3'$ $5'$-monophosphate in skeletal tissue *in vitro. Journal of Biological Chemistry,* **245,** 1520.

Christ, E. J. and Nugteren, D. H. (1970). The biosynthesis and possible function of prostaglandins in adipose tissue. *Biochimica Biophysica Acta,* **218,** 296.

Christlieb, A. R., Dobrinsky, S. J., Lyons, C. J. and Hickler, R. B. (1969). Short term $PGA_1$ infusions in patients with essential hypertension. *Clinical Research,* **17,** 234.

Clegg, P. C. (1966). The effect of prostaglandins on the response of isolated smooth-muscle preparations to sympathomimetic substances. *Memoirs Society for Endocrinology,* **14,** 119.

Clegg, P. C., Hall, W. J. and Pickles, V. R. (1966). The action of ketonic prostaglandins on the guinea pig myometrium. *Journal of Physiology,* (London), **183,** 123.

Coceani, F., Dreifuss, J. J., Puglisi, L. and Wolfe, L. S. (1969). Prostaglandins and membrane function. In: Prostaglandins, Peptides and Amines (ed. P. Mantegazza and E. W. Horton), p. 73, Academic Press, London and New York.

Coceani, F., Pace-Asciak, C., Volta, F. and Wolfe, L. S. (1967). Effect of nerve stimulation on prostaglandin formation and release from the rat stomach. *American Journal of Physiology,* **213,** 1056.

Coceani, F., Pace-Asciak, C. and Wolfe, L. S. (1968). Studies on the effect of nerve stimulation on prostaglandin formation and release in the rat stomach. In: Prostaglandin Symposium of the Worcester Foundation (ed. P. W. Ramwell and J. E. Shaw), p. 39, Interscience, New York.

Coceani, F., Puglisi, L. and Lavers, B. (1971). Prostaglandins and neuronal activity in spinal cord and cuneate nucleus. *Annals of the New York Academy of Sciences,* **180,** 289.

Coceani, F. and Wolfe, L. S. (1965). Prostaglandins in brain and the release of prostaglandin-like compounds from the cat cerebellar cortex. *Canadian Journal of Physiology and Pharmacology,* **43,** 445.

Coceani, F. and Wolfe, L. S. (1966). On the action of prostaglandin $E_1$ and prostaglandins from brain on the isolated rat stomach. *Canadian Journal of Physiology and Pharmacology,* **44**, 933.

Cockrill, J. R., Miller, E. G., Jr. and Kurzrok, R. (1935). The substance in human seminal fluid affecting uterine muscle. *American Journal of Physiology,* **112**, 577.

Cole, B., Robison, G. A. and Hartmann, R. C. (1970). Effects of prostaglandin $E_1$ and theophylline on aggregation and cyclic AMP levels of human blood platelets. *Federation Proceedings,* **29**, 316.

Collier, H. O. J. (1971). Prostaglandins and aspirin. *Nature* (London), **232**, 17.

Crunkhorn, P. and Willis, A. L. (1971). Cutaneous reactions to intradermal prostaglandins. *British Journal of Pharmacology,* **41**, 49.

Curnow, R. T. and Nuttall, F. Q. (1971). Effect of prostaglandin $E_1$ on glycogen metabolism in the metabolism in the rat liver and heart *in vivo. Federation Proceedings,* **30**, 625.

Daniels, E. G., Hinman, J. W., Leach, B. E. and Muirhead, E. E. (1967). Identification of a prostaglandin $E_2$ as the principal vasodepressor lipid of rabbit renal medulla. *Nature* (London), **215**, 1298.

Daugherty, R. M. Jr., Schwinghamer, J. M., Swindall, S. and Haddy, F. J. (1968). The effects of local and systemic infusions of prostaglandin $E_1$ in the skin and muscle vasculature in the dog forelimb. *Journal of Laboratory and Clinical Medicine,* **72**, 869.

Davies, B. N., Horton, E. W. and Withrington, P. G. (1967). The occurrence of prostaglandin $E_2$ in splenic venous blood following nerve stimulation. *Journal of Physiology* (London), **188**, 38P.

Davies, B. N. and Withrington, P. G. (1968). The effects of prostaglandin $E_1$ and $E_2$ on the smooth muscle of the dog spleen and on its responses to catecholamines, angiotensin and nerve stimulation. *British Journal of Pharmacology,* **32**, 136.

Davies, B. N. and Withrington, P. G. (1969). Actions of prostaglandins $A_1$, $A_2$, $E_1$, $E_2$, $F_{1\alpha}$ and $F_{2\alpha}$ on splenic vascular and capsular smooth muscle and their interactions with sympathetic nerve stimulation, catecholamines and angiotensin. In: Prostaglandins, Peptides and Amines (ed. P. Mantegazza and E. W. Horton), p. 53, Academic Press, London.

Davies, B. N. and Withrington, P. G. (1971). Actions of prostaglandin $F_{2\alpha}$ on the splenic vascular and capsular smooth muscle in the dog. *British Journal of Pharmacology,* **41**, 1.

Dekker, A. and Field, J. B. (1970). Correlation of effects of thyrotropin, prostaglandins and ions on glucose oxidation, cyclic-AMP and colloid droplet formation in dog thyroid slices. *Metabolism,* **19**, 453.

Dorp, D. A. van (1971). Recent developments in the biosynthesis and the analysis of prostaglandins. *Annals of the New York Academy of Sciences,* **180**, 181.

DuCharme, D. W., Weeks, J. R. and Montgomery, R. G. (1968). Studies on the mechanism of the hypertensive effect of prostaglandin $F_{2\alpha}$ *Journal of Pharmacology and Experimental Therapeutics,* **160**, 1.

Duda, P., Horton, E. W.. and McPherson, A. (1968). The effects of prostaglandins $E_1$, $E_2$ and $F_{2\alpha}$ on monosynaptic reflexes. *Journal of Physiology,* **196**, 151.

Dunham, E. W. and Zimmerman, B. G. (1970). Release of prostaglandin-like material from dog kidney during nerve stimulation. *American Journal of Physiology,* **219**, 1279.

Eakins, K. (1971). Prostaglandin antagonism by polymeric phosphates of phloretin and related compounds. *Annals of the New York Academy of Sciences,* **180,** 386.

Eakins, K. E. and Karim, S. M. M. (1970). Polyphloretin phosphate: A selective antagonist for prostaglandins $F_{1\alpha}$ and $F_{2\alpha}$. *Life Sciences,* **9,** 1.

Eakins, K. E., Karim, S. M. M. and Miller, J. D. (1970). Antagonism of some smooth muscle actions by polyphloretin phosphate. *British Journal of Pharmacology,* **39,** 556.

Edwards, W. G. Jr., Strong, C. G. and Hunt, J. C. (1969). A vasodepressor lipid resembling prostaglandin $E_2$ ($PGE_2$) in the renal venous blood of hypertensive patients. *Journal of Laboratory and Clinical Medicine,* **74,** 389.

Eglinton, G., Raphael, R. A., Smith, G. N., Hall, W. J. and Pickles, V. R. (1963). The isolation and identification of two smooth muscle stimulants from menstrual fluid. *Nature* (London), **200,** 960.

Eliasson, R. (1959). A comparative study of prostaglandin from human seminal fluid and from prostate gland of sheep. *Acta Physiologica Scandinavica,* **39,** 141.

Eliasson, R. (1966). Mode of action of prostaglandins on the human non-pregnant uterus. *Biochemical Pharmacology,* **15,** 755.

Eliasson, R. and Posse, N. (1960). The effect of prostaglandin on the non-pregnant human uterus *in vivo. Acta Obstetricia et Gynecologica Scandinavica,* **39,** 112.

Eliasson, R. and Posse, N. (1965). Rubin's test before and after intravaginal application of prostaglandin. *International Journal of Fertility,* **10,** 373.

Ellis, L. C. and Baptista, M. H. (1969). Radiation biology of the fetal and juvenile mammal. *U.S. Atomic Energy Commission Div. Techn. Inform.,* p. 963.

Embry, M. P. and Morrison, D. L. (1968). The effect of prostaglandins on the human pregnant myometrium *in vitro. Journal of Obstetrics and Gynaecology of the British Commonwealth,* **75,** 829.

Emerson, T. E. Jr., Kelks, G. W., Daugherty, R. M. Jr. and Hodgman, R. E. (1971). Effects of prostaglandin $E_1$ and $F_{2\alpha}$ on venous return and other parameters in the dog. *American Journal of Physiology,* **220,** 243.

Emmons, P. R., Hampton, J. R., Harrison, M. J. G., Honour, A. J. and Mitchell, J. R. A. (1967). Effect of prostaglandin $E_1$ on platelet behavior *in vitro* and *in vivo. British Medical Journal,* **2,** 468.

Euler, U. S. von. (1934a). A depressor substance in the vesicular gland. *Journal of Physiology* (London), **84,** 21P.

Euler, U. S. von. (1934b). Zur Kenntnis der Pharmakologischen Wirkungen von Nativsekreten und Extrakten männlicher accessorischer Geschlechtsdrüsen. *Naunyn-Schmiedebergs Archiv für experimentelle Pathologie und Pharmakologie,* **175,** 78.

Euler, U. S. von. (1935). Uber die spezifische blutdrucksenkende. Substanz des menschlichen Prostata- und Samen-blasensekretes. *Klinische Wechenschrift,* **14,** 1182.

Euler, U. S. von. (1936). On the specific vasodilating and plain muscle stimulating substances from accessory genital glands in man and certain animals (prostaglandin and vesiglandin). *Journal of Physiology* (London), **88,** 213.

Euler, U. S. von. (1938). Action of adrenaline, acetylcholine and other substances on nerve-free vessels (human placenta). *Journal of Physiology* (London), **93,** 129.

Euler, U. S. von. (1939). Weitere Untersuchungen über Prostaglandin, die physiologisch aktive Substanz gewisser Genitaldrüsen. *Skandinavica Arch. Physiologica,* **81,** 65.

Euler, U. S. von and Eliasson, R. (1967). Prostaglandins. Medicinal Chemistry Monographs, Vol. 8, Academic Press, New York/London.

Fain, J. N. (1967). Adrenergic blockade of hormone-induced lipolysis in isolated fat cells. *Annals of the New York Academy of Sciences, 139, 879.*

Fain, J. N. (1968a). Stimulation by insulin and prostaglandin $E_1$ of glucose metabolism and inhibition of lipolytic action of theophylline on fat cells in the absence of $K^+$. *Endocrinology, 83, 548.*

Fain, J. N. (1968b). Antilipolytic effect of prostaglandin $E_1$ on free fat cells. In: Prostaglandin Symposium of the Worcester Foundation (ed. P. W. Ramwell and J. E. Shaw), p. 67, *Interscience,* New York.

Fassina, G., Carpenedo, F. and Santi, R. (1969). Effect of prostaglandin $E_1$ on isolated short-circuit frog skin. *Life Sciences, 8, 181.*

Fassina, G. and Contessa, A. R. (1967). Digitoxin and prostaglandin $E_1$ as inhibitors of catecholamine-stimulated lipolysis and their interaction with $Ca^{2+}$ in the process. *Biochemical Pharmacology, 16, 1447.*

Feldberg, W. and Myers, R. D. (1966). Appearance of 5-hydroxytryptamine and an unidentified pharmacologically active lipid acid in effluent from perfused cerebral ventricles. *Journal of Physiology* (London), 184, 837.

Ferreira, S. H., Moncada, S. and Vane, J. R. (1971). Indomethacin and aspirin abolish prostaglandin release from the spleen. *Nature New Biology, 231, 237.*

Ferreira, S. H. and Vane, J. R. (1967). Prostaglandins: their disappearance from and release into the circulation. *Nature* (London), 216, 868.

Ferri, S., Galatulas, I. and Piccinini, F. (1965). Azione della prostaglandina $E_1$ sulla coagulazione del sangue. *Bolletino della societa italiana di biologica sperimentale,* 41, 1243.

Field, J., Dekker, A., Zor, U. and Kaneko, T. (1971). *In vitro* effects of prostaglandins on thyroid gland metabolism. *Annals of the New York Academy of Sciences,* 180, 278.

Fischer, T. V. (1967). Local uterine regulation of the corpus luteum. *American Journal of Anatomy,* 121, 425.

Flack, J. D., Jessup, R. and Ramwell, P. W. (1969). Prostaglandin stimulation of rat corticosteroidogenesis. *Science,* 163, 691.

Fredholm, B. B., Oberg, B. and Rosell, S. (1970a). Effects of vasoactive drugs on circulation in canine subcutaneous adipose tissue. *Acta Physiologica Scandinavica,* 79, 564.

Fredholm, B. B. and Rosell, S. (1970). Effects of prostaglandin $E_1$ in canine subcutaneous adipose tissue *in situ. Acta Physiologica Scandinavica,* 80, 450.

Fredholm, B. B., Rosell, S. and Strandberg, K. (1970b). Release of prostaglandin-like material from canine subcutaneous adipose tissue by nerve stimulation. *Acta Physiologica Scandinavica,* 79, 18A.

Fried, J., Lin, C., Mehra, M., Kao, W. and Dalven, P. (1971). Synthesis and biological activity of prostaglandins and prostaglandin antagonists. *Annals of the New York Academy of Sciences,* 180, 38.

Fried, J., Santhanakrishnan, T. S., Himizu, J., Lin, C. H. and Ford, S. H. (1969). Prostaglandin antagonists: Synthesis and smooth muscle activity. *Nature* (London), 233, 208.

Fuchs, F., Prieto, M. and Marcus, S. (1971). Effect of prostaglandins on uterine activity in pregnant rhesus monkeys. *Annals of the New York Academy of Sciences,* 180, 531.

Giles, T. D., Quiroz, A. C. and Burch, G. E. (1969). The effects of prostaglandins $E_1$ on the systemic and pulmonary circulations of intact dogs. The influence of urethane and pentobarbital anesthesia. *Experientia,* **25**, 1056.

Glaviano, V. and Masters, T. (1971). Inhibitory action of intracoronary prostaglandin $E_1$ on myocardial lipolysis. *American Journal of Physiology,* **220**, 1187.

Giroud, J. P. and Willoughby, D. A. (1970). The interrelations of complement and prostaglandin-like substance in acute inflammation. *Journal of Pathology,* **101**, 241.

Goldblatt, M. W. (1933). A depressor substance in seminal fluid. *Journal of the Society for Chemistry and Industry,* London, **52**, 1056.

Goldblatt, M. W. (1935). Properties of human seminal plasma. *Journal of Physiology,* (London), **84**, 208.

Grantham, J. J. and Orloff, J. (1968). Effect of prostaglandin $E_1$ on the permeability response of the isolated collecting tubule to vasopressin, adenosine 3', 5'-monophosphate and theophylline. *Journal of Clinical Investigation,* **47**, 1154.

Greenberg, R. A. and Sparks, H. V. (1969). Prostaglandins and consecutive vascular segments of the canine hindlimb. *American Journal of Physiology,* **216**, 567.

Gutknecht, G. D., Cornette, J. C. and Pharriss, B. B. (1969). Antifertility properties of prostaglandin $F_{2\alpha}$ *Biology of Reproduction,* **1**, 367.

Gutknecht, G. D., Wyngarden, L. J. and Pharriss, B. B. (1971). The effect of prostaglandin $F_{2\alpha}$ on ovarian and plasma progesterone levels in the pregnant hamster. *Proceedings of the Society for Experimental Biology and Medicine,* **136**, 1151.

Haessler, H. A. and Crawford, J. D. (1966). Lipolysis in homogenates of adipose tissue: An inhibitor found in fat from obese rats. *Science* (New York), **154**, 909.

Haessler, H. A. and Crawford, J. D. (1967). Insulin-like inhibition of lipolysis and stimulation of lipogenesis by prostaglandin $E_1$ ($PGE_1$). *Journal of Clinical Investigation,* **46**, 1065.

Hamberg, M. (1969). Biosynthesis of prostaglandins in the renal medulla of the rabbit. *FEBS Letters,* **5**, 127.

Hamberg, M. (1968). Metabolism of prostaglandins in rat liver mitochondria. *European Journal of Biochemistry,* **6**, 135.

Hargrove, J. L., Johnson, J. M. and Ellis, L. C. (1971). Prostaglandins $E_1$ induced inhibition of rabbit testicular contractions *in vitro. Proceedings of the Society for Experimental Biology and Medicine,* **136**, 958.

Hauge, A., Lunde, P. K. M. and Waaler, B. A. (1967). Effects of prostaglandin $E_1$ and adrenaline on the pulmonary vascular resistance (PVR) in isolated rabbit lungs. *Life Sciences,* **6**, 673.

Hawkins, D. F. (1968). Relevance of prostaglandin to problems of human subfertility. In: Prostaglandin Symposium of the Worcester Foundation (ed. P. W. Ramwell and J. E. Shaw), p. 1, Interscience, New York.

Hawkins, D. F., Jessup, R. and Ramwell, P. W. (1968). Effect of ovarian hormones on response of the isolated rat uterus to prostaglandins. In: Prostaglandin Symposium of the Worcester Foundation (ed. P. W. Ramwell and J. E. Shaw), p. 11, Interscience, New York.

Hedqvist, P. (1970). Studies on the effect of prostaglandins $E_1$ and $E_2$ on the sympathetic neuromuscular transmission in some animal tissues. *Acta Physiologica Scandinavica,* Suppl. 345, 1.

Hedqvist, P. (1971). Prostaglandin E compounds and sympathetic neuromuscular transmission. *Annals of the New York Academy of Sciences,* **180**, 410.

Hedqvist, P. and Brundin, J. (1969). Inhibition of prostaglandin $E_1$ of noradrenaline release and of effector responses to nerve stimulation in the cat spleen. *Life Sciences,* **8**, 389.

Hedwall, P. R., Abdel-Sayed, W., Schmid, P. G. and Abboud, F. M. (1970). Selective interaction between prostaglandin $E_1$ ($PGE_1$) and adrenergic stimuli. *Circulation 42* Suppl. III, 89.

Hickler, R. B., Lauler, D. P., Saravis, C. A., Vagnucci, A. I., Steiner, G. and Thorn, G. W. (1964). Vasodepressor lipid from the renal medulla. *Journal of the Canadian Medical Association,* **90**, 280.

Higgins, C., Vatner, S., Franklin, D. and Braunwald, E. (1970). Augmentation of coronary blood flow and cardiac output in conscious dogs by intravenous prostaglandin $A_1$. *Circulation 42* Suppl. III, 123.

Hillier, K. and Karim, S. M. M. (1968). Effects of prostaglandins $E_1$, $E_2$, $F_{1\alpha}$ and $F_{2\alpha}$ on isolated human umbilical and placental blood vessels. *Journal of Obstetrics and Gynaecology of the British Commonwealth,* **75**, 667.

Hodgman, R. E., Jelke, G. W., Swindall, S. and Daugherty, R. M. Jr. (1970). Effects of local infusion of $PGF_{2\alpha}$ on the skin and muscle vasculature of the dog forelimb. *Clinical Research,* **18**, 312.

Hoffer, B. J., Siggins, G. R. and Bloom, F. E. (1969). Prostaglandins $E_1$ and $E_2$ antagonize norepinephrine effects on cerebellar Purkinje cells: Microelectrophoretic study. *Science,* **166**, 1418.

Hollenberg, M., Walker, R. S. and McCormick, D. P. (1968). Cardiovascular responses to intracoronary infusion of prostaglandin $E_1$, $F_{1\alpha}$ and $F_{2\alpha}$. *Archives internationales de pharmacodynamie et de thérapie,* **174**, 66.

Holmes, S. W. (1965). Prostaglandin $E_1$, fatty acids and microbial growth. *Nature* (London), **206**, 405.

Holmes, S. W. and Horton, E. W. (1967). The nature and distribution of prostaglandins in the central nervous system of the dog. *Journal of Physiology,* (London), **191**, 134P.

Holmes, S. W., Horton, E. W. and Main, I. H. M. (1963). The effect of prostaglandin $E_1$ on responses of smooth muscle to catecholamines, angiotensin and vasopressin. *British Journal of Pharmacology,* **21**, 538.

Horton, E. W. (1964). Actions of prostaglandins $E_1$, $E_2$ and $E_3$ on the central nervous system. *British Journal of Pharmacology,* **22**, 189.

Horton, E. W. (1969). Hypotheses on physiological roles of prostaglandins. *Physiological Reviews,* **49**, 122.

Horton, E. W. and Jones, R. L. (1969). Prostaglandins $A_1$, $A_2$ and 19-hydroxy $A_1$; their actions on smooth muscle and their inactivation on passage through the pulmonary and hepatic portal vascular bed. *British Journal of Pharmacology,* **37**, 705.

Horton, E. W. and Main, I. H. M. (1963). A comparison of the biological activities of four prostaglandins. *British Journal of Pharmacology,* **21**, 182.

Horton, E. W. and Main, I. H. M. (1965). A comparison of the actions of prostaglandins $F_{2\alpha}$ and $E_1$ on smooth muscle. *British Journal of Pharmacology,* **24**, 470.

Horton, E. W. and Main, I. H. M. (1966). The identification of prostaglandins in central nervous tissues of the cat and the fowl. *Journal of Physiology* (London), 185, 36P.

Horton, E. W. and Main, I. H. M. (1967). Further observations on the central nervous actions of prostaglandins $F_{2\alpha}$ and $E_1$. *British Journal of Pharmacology,* 30, 568.

Horton, E. W., Main, I. H. M. and Thompson, C. J. (1965). Effects of prostaglandins on the oviduct, studied in rabbits and ewes. *Journal of Physiology* (London), 180, 514.

Hyman, A. L. (1969). The active responses of pulmonary veins in intact dogs to prostaglandins $F_{2\alpha}$ and $E_1$. *Journal of Pharmacology and Experimental Therapeutics,* 165, 267.

Jackson, R. T. (1970). Prostaglandin $E_1$ as a nasal constrictor in normal human volunteers. *Current Therapeutic Research,* 12, 711.

Jacobson, E. D. (1970). Comparison of prostaglandin $E_1$ and norepinephrine on the gastric mucosal circulation. *Proceedings of the Society for Experimental Biology & Medicine,* 133, 516.

Johnston, H. H., Herzog, J. P. and Lauler, D. P. (1967). Effect of prostaglandin $E_1$ on renal hemodynamics, sodium and water excretion. *American Journal of Physiology,* 213, 939.

Juhlin, L. and Michaelsson, G. (1969). Cutaneous vascular reaction to prostaglandins in healthy subjects and in patients with urticaria and atopic dermatitis. *Acta dermato-venereologica,* 49, 251.

Kadar, D. and Sunahara, F. A. (1969). Inhibition of prostaglandin effects by ouabain in the canine vascular tissue. *Canadian Journal of Physiology and Pharmacology,* 47, 871.

Kadowitz, P. J., Sweet, C. S. and Brody, M. J. (1971). Potentiation of adrenegic venomotor responses by angiotensin, prostaglandin $F_{2\alpha}$ and cocaine. *Journal of Pharmacology and Experimental Therapeutics,* 176, 167.

Kaley, G. and Weiner, R. (1971). Prostaglandin $E_1$: A potential mediator of the inflammatory response. *Annals of the New York Academy of Sciences,* 180, 338.

Kaneko, T., Zor, U. and Field, J. B. (1969). Thyroid-stimulating hormones and prostaglandin $E_1$ stimulation of cyclic 3' 5' AMP in thyroid slices. *Science,* 163, 1062.

Kaplan, H. R., Grega, G. J., Sherman, G. P. and Buckley, J. P. (1969). Central and reflexogenic cardiovascular actions of prostaglandin $E_1$. *International Journal of Neuropharmacology,* 8, 15.

Karim, S. M. M. (1966). Identification of prostaglandins in human amniotic fluid. *Journal of Obstetrics and Gynaecology of the British Commonwealth,* 73, 903.

Karim, S. M. M. (1967). The identification of prostaglandins in human umbilical cord. *British Journal of Pharmacology,* 29, 230.

Karim, S. M. M. (1971). Action of prostaglandin in the pregnant woman. *Annals of the New York Academy of Sciences,* 180, 483.

Karim, S. M. M. and Devlin, J. (1967). Prostaglandin content of amniotic fluid during pregnancy and labour. *Journal of Obstetrics and Gynaecology of the British Commonwealth,* 74, 230.

Karim, S. M. M. and Filshie, G. M. (1970). Therapeutic abortion using prostaglandin $F_{2\alpha}$ *Lancet,* 1, 157.

Karim, S. M. M., Hillier, K., Trussell, R. R., Patel, R. C. and Tamusauge, S. (1970). Induction of labour with prostaglandin $E_2$. *Journal of Obstetrics and Gynaecology of the British Commonwealth,* 77, 200.

Karim, S. M. M., Trussell, R. R., Hillier, K. and Patel, R. C. (1969). Induction of labour with prostaglandin $F_{2\alpha}$. *Journal of Obstetrics and Gynaecology of the British Commonwealth,* 76, 769.

Karlson, S. (1959). The influence of seminal fluid on the motility of the nonpregnant human uterus. *Acta Obstetricia et Gynecologica Scandinavica,* 38, 503.

Katori, M., Takeda, K. and Imai, S. (1970). Effects of prostaglandin $E_1$ and $F_{1\alpha}$ on the heart-lung preparation of the dog. *Tohoku Journal of Experimental Medicine,* 101, 67.

Katsuki, S., Onomae, T., Ino, K. and Ito, A. (1969). The effects of prostaglandin $E_1$ ($PGE_1$) on the brain circulation (in Japanese). In: The Prostaglandins, Symposium, 20 Sept. 1968, Kyoto, pp. 83-85, Ono Pharmaceutical Co., Osaka.

Kayaalp, S. O. and Türker, R. K. (1968). Effect of hemicholinium (HC-3) on the catecholamine releasing action of prostaglandin $E_1$. *European Journal of Pharmacology,* 3, 139.

Khairallah, P. A., Page, I. H. and Türker, R. K. (1967). Some properties of prostaglandin $E_1$ action of muscle. *Archives internationales de pharmacodynamie et de Thérapie,* 169, 328.

Kirton, K. T., Duncan, G., Oesterling, T. and Forbes, A. (1971). Prostaglandins and reproduction in the rhesus monkey. *Annals of the New York Academy of Sciences,* 180, 445.

Kirton, K. T., Pharriss, B. B. and Forbes, A. D. (1970). Luteolytic effects of prostaglandin $F_{2\alpha}$ in primates. *Proceedings of the Society for Experimental Biology and Medicine,* 133, 314.

Kischer, C. W. (1967). Effects of specific prostaglandins on development of chick embryo skin and down feather organ *in vitro. Developmental Biology,* 16, 203.

Kischer, C. W. (1969). Accelerated maturation of chick embryo skin treated with a prostaglandin ($PGB_1$). An electron microscopic study. *American Journal of Anatomy,* 124, 491.

Klaus, W. and Piccinini, F. (1967). Uber die Wirkung von Prostaglandin $E_1$ auf den Ca-Haushalt isolierter Meerschweichenherzen. *Experientia* (Basel), 23, 556.

Klein, D. C. and Raisz, L. G. (1970). Prostaglandins: Stimulation of bone resorption in tissue culture. *Endocrinology,* 86, 1436.

Kloeze, J. (1967). Influence of prostaglandins on platelet adhesiveness and platelet aggregation. In: Prostaglandins (ed. S. Bergström and B. Samuelsson), p. 241, Almqvist Wiksell, Stockholm.

Kloeze, J. (1969). Relationship between the chemical structure and platelet-aggregation activity of prostaglandins. *Biochemica Biophysica Acta,* 187, 285.

Kloeze, J. (1970a). Influence of prostaglandins $E_1$ and $E_2$ on coagulation of rat blood. *Experientia,* 26, 307.

Kloeze, J. (1970b). Prostaglandins and platelet aggregation *in vivo.* I. Influence of $PGE_1$ $\omega$-homo-$PGE_1$ on transient thrombocytopenia and of $PGE_1$ on the $LD_{50}$ of ADP. *Thrombosis et diathesis haemorrhagica,* 23, 286.

Kloeze, J. (1970c). Prostaglandins and platelet aggregation *in vivo.* II. Influence of $PGE_1$ and $PGF_{1\alpha}$ on platelet thrombus formation induced by an electric stimulus in veins on the rat brain surface. *Thrombosis et diathesis haemorrhagica,* 23, 293.

Krnjevic, K. (1965). Actions of drugs on single neurones in the cerebral cortex. *British Medical Bulletin,* **21**, 10.

Kuehl, F. A., Humes, J. L., Tarnoff, J., Cirillo, V. J. and Ham, E. A. (1970a). Prostaglandin receptor site: Evidence for an essential role in the action of luteinizing hormone. *Science,* **169**, 883.

Kuehl, K. A., Patanelli, D. J., Tarnoff, J. and Humes, J. L. (1970b). Testicular adenyl cyclase: Stimulation by the pituitary gonadotrophines. *Biology of Reproduction,* **2**, 154.

Kunze, H. and Vogt, W. (1971). Significance of phospholipase A for prostaglandin formation. *Annals of the New York Academy of Sciences,* **180**, 123.

Kuo, J. F. and Greengard, P. (1969). Cyclic nucleotide-dependent protein kinase IV. Widespread occurrence of adenosine $3',5'$-monophosphate-dependent protein kinase in various tissues and phyla of the animal kingdom. *Proceedings of the National Academy of Science, USA,* **64**, 1349.

Kupiecki, F. P. (1967). Effects of prostaglandin $E_1$ on lipolysis and plasma free fatty acids in the fasted rat. *Journal of Lipid Research,* **8**, 577.

Kurzrok, R. and Lieb, C. C. (1930). Biochemical studies of human semen. II. The action of semen on the human uterus. *Proceedings of the Society for Experimental Biology and Medicine,* **28**, 268.

Lavery, H. A., Lowe, R. D. and Scroop, G. C. (1970). Cardiovascular effects of prostaglandins mediated by the central nervous system of the dog. *British Journal of Pharmacology,* **39**, 511.

Lee, J. B. (1968). Cardiovascular implications of the renal prostaglandins. In: Prostaglandin Symposium of the Worcester Foundation (ed. P. W. Ramwell and J. E. Shaw), p. 131, Interscience, New York.

Lee, J. B., Covino, B. G., Takman, B. H. and Smith, E. R. (1965). Renomedullary vasodepressor substance, medullin: Isolation, chemical characterization and physiological properties. *Circulation Research,* **17**, 57.

Lee, J. B., McGiff, J. C., Kannegiesser, H., Aykent, Y. Y., Mudd, J. G. and Frawley, T. F. (1971). Prostaglandin $A_1$: Antihypertensive and renal effects. *Annals of Internal Medicine,* **74**, 703.

Lindner, H. R. and Zmigrod, A. (1967). Microdetermination of progestins in rat ovaries. Progesterone and 20α-hydroxy-pregn-4-en-3-one content during pro-oestrus, oestrus and pseudopregnancy. *Acta Endocrinologica,* **56**, 16.

Lippmann, W. (1969). Inhibition of gastric acid secretion in the rat by synthetic prostaglandins. *Journal of Pharmacy & Pharmacology,* **21**, 335.

Lippman, W. (1970). Inhibition of gastric acid secretion by a potent synthetic prostaglandin. *Journal of Pharmacy & Pharmacology,* **22**, 65.

Lipson, L. C. and Sharp, G. W. G. (1971). Effect of prostaglandin $E_1$ on sodium transport and osmotic water flow in the toad bladder. *American Journal of Physiology,* **220**, 1046.

Lipson, L. C., Hynie, S. and Sharp, G. W. G. (1971). Effect of prostaglandin $E_1$ on osmotic water flow and sodium transport in the toad bladder. *Annals of the New York Academy of Sciences,* **180**, 261.

MacLeod, R. M. and Lehmeyer, J. E. (1970). Release of pituitary growth hormone by prostaglandins and dibutyryl adenosine cyclic $3',5'$-monophosphate in the absence of protein synthesis. *Proceedings of the National Academy of Sciences,* **67**, 1172.

MacLeod, R. M., Lehmeyer, J. E. and Frontham, E. H. (1971). Stimulation of growth hormone release by prostaglandin and dibutyryl cyclic AMP in pituitary glands of tumor-bearing rats. *Federation Proceedings,* **30**, 533.

Mandel, L. R. and Kuehl, F. A. Jr. (1967). Lipolytic action of 3,3'5-tri-iodo-l-thyronine, a cyclic AMP phosphodiesterase inhibitor. *Biochemical and Biophysical Research Communications,* **28**, 13.

Mannaioni, P. F. (1970). Influence of bradykinin and prostaglandin $E_1$ on the uptake and release of histamine by murine neoplastic mast cells *in vitro. Biochemical Pharmacology,* **19**, 1159.

Mantegazza, P. (1965). La prostaglandina $E_1$ come sostanza sensibilizzatrice per il calcio a livello del cuore isolato di cavia. *Atti della Accademia lombarda,* **20**, 66.

Mark, A. L., Schmid, P. G., Eckstein, J. W. and Wendling, M. G. (1971). Venous responses to prostaglandin $F_{2\alpha}$. *American Journal of Physiology,* **220**, 222.

Marquis, N. R., Becker, J. A. and Vigdahl, R. L. (1970). Platelet aggregation III. An epinephrine induced decrease in cyclic AMP synthesis. *Biochemistry Biophysics Research Communications,* **39**, 783.

Marquis, N. R., Vigdahl, R. L. and Tavormina, P. A. (1969). Platelet aggregation. I. Regulation by cyclic AMP and Prostaglandin $E_1$. *Biochemical Biophysical Research Communications,* **36**, 965.

Marrazzi, M. A. and Matschinsky, M. A. (1971). Reactions and binding sites of 15-OH-prostaglandin dehydrogenase (PGDH). *Pharmacologist,* **13**, 292.

Marsh, J. M. (1970). The stimulating effect of prostaglandin $E_2$ on adenyl cyclase in the bovine corpus luteum. *FEBS Letters,* **7**, 283.

Marsh, J. M. (1971). The effect of prostaglandins on the adenyl cyclase of the bovine corpus luteum. *Annals of the New York Academy of Sciences,* **180**, 416.

Maxwell, G. M. (1967). The effect of prostaglandin $E_1$ upon the general and coronary hemodynamics and metabolism of the intact dog. *British Journal of Pharmacology,* **31**, 162.

Mayer, H. E., Abboud, F. M., Schmid, P. G. and Mark, A. L. (1970). Release of norephinephrine by prostaglandin $E_1$. *Clinical Research,* **18**, 594.

McCracken, J. A., Glew, M. E. and Scaramuzzi, R. J. (1970). Corpus luteum regression induced by prostaglandin $F_{2\alpha}$ *Journal of Clinical Endocrinology,* **30**, 544.

McCracken, J. (1971). Prostaglandin $F_{2\alpha}$ and corpus luteum regression. *Annals of the New York Academy of Sciences,* **180**, 456.

McGiff, J. C., Crowshaw, K., Terragno, N. A., Lonigro, A. J., Strand, J. C., Williamson, M. A., Ng, K. K. F. and Lee, J. B. (1969a). Release of prostaglandin-like substances during acute renal ischemia. *Circulation 40,* Suppl. III, 144.

McGiff, J. C., Terragno, N. A., Strand, J. C., Lee, J. B., Lonigro, A. J. and Ng, K. K. F. (1969b). Selective passage of prostaglandins across the lung. *Nature* (London), **223**, 742.

Micheli, H. (1969). Factors modifying the effect of prostaglandin $E_1$ on lipolysis in adipose tissue. In: Drugs Affecting Lipid Metabolism (ed. W. L. Holmes, L. A., Carlson and R. Paoletti), p. 75, Plenum Press, London.

Micheli, H., Carlson, L. A. and Hallberg, D. (1969). Comparison of lipolysis in human subcutaneous and omental adipose tissue with regard to effects of noradrenaline, theophylline, prostaglandin $E_1$ and age. *Acta chirurgica Scandinavica,* **135**, 663.

Micheli, H. (1970). Lipolysis in rabbit, dog and human adipose tissue. *Acta Universitatis Upsalla,* **67**, 1.

Mills, D. C. B. and Smith, J. B. (1971). The influence of platelet aggregation of drugs that affect the accumulation of adenosine $3' : 5'$ cyclic monophosphate in platelets. *Biochemical Journal*, **121**, 185.

Milton, A. S. and Wendlandt, S. (1970). A possible role for prostaglandin $E_1$ as a modulator for temperature regulation in the central nervous system of the cat. *Journal of Physiology*, **207**, 76P.

Moskowitz, J., Harwood, J. P., Reid, W. D. and Krishna, G. (1971). The interaction of norepinephrine and prostaglandin $E_1$ on the adenyl cyclase system of human and rabbit blood platelet. *Biochimica et Biophysica Acta*, **230**, 279.

Mühlbachová, E., Sólyom, A. and Puglisi, L. (1967). Investigations on the mechanism of the prostaglandin $E_1$ antagonism to norepinephrine and theophylline-induced lipolysis. *European Journal of Pharmacology*, **1**, 321.

Muirhead, E. E., Brooks, B., Kosinski, M., Daniels, E. G. and Hinman, J. W. (1966). Renomedullary antihypertensive principle in renal hypertension. *Journal of Laboratory and Clinical Medicine*, **67**, 778.

Muirhead, E. E., Daniels, E. G., Booth, E., Freyburger, W. A. and Hinman, J. W. (1965). Renomedullary vasodepression and antihypertensive function. *Archives of Pathology*, **80**, 43.

Muirhead, E. E., Leach, B. E., Brown, G. B., Daniels, E. G. and Hinman, J. W. (1967). Antihypertensive effect of prostaglandin $E_2$ ($PGE_2$) in renovascular hypertension. *Journal of Laboratory and Clinical Medicine*, **70**, 986.

Mürer, E. H. (1971). Effect of prostaglandin $E_1$ on clot retraction. *Nature* (London), **229**, 113.

Murphy, G. P., Hesse, V. E., Evers, J. L., Hobika, G., Mostert, J. W., Szolnoky, A., Schoonees, R., Abramczyk, J. and Grace, J. T. (1970). The renal and cardiodynamic effects of prostaglandins ($PGE_1$, $PGA_1$) in renal ischemia. *Journal of Surgical Research*, **10**, 533.

Najak, Z., Hillier, K. and Karim, S. M. M. (1970). The action of prostaglandins on the human isolated non-pregnant cervix. *Journal of Obstetrics and Gynaecology of the British Commonwealth*, **77**, 701.

Nakano, J. (1966). Effect of changes in coronary arterial blood flow on the myocardial contractile force. *Japanese Heart Journal*, **7**, 78.

Nakano, J. (1968a). Effect of prostaglandins $E_1$, $A_1$ and $F_{2\alpha}$ on cardiovascular dynamics in dogs. In: Prostaglandin Symposium of the Worcester Foundation (ed. P. W. Ramwell and J. E. Shaw), p. 201, Interscience, New York.

Nakano, J. (1968b). Effects of prostaglandins $E_1$, $A_1$ and $F_{2\alpha}$ on the coronary and peripheral circulations. *Proceedings of the Society for Experimental Biology and Medicine*, **127**, 1160.

Nakano, J. (1969). Cardiovascular effect of a prostaglandin isolated from a gorgonian *Plexaura homomalla*. *Journal of Pharmacy and Pharmacology*, **21**, 782.

Nakano, J. (1970a). Metabolism of prostaglandin $E_1$ in kidney and lung. *Federation Proceedings*, **29**, 746.

Nakano, J. (1970b). Metabolism of prostaglandin $E_1$ in dog kidneys. *British Journal of Pharmacology*, **40**, 317.

Nakano, J. (1971). Effects of the metabolites of prostaglandin $E_1$, on the systemic and peripheral circulations in dogs. *Proceedings of the Society for Experimental Biology and Medicine*, **136**, 1265.

Nakano, J. (1972). Relationship between chemical structure of prostaglandins and their vasoactivities in dogs. *British Journal of Pharmacology*, **44**, 63.

Nakano, J. (1972b). Cardiovascular actions of prostaglandins. In: Prostaglandins (ed. P. W. Ramwell and J. E. Shaw), Plenum Press, New York. (in press).

Nakano, J., Änggård, E. and Samuelsson, B. (1969). 15-hydroxy-prostanoate dehydrogenase. Prostaglandins as substrate and inhibitors. *European Journal of Biochemistry,* 11, 386.

Nakano, J. and Cole, B. (1969). Effects of prostaglandins $E_1$ and $F_{2\alpha}$ on systemic, pulmonary and splanchnic circulations in dogs. *American Journal of Physiology,* · 217, 222.

Nakano, J., Cole, B. and Ishii, T. (1968a). Effects of disodium EDTA on the cardiovascular responses to prostaglandin $E_1$. *Experientia,* 24, 808.

Nakano, J., Ishii, T. and Gin, A. C. (1968b). Effect of prostaglandins $E_1$, $A_1$ and $F_{2\alpha}$ on norepinephrine-induced lipolysis. *Clinical Research,* 16, 30.

Nakano, J. and Kessinger, J. M. (1970). Effects of 8-isoprostaglandin $E_1$ on the systemic and pulmonary circulations in dogs. *Proceedings of the Society for Experimental Biology and Medicine,* 133, 1314.

Nakano, J. and McCurdy, J. R. (1967a). Cardiovascular effects of prostaglandin $E_1$. *Journal of Pharmacology & Experimental Therapeutics,* 156, 538.

Nakano, J. and McCurdy, J. R. (1967b). Effects of prostaglandin $E_1$ ($PGE_1$) and $A_1$ ($PGA_1$) on the systemic venous return and pulmonary circulation. *Clinical Research,* 15, 409.

Nakano, J. and McCurdy, J. R. (1968). Hemodynamic effects of prostaglandins $E_1$, $A_1$ and $F_{2\alpha}$ in dogs. *Proceedings of the Society of Experimental Biology & Medicine,* 128, 39.

Nakano, J., Perry, M. and Denton, D. (1968c). Effect of prostaglandin $E_1$ ($PGE_1$), $A_1$ ($PGA_1$) and $F_{2\alpha}$ ($PGF_{2\alpha}$) on the peripheral circulation. *Clinical Research,* 16, 110.

Nakano, J. and Prancan, A. V. (1971). Metabolic degradation of prostaglandin $E_1$ in rat plasma and in rat brain, heart, lung, kidney and testicle homogenates. *Journal of Pharmacy and Pharmacology,* 23, 231.

Nakano, J., Prancan, A. V. and Kessinger, J. M. (1971). Effect of prostaglandins $E_1$ and $A_1$ on the gastric circulation in dogs. *Clinical Research,* 19, 399.

Neill, J. D., Johansson, E. D. B. and Knobil, E. (1969). Failure of hysterectomy to influence the normal pattern of cyclic progesterone secretion in the rhesus monkey. *Endocrinology,* 84, 464.

Nutter, D. O. and Crumly, H. (1970). Coronary-myocardial responses to prostaglandins $E_1$ and $A_1$. *Circulation,* 42, Suppl. III, 124.

Nutting, E. F. and Cammarara, P. S. (1969). Effects of prostaglandins on fertility in female rats. *Nature* (London), 222, 287.

Onaya, T. and Solomon, D. H. (1970). Stimulation by prostaglandin $E_1$ of endocytosis and glucose oxidation in canine thyroid slices. *Endocrinology,* 86, 423.

Orloff, J. and Grantham, J. (1967). The effect of prostaglandin ($PGE_1$) on the permeability response of rabbit collecting tubules to vasopressin. In: Prostaglandins (ed. S. Bergström and B. Samuelsson), p. 143, Almqvist and Wiksell, Stockholm.

Orloff, J. and Handler, J. (1967). The role of adenosine $3',5'$-phosphate in the action of antidiuretic hormone. *American Journal of Medicine,* 42, 757.

Orloff, J., Handler, J. S. and Bergström, S. (1965). Effect of prostaglandin ($PGE_1$) on the permeability response of the toad bladder to vasopressin, theophylline and adenosine $3',5'$-monophosphate. *Nature* (London), **205**, 397.

Paoletti, R., Lentati, R. L. and Korolkiewicz, Z. (1967). Pharmacological investigations on the prostaglandin $E_1$ effect on lipolysis. In: Prostaglandins (ed. S. Bergström and B. Samuelsson), p. 147, Almqvist and Wiksell, Stockholm.

Paton, D. M. and Daniel, E. E. (1967). On the contractile response of the isolated rat uterus to prostaglandin $E_1$. *Canadian Journal of Physiology and Pharmacology*, **45**, 795.

Peng, T. C., Six, K. M. and Munson, P. L. (1970). Effects of prostaglandin $E_1$ on the hypothalamus hypophyseal-adrenocortical axis in rats. *Endocrinology*, **86**, 202.

Petersen, M. J. and Edelman, I. S. (1964). Calcium inhibition of the action of vasopressin on the urinary bladder of the toad. *Journal of Clinical Investigation*, **43**, 583.

Petersen, M. J., Patterson, C. and Ashmore, J. (1968). Effects of antilipolytic agents on dibutyryl cyclic AMP induced lipolysis in adipose tissue. *Life Sciences*, **7**, 551.

Pharriss, B. B. (1970). The possible vascular regulation of luteal function. *Perspectives in Biology and Medicine*, **13**, 434.

Pharriss, B. B. (1971). Prostaglandin induction of luteolysis. *Annals of the New York Academy of Sciences*, **180**, 436.

Pharriss, B. B., Cornette, J. C. and Gutnecht, G. D. (1970). Vascular control of luteal steroidogenesis. *Journal of Reproduction and Fertility*, Suppl. 10, 97.

Pharriss, B. B. and Wyngarden, L. J. (1969). The effect of $PGF_{2\alpha}$ on the progesterone content of the ovaries from pseudopregnant rats. *Proceedings of the Society for Experimental Biology and Medicine*, **130**, 92.

Pharriss, B. B., Wyngarden, L. J. and Gutknecht, G. D. (1968). Biological interactions between prostaglandins and luteotropins in the rat. In: Gonadotropins (ed. E. Rosenberg), p. 121, Geron-X, inc., Los Altos, Calif.

Piccinini, F., Pomarelli, P. and Chiarra, A. (1969). Further investigations on the mechanism of the inotropic action of prostaglandin $E_1$ in relation to the ion balance in the frog heart. *Pharmacological Research Communications*, **1**, 381.

Pickles, V. R. (1959). Myometrial responses to the menstrual plain-muscle stimulant. *Journal of Endocrinology*, **19**, 150.

Pickles, V. R. and Hall, W. J. (1963). Some physiological properties of the 'menstrual stimulant' substances $A_1$ and $A_2$. *Journal of Reproduction and Fertility*, **6**, 315.

Pickles, V. R., Hall, W. J., Best, F. A. and Smith, G. N. (1965). Prostaglandins in endometrium and menstrual fluid from normal and dysmenorrhoeic subjects. *Journal of Obstetrics and Gynaecology of the British Commonwealth*, **72**, 185.

Pickles, V. R., Hall, W. J., Glegg, P. C. and Sullivan, T. J. (1966). Some experiments on the mechanism of action of prostaglandins on the guinea-pig and rat myometrium. *Memoirs of the Society for Endocrinology*, **14**, 89.

Pike, J. E., Kupiecki, F. P. and Weeks, J. R. (1967). Biological activity of the prostaglandins and related analogs. In: Prostaglandins (ed. S. Bergström and B. Samuelsson), p. 161, Almqvist and Wiksell, Stockholm.

Ramwell, P. W. and Shaw, J. E. (1966). Spontaneous and evoked release of prostaglandins from the cerebral cortex of anesthetized cats. *American Journal of Physiology*, **211**, 125.

Ramwell, P. W. and Shaw, J. E. (1967). Prostaglandin release from tissues by drug, nerve and hormone stimulation. In: Prostaglandins (ed. S. Bergström and B. Samuelsson), p. 283, Almqvist and Wiksell, Stockholm.

Ramwell, P. W. and Shaw, J. E. (1968). Prostaglandin inhibition of gastric secretion. *Journal of Physiology* (London), **195**, 34P.

Ramwell, P. W. and Shaw, J. E. (1970). Biological significance of the prostaglandins. *Recent Progress in Hormone Research*, **26**, 139.

Ramwell, P. W., Shaw, J. E., Corey, E. J. and Andersen, N. (1969). Biological activity of synthetic prostaglandins. *Nature* (London), **221**, 1251.

Ramwell, P. W., Shaw, J. E., Douglas, W. W. and Poisner, A. M. (1966a). Efflux of prostaglandin from adrenal glands stimulated with acetylcholine. *Nature* (London), **210**, 273.

Ramwell, P. W., Shaw, J. E. and Jessup, R. (1966b). Spontaneous and evoked release of prostaglandins from frog spinal cord. *American Journal of Physiology*, **211**, 998.

Ramwell, P. W., Shaw, J. E. and Kucharski, J. (1965). Prostaglandin release from the rat phrenic nerve-diaphragm preparation. *Science* (New York), **149**, 1390.

Rizack, M. A. (1961). An epinephrine-sensitive lipolytic activity in adipose tissue. *Journal of Biological Chemistry*, **236**, 657.

Robert, A., Nezamis, J. E. and Phillips, J. P. (1968a). Effect of prostaglandin $E_1$ on gastric secretion and ulcer formation in the rat. *Gastroenterology*, **55**, 481.

Robison, G. A., Arnold, A. and Hartmann, R. C. (1969). Divergent effects of epinephrine and prostaglandin $E_1$ on the level of cyclic AMP in human blood platelets. *Pharmacological Research Communications*, **1**, 325.

Robison, G. A., Butcher, R. W. and Sutherland, E. W. (1967). Adenyl cyclase as an adrenergic receptor. *Annals of the New York Academy of Sciences*, **139**, 703.

Robison, G., Cole, B., Arnold, A. and Hartmann, R. (1971). Effects of prostaglandins on function and cyclic AMP levels of human blood platelets. *Annals of the New York Academy of Sciences*, **180**, 324.

Ruddon, R. W. and Johnson, J. M. (1967). The effect of prostaglandins on protein and nucleic acid synthesis in a cell-free system. *Life Sciences*, **6**, 1245.

Sabatini-Smith, S. (1970). Action of prostaglandins $E_1$ and $F_{2\alpha}$ on calcium flux in the isolated guinea-pig atria and fragmented cardiac sarcoplasmic reticulum. *Pharmacologist*, **12**, 239.

Said, S. I. (1968). Some respiratory effects of prostaglandins $E_2$ and $F_{2\alpha}$. In: Prostaglandin Symposium of the Worcester Foundation (ed. P. W. Ramwell and J. E. Shaw), p. 207, Interscience, New York.

Samuelsson, B. (1964). Identification of a smooth muscle-stimulating factor in bovine brain. *Biochimica et Biophysica Acta*, **84**, 218.

Samuelsson, B. (1970). Biosynthesis and metabolism of prostaglandins. *Proceedings of the 4th International Congress of Pharmacology*, **4**, 12. Karger, Basel/New York.

Samuelsson, B., Granström, E., Green, K. and Hamberg, M. (1971). Metabolism of prostaglandins. *Annals of the New York Academy of Sciences*, **180**, 138.

Sandberg, F., Ingelman-Sundberg, A., Lindgren, L. and Ryden, G. (1962). *In vitro* effects of prostaglandin on different parts of the human fallopian tube. *Nature* (London), **193**, 781.

Sandberg, F., Ingelman-Sundberg, A. and Ryden, G. (1963). The specific effect of prostaglandin on different parts of the human fallopian tube. *Journal of Obstetrics and Gynaecology of the British Commonwealth*, **70**, 130.

Sandberg, F., Ingelman-Sundberg, A. and Ryden, G. (1964). The effect of prostaglandin $E_2$ and $E_3$ on the human uterus and fallopian tubes *in vitro*. *Acta Obstetrica et Gynecologica Scandinavica,* **43**, 95.

Sandberg, F., Ingelman-Sundberg, A. and Ryden, G. (1965). The effect of prostaglandin $F_{1\alpha}$, $F_{1\beta}$, $F_{2\alpha}$ and $F_{2\beta}$, on the human uterus and the fallopian tubes *in vitro*. *Acta Obstetrica et Gynecologica Scandinavica,* **44**, 585.

Sanner, J. H., Rozek, L. F. and Cammarata, P. S. (1968). Comparative smooth muscle and cardiovascular actions of prostaglandins $E_2$, $F_{2\alpha}$ and $F_{2\beta}$. In: Prostaglandin Symposium of the Worcester Foundation (ed. P. W. Ramwell and J. E. Shaw), p. 215, Interscience, New York.

Sanner, J. H. (1969). Antagonism of prostaglandin $E_2$ by 1-acetyl-2-(8-chloro-10,11-dihydro-dibenz (b,f)-(1,4)-oxazepine-10-carbonyl-hydrazine (SC-19220). *Archives internationales de pharmacodynamie et de thérapie,* **180**, 46.

Sanner, J. H. (1971). Prostaglandin inhibition with a dibenzoxazepine hydrazide derivative and morphine. *Annals of the New York Academy of Sciences,* **180**, 396.

Saruta, T. and Kaplan, N. M. (1971). The effects of prostaglandins upon beef adrenal steroidogenesis. *Clinical Research,* **19**, 69.

Schofield, J. G. (1970). Prostaglandins $E_1$ and the release of growth hormone *in vitro*. *Nature* (London), **228**, 179.

Schweppe, J. S. and Jungmann, R. A. (1970). Prostaglandins: The inhibition of hepatic cholesterol ester synthetase in the rat. *Proceedings of the Society for Experimental Biology and Medicine,* **133**, 1307.

Scott, R. E. (1970). Effects of prostaglandins, epinephrine and NaF on human leucocyte, platelet and liver adenyl cyclase. *Blood,* **35**, 514.

Sekhar, N. C. (1970). Effect of eight prostaglandins on platelet aggregation. *Journal of Medicinal Chemistry,* **13**, 39.

Sekhar, N. C., Weeks, J. R. and Kupiecki, F. P. (1968). Antithrombotic activity of a new prostaglandin, 8-iso-$PGE_1$. *Circulation,* **38**, Suppl. VI, 23.

Shaw, J. E. (1966). Prostaglandin release from adipose tissue *in vitro* evoked by nerve stimulation or catecholamines. *Federation Proceedings,* **25**, 770.

Shehadeh, Z., Price, W. E. and Jacobson, E. D. (1969). Effects of vasoactive agents on intestinal blood flow and motility in the dog. *American Journal of Physiology,* **216**, 386.

Shio, H., Plasse, A. M. and Ramwell, P. W. (1970). Platelet swelling and prostaglandins. *Microvascular Research,* **2**, 294.

Siggins, G., Hoffer, B. and Bloom, F. (1971). Prostaglandin-norepinephrine interactions in brain: Microelectrophoretic and histochemical correlates. *Annals of the New York Academy of Sciences,* **180**, 302.

Smith, E. R., McMorrow, J. V. Jr., Covino, B. G. and Lee, J. B. (1968). Studies on the vasodilator action of prostaglandin $E_1$. In: Prostaglandin Symposium of the Worcester Foundation (ed. P. W. Ramwell and J. E. Shaw), p. 259, Interscience, New York.

Smith, J. B. and Willis, A. L. (1971). Selective inhibition of synthesis of prostaglandins in human platelets. *Nature New Biology,* **231**, 235.

Sobel, B. E. and Robison, A. K. (1969). Activation of guinea pig myocardial adenyl cyclase by prostaglandins. *Circulation,* **40**, Suppl. III, 189.

Solomon, L. M., Juhlin, L. and Kirschenbaum, M. B. (1968). Prostaglandin on cutaneous vasculature. *Journal of Investigative Dermatology,* **51**, 280.

Sólyóm, A., Puglisi, L. and Mühlvachová, E. (1967). Effect of *in vitro* theophylline and prostaglandin $E_1$ on free fatty acid release and on triglyceride synthesis in rat adipose tissue. *Biochemical Pharmacology,* 16, 521.

Speroff, L. and Ramwell, P. W. (1970a). Prostaglandins in reproductive physiology. *American Journal of Obstetrics and Gynecology,* 107, 1111.

Speroff, L. and Ramwell, P. W. (1970b). Prostaglandin stimulation of *in vitro* progesterone synthesis. *Journal of Clinical Endocrinology & Metabolism,* 30, 345.

Steinberg, D. (1967). Prostaglandins as adrenergic antagonists. *Annals of the New York Academy of Sciences,* 139, 897.

Steinberg, D. and Pittman, R. (1966). Depression of plasma FFA levels in unanesthetized dogs by single intravenous doses of prostaglandin $E_1$. *Proceedings of the Society for Experimental Biology and Medicine,* 123, 192.

Steinberg, D., Vaughan, M., Nestel, P. and Bergström, S. (1963). Effects of prostaglandin E opposing those of catecholamines on blood pressure and on triglyceride breakdown in adipose tissue. *Biochemical Pharmacology,* 12, 764.

Steinberg, D. and Vaughan, M. (1967). *In vitro* and *in vivo* effects of prostaglandins on free fatty acid metabolism. In: Prostaglandins (ed. S. Bergström and B. Samuelsson), p. 109, Almqvist and Wiksell, Stockholm.

Steinberg, D., Vaughan, M., Nestel, P. J., Strand, O. and Bergström, S. (1964). Effects of the prostaglandins on hormone-induced mobilization of free fatty acids. *Journal of Clinical Investigations,* 43, 1533.

Stock, K., Aulich, A. and Westermann, E. (1968). Studies on the mechanism of antilipolytic action of prostaglandin $E_1$. *Life Sciences,* 7, 113.

Stock, K., Böhle, E. and Westermann, E. (1967). Differential effects of prostaglandin $E_1$ on lipolysis. *Progress in Biochemical Pharmacology,* 3, 122.

Stock, K. and Westermann, E. (1966). Competitive and non-competitive inhibition of lipolysis by $\alpha$- and $\beta$-adrenergic blocking agents, methoxamine derivatives and prostaglandin $E_1$. *Life Sciences,* 5, 1667.

Stovall, R. and Jackson, R. T. (1967). Prostaglandins and nasal blood flow. *Annals of Otology, Rhinology and Laryngology,* 76, 1051.

Strong, C. G. and Bohr, D. F. (1967). Effects of prostaglandins $E_1$, $E_2$, $A_1$ and $F_{1\alpha}$ on isolated vascular smooth muscle. *American Journal of Physiology,* 213, 725.

Strong, C. G., Boucher, R., Nowaczynski, W. and Genest, J. (1966). Renal vasodepressor lipid. *Proceedings of Staff Meetings, Mayo Clinic,* 1, 433.

Sussman, K. E. and Vaughan, G. D. (1967). Insulin release after ACTH, glucagon, and adenosine $3',5'$ phosphate cyclic AMP in the perfused isolated rat pancreas. *Diabetes,* 16, 449.

Suzuki, T., Abiko, Y. and Funaki, T. (1969). Effects of prostaglandin $E_1$ on the cardiovascular system in dogs. *Folia Pharmacologia Japonica,* 65, 1.

Sullivan, T. J. (1966). Response of the mammalian uterus to prostaglandins under differing hormonal conditions. *British Journal of Pharmacology,* 26, 678.

Tobian, L. and Viets, J. (1970). Potentiation of *in vitro* norepinephrine vasoconstriction with prostaglandin $E_1$. *Federation Proceedings,* 29, 387.

Turtle, J. R., Littleton, G. K. and Kipnis, D. M. (1967). Stimulation of insulin secretion by theophylline. *Nature* (London), 213, 727.

Tuttle, R. S. and Skelly, M. M. (1968). Interactions of prostaglandin $E_1$ and ouabain on contractility of isolated rabbit atria and intracellular cation concentration. In: Prostaglandin Symposium of the Worcester Foundation (ed. P. W. Ramwell and J. E. Shaw), p. 309, Interscience, New York.

Vale, W., Rivier, C. and Guillemin, R. (1971). A 'prostaglandin receptor' in the mechanisms involved in the secretion of anterior pituitary hormones. *Federation Proceedings*, **30**, 363.

Vander, A. J. (1968). Direct effects of prostaglandin on renal function and renal release in anesthetized dog. *American Journal of Physiology*, **214**, 218.

Vane, J. R. (1969). The release and fate of vasoactive hormones in the circulation. *British Journal of Pharmacology*, **35**, 209.

Vane, J. R. (1971). Inhibition of prostaglandin synthesis as a mechanism of action for aspirin-like drugs. *Nature New Biology*, **231**, 232.

Vaughan, M. (1964). Effect of pitressin on lipolysis and on phosphorylase activity in rat adipose tissue. *American Journal of Physiology*, **207**, 1166.

Vaughan, M. (1967). An effect of prostaglandin $E_1$ on glucose metabolism in rat adipose tissue. In: Prostaglandins (ed. S. Bergström and B. Samuelsson), p. 139, Almqvist and Wiksell, Stockholm.

Vergroesen, A. J. and DeBoer, J. (1968). Effects of prostaglandins $E_1$ and $F_{1\alpha}$ on isolated frog and rat hearts in relation to the potassium-calcium ratio of the perfusion fluid. *European Journal of Pharmacology*, **3**, 171.

Vergroesen, A. J., DeBoer, J. and Gottenbos, J. J. (1967). Effects of prostaglandins on perfused isolated rat hearts. In: Prostaglandins (ed. S. Bergström and B. Samuelsson), p. 211, Almqvist and Wiksell, Stockholm.

Vigdahl, R. L. and Marquis, N. R. (1970). Cyclic AMP mediated inhibition of platelet aggregation by vasodilators. *Circulation*, **42**, Suppl. III, 50.

Vigdahl, R. L., Marquis, N. R. and Tavormina, P. A. (1969). Platelet aggregation II. Adenyl cyclase, prostaglandin $E_1$ and calcium. *Biochemical & Biophysical Research Communications*, **37**, 409.

Viguera, M. G. and Sunahara, F. A. (1969). Microcirculatory effects of prostaglandins. *Canadian Journal of Physiology and Pharmacology*, **47**, 627.

Vilhardt, H. and Hedqvist, P. (1970). A possible role of prostaglandin $E_2$ in the regulation of vasopressin secretion in rats. *Life Sciences*, **9**, 825.

Vogt, W., Meyer, U., Kunze, H., Lufft, E. and Babilli, S. (1969). Entstehung von SRS-C in der durchstromten Meerschweinchenlunge durch Phospholipase A. Identifizierung mit prostaglandin. *Naunyn-Schmiedebergs Archiv für experimentalle Pathologie und Pharmakologie*, **262**, 124.

Waitzman, M. B. (1970). Pupil size and ocular pressure after sympathectomy and prostaglandin-catecholamine treatment. *Experimental Eye Research*, **10**, 219.

Waitzman, M. B. and King, C. D. (1967). Prostaglandin influences on intraocular pressure and pupil size. *American Journal of Physiology*, **212**, 329.

Weeks, J. R., Sekhar, N. C. and DuCharme, D. W. (1969). Relative activity of prostaglandins $E_1$, $A_1$, $E_2$ and $A_2$ on lipolysis, platelet aggregation, smooth muscle and the cardiovascular system. *Journal of Pharmacy and Pharmacology*, **21**, 103.

Weeks, J. R. and Walk, R. A. (1967). Reduction of variability between replicates in assay of hormone stimulated lipolysis. *Pharmacologist*, **9**, 254.

Weeks, J. R., Sekhar, N. C. and Kupiecki, P. K. (1968). Pharmacological profile of a new prostaglandin, 8-iso-prostaglandin $E_1$. *Pharmacologist*, **10**, 212.

Weeks, J. R. and Wingerson, F. (1964). Cardiovascular action of prostaglandin $E_1$ evaluated using unanesthetized relatively unrestrained rats. *Federation Proceedings*, **23**, 327.

Weiner, R. and Kaley, G. (1969). Influence of prostaglandin $E_1$ on the terminal vascular bed. *American Journal of Physiology*, **217**, 563.

Wennmalm, Å. and Hedqvist, P. (1970). Prostaglandin $E_1$ as inhibitor of the sympathetic neuroeffector system in the rabbit heart. *Life Sciences*, **9**, 931.

White, R. P., Denton, I. C. and Robertson, J. T. (1971). Differential effects of prostaglandins $A_1$, $E_1$ and $F_{2\alpha}$ on cerebrovascular tone in dogs and rhesus monkey. *Federation Proceedings*, **30**, 625.

Willebrands, A. F. and Tasseron, S. J. A. (1968). Effect of hormones on substrate preference in isolated rat heart. *American Journal of Physiology*, **215**, 1089.

Willis, A. L. (1969). Parallel assay of prostaglandin-like activity in rat inflammatory exudate by means of cascade superfusion. *Journal of Pharmacy & Pharmacology*, **21**, 126.

Willoughby, D. A. (1968). Effects of prostaglandins $PGF_{2\alpha}$ and $PGE_1$ on vascular permeability. *Journal of Pathology and Bacteriology*, **96**, 381.

Wilson, D. E. and Levine, R. A. (1969). Decreased canine gastric mucosal blood flow induced by prostaglandin $E_1$: A mechanism for its inhibitory effect on gastric secretion. *Gastroenterology*, **56**, 1268.

Wiqvist, N. and Bygdeman, M. (1970). Induction of therapeutic abortion with intravenous prostaglandin $F_{2\alpha}$. *Lancet*, **1**, 889.

Wolfe, S. M. and Shulman, N. R. (1969). Adenyl cyclase activity in human platelets. *Biochemical and Biophysical Research Communications*, **35**, 265.

Wolfe, S. M. and Shulman, N. R. (1970). Inhibition of platelet energy production and release reaction by $PGE_1$, theophylline and cAMP. *Biochemical Biophysical Research Communications*, **41**, 128.

Zetler, G. and Wiechell, H. (1969). Pharmakologisch aktive Lipide in Extrakten aus Tube und Ovar des Menschen. *Naunyn-Schmiedebergs Archiv für experimentelle Pathologie und Pharmakologie*, **265**, 101.

Zieve, P. D. and Greenough, W. B., III (1969). Adenyl cyclase in human platelets: Activity and responsiveness. *Biochemical and Biophysical Research Communications*, **35**, 462.

Zor, U., Bloom, G., Lowe, I. P. and Field, J. B. (1969a). Effects of theophylline, prostaglandin $E_1$ and adrenergic blocking agents on TSH stimulation of thyroid intermediary metabolism. *Endocrinology*, **84**, 1082.

Zor, U., Kaneko, T., Lowe, I. P., Bloom, G. and Field, J. B. (1969b). Effect of thyroid stimulating hormone and prostaglandins on thyroid adenyl cyclase activation and cyclic 3'5'-adenosine monophosphate. *Journal of Biological Chemistry*, **244**, 5189.

Zor, U., Kaneko, T., Schneider, H. P. G., McCann, S. M. and Field, J. B. (1970). Further studies of stimulation of anterior pituitary cyclic adenosine 3'5'-monophosphate by hypothalamic extract and prostaglandins. *Journal of Biological Chemistry*, **245**, 2883.

# CHAPTER III

# Distribution and Metabolism

Priscilla J. Piper

## Distribution

Prostaglandins are described as being 'ubiquitous among mammalian tissues' (Bergström, Carlson and Weeks, 1968) and can be extracted from most animal tissues.

The history of prostaglandins goes back to 1930 when two New York gynaecologists observed that fresh human semen causes either strong contractions or relaxations of the human uterus (Kurzrok and Lieb, 1930). A few years later Goldblatt (1935) and von Euler (1934, 1935) independently observed the smooth muscle stimulating activity of human seminal plasma. Von Euler found similar activity in the seminal fluid of some other animals and he gave the name 'prostaglandin' to acid lipids which contract smooth muscle and which were derived from extracts of sheep vesicular glands (von Euler, 1935).

### Extraction

Human seminal plasma contains the highest concentration and number of prostaglandins yet isolated from a single source. Thirteen different prostaglandins have been isolated ($E_1$, $E_2$, $E_3$, $F_{1\alpha}$, $F_{2\alpha}$, $A_1$, $A_2$, $B_1$, $B_2$ and 19 hydroxy $A_1$, $A_2$, $B_1$ and $B_2$) (Hamberg and Samuelsson, 1966; Bygdeman and Samuelsson, 1966). Seminal fluid from monkey, ram, rabbit (Horton and Thompson, 1964) and goat (Eliasson, 1959) also contains prostaglandins but that of stallion, bull and boar contains none (von Euler, 1937). Ram semen contains five prostaglandins, $E_1$, $E_2$, $E_3$, $F_{1\alpha}$, $F_{2\alpha}$ (Bygdeman and Holmberg, 1966; Hamberg and Samuelsson, 1967) and the ram vesicular gland is a good source of prostaglandins. The enzyme system from this gland can be used for laboratory conversion of fatty acids into prostaglandins (van Dorp, Beerthuis, Nugteren and Vonkeman, 1964a). No prostaglandins are present in the male accessory glands of bull, bear, dog, cat, rabbit, guinea-pig, hamster, rat, mouse, ferret or elk (Eliasson, 1959; Horton and Thompson, 1964; von Euler and Hammerström, 1937).

Prostaglandins also occur in the female reproductive tract and are found in the endometrium and in menstrual fluid (Pickles, Hall, Best and Smith, 1965; Hall, 1966). Two of the principal smooth muscle-stimulating substances in menstrual fluid are prostaglandin $E_2$ and $F_{2\alpha}$. Prostaglandins $E_1$, $E_2$, $F_{1\alpha}$ and $F_{2\alpha}$ are also present in human amniotic fluid and in extracts of blood vessels of the umbilical cord (Karim, 1966; Karim and Devlin, 1967; Karim, 1967). Ovaries of cows and pigs and testes of the ram contain relatively little prostaglandin-like activity (von Euler and Hammerström, 1937). Extracts of rabbit renal medulla contain prostaglandins $E_2$, $F_{2\alpha}$ and $A_2$ (Hickler, Birbari, Quershi and Karnovsky, 1966; Crowshaw and Szyik, 1970; Crowshaw, 1971) but prostaglandins $F_{2\alpha}$ and $A_2$ may be formed by dehydration of prostaglandin $E_2$ during extraction (Strong, Boucher, Nowaczynski and Genest, 1966). Karim, Sandler and Williams (1967) were unable to detect prostaglandins in extracts of human kidney.

Prostaglandins occur in many other tissues including lungs from cattle (Samuelsson, 1964a), sheep, pigs (Bergström, Dressler, Krabisch, Ryhage and Sjövall, 1962), guinea-pigs (Änggård, 1965), cat, rat, rabbit, chicken (Karim, Hillier and Devlin, 1968) and man (Karim, *et al.*, 1967). With the exception of the cat, lung tissue contains more prostaglandin of the F series, particularly $F_{2\alpha}$.

Extracts of central nervous tissue from various species contain prostaglandins of the E and F series (Table 1, modified from Horton, 1969).

Table 1

Prostaglandins detected

| *Species (whole brain)* | $E_1$ | $E_2$ | $F_{1\alpha}$ | $F_{2\alpha}$ | |
|---|---|---|---|---|---|
| Cat | | | | + | Coceani and Wolfe, 1965; Wolfe, Coceani and Pace-Asciak, 1967 |
| Dog | + | + | + | + | Holmes and Horton, 1968a |
| Rabbit | | + | | + | Hopkin, Horton and Whittaker, 1968 |
| Mouse | | | | + | Holmes and Horton, 1968b |
| Rat (cortex) | | | | + | Kataoka, Ramwell and Jessup, 1967 |
| Ox | | | | + | Samuelsson, 1964a |
| Chicken | | + | | + | Horton and Main, 1967 |

There is no clear regional variation of the four prostaglandins extracted from dog brain so they cannot be associated with specific pathways in the central nervous system (Horton, 1969).

Prostaglandins can be extracted from the irides of rabbits, cats, ox (Posner, 1970) and sheep (Änggård and Samuelsson, 1964). The material extracted from the rabbit iris, first known as irin (Ambache, 1957), is probably a mixture of $PGE_2$ and $F_{2\alpha}$ (Änggård and Samuelsson, 1964; Ambache, Brummer, Rose and Whiting, 1966).

Small amounts of prostaglandin-like material are found in extracts of sheep intestine (Von Euler and Hammerström, 1937) and darmstöff (obtained from frog intestine) contains a mixture of prostaglandins $E_1$ and $F_{1\alpha}$ (Suzuki and Vogt, 1965). Prostaglandins may be extracted from superfusates of the serosal surface of the unstimulated rat stomach (Coceani, Pace-Asciak, Volta and Wolfe, 1967a) and prostaglandin $E_2$ occurs in extracts of the human stomach (Bennett, Murray and Wyllie, 1968). Extracts of cat adrenal glands contain prostaglandin $F_{1\alpha}$, most of the prostaglandin being present in extracts of the cortex (Ramwell, Shaw, Douglas and Poisner, 1966). The distribution of prostaglandins in human tissues is summarized in Table 2 (from Karim *et al.*, 1967). Recently mouse tumours have been shown to contain concentrations of $PGE_2$ which are only exceeded by that contained in human seminal plasma (Maddox and Sykes, 1972).

A prostaglandin has been detected outside the vertebrate species mentioned, 15-R prostaglandin $A_2$ and the 15-acetyl derivative of its methyl ester occur in the air dried cortex of the gorgonian *Plexaura homonalla,* a species of coral found in the Caribbean (Weinheimer and Spraggins, 1969).

Table 2
Distribution of Prostaglandins in Human Tissue

| Tissue | Specimen number | $E_1$ | $E_2$ | $F_{1\alpha}$ | $F_{2\alpha}$ |
|---|---|---|---|---|---|
| Thyroid | 1 | – | 4.5 | – | 50.0 |
| | 2 | – | – | – | 100.0 |
| | 3 | – | 24.5 | – | – |
| | 4 | – | 12.5 | – | 25.0 |
| | 5 | – | 3.5 | – | 4.0 |
| Pancreas | 1 | – | 0.75 | – | 2.0 |
| | 2 | – | – | – | – |
| | 3 | – | 1.5 | – | 7.5 |
| | 4 | – | 0.3 | – | 0.8 |
| Adrenal cortex | 1 | – | 2.5 | – | 3.0 |
| | 2 | – | 3.0 | – | 6.3 |

Table 2–*cont.*

| Tissue | | Prostaglandins | | | |
|---|---|---|---|---|---|
| | | $E_1$ | $E_2$ | $F_{1\alpha}$ | $F_{2\alpha}$ |
| Adrenal medulla | 1 | — | 45.0 | — | 25.5 |
| | 2 | — | 22.5 | — | 64.0 |
| | 3 | — | — | — | 34.0 |
| Thymus Infant | 1 | 11.3 | — | — | — |
| Infant | 2 | 19.5 | — | — | — |
| Adult | 3 | 9.0 | — | — | — |
| Parotid gland | 1 | — | 0.5 | — | 2.5 |
| | 2 | — | 5.0 | — | 0.5 |
| Submandibular salivary gland | 1 | — | 5.5 | — | 1.0 |
| | 2 | — | 10.0 | — | — |
| | 3 | — | 1.0 | — | — |
| Cardiac muscle | 1 | — | 2.25 | — | — |
| | 2 | — | 3.50 | — | — |
| Rectus abdominis muscle | 1 | — | 1.0 | — | — |
| | 2 | — | 10.5 | — | — |
| Psoas muscle | 1 | — | 1.9 | — | — |
| | 2 | — | 1.3 | — | — |
| Cervical sympathetic chain | 1 | — | 1.9 | — | 4.0 |
| | 2 | — | 3.0 | — | 3.9 |
| | 3 | — | 15.0 | — | — |
| Vagus nerve | 1 | — | 5.3 | — | 5.0 |
| | 2 | — | 3.1 | — | 9.4 |
| Phrenic nerve | 1 | 10.5 | — | — | — |
| Brachial plexus | 1 | — | 2.0 | — | 4.2 |
| | 2 | — | 1.6 | — | 3.9 |
| Bronchi | 1 | — | 4.5 | — | 1.0 |
| | 2 | — | 7.8 | — | 2.5 |
| Lung parenchyma | 1 | — | 2.4 | — | 50.0 |
| | 2 | — | 1.3 | — | 12.4 |

The figures refer to concentrations in ng/g tissue.
A dash indicates that prostaglandins were not detected.

Reproduced from Karim, Sandler and Williams (1967) with permission of the authors and publisher.

*Release*

The fact that prostaglandins can be extracted from a tissue does not necessarily mean that they have a physiological role in that tissue. To demonstrate such a role for prostaglandins it is first of all important to detect the release of prostaglandins when a tissue is stimulated in some physiological way. For instance when the dog spleen is stimulated to contract, large amounts of prostaglandin $E_2$ and $F_{2\alpha}$ (up to $10 \mu g/min$ assayed as prostaglandin $E_2$) are released but less than $1 \mu g$ can be extracted from the resting organ (Gilmore, Vane and Wyllie, 1968). Many tissues, including lungs, adrenals, stomach and intestine, release more prostaglandins when stimulated than they contain (see Ramwell and Shaw, 1970). 'Thus the provocation of prostaglandin release in these instances should be regarded as provocation of prostaglandin synthesis followed by release' (Piper and Vane, 1971).

A basal release of prostaglandins may be detected from many vertebrate tissues and increased release readily occurs in response to stimulation as shown in Table 3 (modified from Piper and Vane, 1971). Prostaglandins can be released as well as extracted from the urogenital tract. Karim (1968) showed that prostaglandin $F_{2\alpha}$ appears in maternal venous blood during labour and Karim and Devlin (1967) and Karim and Hillier (1970) found that there are high concentrations of $PGE_2$ and $PGF_{2\alpha}$ in amniotic fluid during spontaneous abortion but were uncertain

Table 3
Release of Prostaglandins by Various Stimuli

| Species | Tissue | Stimulus | Reference |
|---|---|---|---|
| Rabbit | Eye (ant. chamber) | Mechanical | Ambache *et al.* (1965) |
| | Spleen | Adrenaline, Noradrenaline | Vane & Willis |
| | | Serotonin | (unpublished) |
| | Epigastric fat pad | Hormones | Lewis & Matthews (1969) |
| | Leucocytes | Phagocytosis | Higgs & Youlton (1972) |
| Cat | Somatosensory cortex | Neural, analeptics etc. | Ramwell & Shaw (1966) |
| | | Reticular formation | Bradley *et al.* (1969) |
| | Spleen | Catecholamines | Pojda, Vane & Willis |
| | | | (unpublished) |
| | Adrenal gland | Acetylcholine | Ramwell, Shaw, Douglas & Poisner (1966) |
| Dog | Spleen | Neural | Davies *et al.* (1968) |
| | | Neural, Catecholamines | Ferreira & Vane (1967) |
| | | Neural, Colloids | Gilmore *et al.* (1968) |
| | Bladder | Distension | Gilmore (1968) |
| | Cerebral ventricles | Serotonin | Holmes (1970) |
| | Kidney | Ischaemia | McGiff *et al.* (1970) |

Table 3—*cont.*

| Species | Tissue | Stimulus | Reference |
|---------|--------|----------|-----------|
| Rat | Phrenic diaphragm | Neural, biogenic amines | Ramwell *et al.* (1965) |
| | | | Laity (1969) |
| | Epididymal fat pad | Neural, biogenic amines | Shaw & Ramwell (1968b) |
| | Stomach | Neural, stretch | Bennett *et al.* (1967) |
| | | Neural | Coceani *et al.* (1967a, b) |
| | | Neural, secretagogues | Shaw & Ramwell (1968a) |
| | Skin | Inflammation | Willis (1969) |
| | Liver | Glucagon | Dawson & Ramwell (unpublished) |
| | Lung | Air embolus | Alabaster & Bakhle (1970) |
| | | Infusion of particles | Lindsey & Willie (1970) |
| Guinea-pig | Lung (whole perfused) | Anaphylaxis | Piper & Vane (1969a, b) |
| | | Particles | Lindsey & Wyllie (1970) |
| | | | Palmer, Piper & Vane (1970b) |
| | | | Piper & Vane (1971) |
| | | Phospholipase A | Vogt, Meyer, Kunze, Lufft & Babilli (1969) |
| | | Histamine | Alabaster & Bakhle (unpublished) |
| | | Tryptamine, serotonin | Alabaster & Bakhle (1970) |
| | | Massage | Piper & Vane (1971) |
| | | Distension | Berry, Edmonds & Wyllie (1970) |
| | | Air embolus | Piper & Vane (1971) |
| | Lung (chopped) | Stirring | Palmer, Piper & Vane (1970a) |
| | | | Piper & Vane (1971) |
| | Uterus | Distension | Poyser *et al.* (1971) |
| Human | Thyroid | Medullary carcinoma | Williams *et al.* (1968) |
| | Uterus | Parturition | Karim (1968) |
| | | Distension | Horton *et al.* (1971) |
| | Platelets | Thrombin | Smith & Willis (1970) |
| | Skin | Inflammation | Greaves, McDonald-Gibson & Søndergaard (1971) |
| | Lung (chopped) | Anaphylaxis | Piper & Walker (1972) |
| | | Agitation | (to be published) |
| Frog | Intestine | Distilled water | Vogt & Distelkotter (1967) |
| | Skin | Isoprenaline | Ramwell & Shaw (1970) |
| | Spinal cord | Neural, analeptic | Ramwell *et al.* (1966) |

of their origin. However, Horton, Thompson, Jones and Poyser (1971) and Poyser, Horton, Thompson and Los (1971) have shown that prostaglandin $F_{2\alpha}$ is released when the uterus of rabbit or guinea-pig is stretched. Distension of the bladder of an anaesthetized dog similarly causes release of prostaglandin-like material into the blood (Gilmore, 1968).

Release of prostaglandins occurs from isolated perfused lungs from guinea-pigs and rats and also from chopped lung tissue from the guinea-pig. Prostaglandins $E_2$ and $F_{2\alpha}$ are released from isolated perfused lungs of guinea-pigs (previously sensitized to ovalbumen) when the lungs are challenged (Piper and Vane, 1969a, b). Infusion of suspensions of particles such as Sephadex G10 into guinea-pig or rat lungs causes release of prostaglandins (Lindsey and Wyllie, 1970; Palmer, Piper and Vane, 1970b, Piper and Vane, 1971) and air embolus in guinea-pig and rat lungs also leads to release of prostaglandin-like material as does an infusion of histamine, tryptamine and serotonin (Alabaster and Bakhle, 1970). Repeated inflation of guinea-pig isolated perfused lungs with fairly large volumes of air causes release of prostaglandins (Berry, Edmonds and Wyllie, 1971) as does gentle massage of the external surface of the lungs (Piper and Vane, 1971). Injection of phospholipase A into guinea-pig perfused lungs releases SRS-C which contains prostaglandins (Vogt, Meyer, Kunze, Lufft and Babilli, 1969). When chopped lung tissue from guinea-pig is superfused, agitation of the lung tissue releases prostaglandins into the effluent (Palmer, Piper and Vane, 1970a).

Release of prostaglandins $E_2$ and $F_{2\alpha}$ has been shown from spleen of rabbit (Vane and Willis, unpublished), cat (Pojda, Vane and Willis, unpublished; Willis, 1971; Ferreira and Moncada, 1971) and dog (Davies, Horton and Withrington, 1968; Ferreira and Vane, 1967; Gilmore *et al.,* 1968; Ferreira, Moncada and Vane, 1971). Stimulation of the splanchnic nerves of dog isolated spleens perfused with either blood or Krebs solution leads to a contraction of the splenic capsule and a release of prostaglandins $E_2$ and $F_{2\alpha}$ into the venous effluent (Davies, Horton and Withrington, 1968; Ferreira and Vane, 1967; Gilmore *et al.,* 1968). Injection or infusion of catecholamines into isolated perfused spleens from rabbit, cat and dog also cause contraction of the spleen and release of prostaglandins (Vane and Willis, unpublished; Willis, 1971; Pojda, Vane and Willis, unpublished; Ferreira and Vane, 1967). Gilmore, Vane and Wyllie (1969) showed that these same two prostaglandins are released from dog isolated perfused spleens when colloidal suspensions of particles are injected; in this instance release of prostaglandins occurs in the absence of contraction of the splenic capsule. Prostaglandins are also released from cat perfused liver by administration of glucagon (Dawson and Ramwell, unpublished). Smith and Willis (1970) found that human platelets aggregated by thrombin release prostaglandins $E_2$ and $F_{2\alpha}$.

Prostaglandins can be released from nervous tissue of various species. Prostaglandins of the E and F series are released from cat somatosensory cortex in response to stimulation of sensory nerves, administration of analeptic drugs (Ramwell and Shaw, 1966) and electro-cortical arousal caused by stimulation of the reticular formation (Bradley, Samuels and Shaw, 1969). In the dog infusion of serotonin into the lateral ventricles causes release of prostaglandin E into the ventricles (Holmes, 1970). Prostaglandins are also released from the frog spinal cord either by nerve stimulation or analeptic drugs (Ramwell, Shaw and Jessup, 1966).

Prostaglandins are released from the rat phrenic nerve-diaphragm preparation in response to stimulation of the phrenic nerve and administration of catecholamines (Ramwell, Shaw and Kucharski, 1965; Laity, 1969).

Mechanical stimulation of the rabbit eye causes release of prostaglandins $E_2$ and $F_{2\alpha}$ into fluid perfusing the anterior chamber (Änggård and Samuelsson, 1964; Ambache *et al.*, 1966).

Prostaglandins are released from the mucosal and serosal surfaces of the rat stomach. Coceani *et al.*, 1967a and Coceani, Pace-Asciak, Volta and Wolfe, 1967b, demonstrated the release of prostaglandin $E_2$ and $F_{2\alpha}$ into the fluid in contact with the serosal surface of isolated intact stomachs from rats in response to either transmural or vagal stimulation. Bennett, Friedman and Vane (1967) showed that prostaglandin $E_1$ is released into the lumen of a similar preparation of rat stomach when the pressure of fluid in the stomach is raised or the stomach is stimulated either transmurally or via the vagus. Prostaglandin-like activity can also be detected when isolated strips of the pyloric portion of a rat stomach are stretched. Shaw and Ramwell (1968a) found that either vagal stimulation or administration of secretagogues released prostaglandins $E_1$, $E_2$ and $F_{1\alpha}$ from rat stomach *in vivo.*

Prostaglandin release also occurs from the skin of frog, rat and man. Ramwell and Shaw (1970) found that application of isoprenaline to the inside of superfused frog skin increases the efflux of prostaglandins $E_1$ and $E_2$ from the outside surface of the skin. The release of prostaglandins from rat and human skin is associated with inflammatory conditions. Willis (1969) found that prostaglandins are present in the exudate from carageenin-air blebs in the skin of rats and Greaves, Søndergaard and McDonald-Gibson (1971) have found prostaglandins $E_1$, $E_2$, $F_{1\alpha}$ and $F_{2\alpha}$ in the effluent from the perfused skin of patients with allergic eczema.

Adipose tissue releases prostaglandins when stimulated by various methods. Prostaglandins $E_1$, $E_2$ and $F_{1\alpha}$ are released when rat epididymal fat pads are incubated with noradrenaline and other lipolytic drugs or when the nerves to the fat pads are stimulated (Shaw and Ramwell, 1968b). Adrenocorticotrophic hormone, $\beta$-melanocyte stimulating hormone, porcine growth hormone or glucagon cause release of prostaglandins from rabbit epigastric fat pads (Lewis and Matthews, 1969).

Stimulation of cat adrenal glands with acetylcholine leads to release of prostaglandin $F_{1\alpha}$ together with catecholamines and ATP metabolites (Ramwell *et al.,* 1966). The amount of prostaglandin released on stimulation exceeds the amount that can be extracted from the resting gland.

Williams, Karim and Sandler (1968) found a higher concentration of prostaglandins in medullary carcinoma of the human thyroid than in normal thyroid glands and identified prostaglandins $E_2$ and $F_{2\alpha}$ in the venous blood draining the tumour.

Thus prostaglandin release occurs from a wide variety of tissues from a number of species in response to stimuli varying from physiological to pathological. The only common link connecting these various types of prostaglandin release is distortion or damage of cell membranes (Piper and Vane, 1971). The exact site of origin of prostaglandins has not been located but they may be derived from the lipids of the cell membrane.

## Metabolism

### Synthesis

The primary prostaglandins all have the same basic chemical structure and differ only in their degree of unsaturation. These 20 carbon acidic lipids are formed enzymically, by prostaglandin synthetase, from the essential fatty acids (see also Chapter I). Biosynthesis of prostaglandins has been demonstrated in homogenates of sheep vesicular glands (van Dorp *et al.,* 1964a; Bergström, Danielsson, Klenberg and Samuelsson, 1964a; Bergström, Danielsson and Samuelsson, 1964b), bovine seminal vesicles (Wallach, 1965), lung of guinea-pig (Änggård and Samuelsson, 1965; van Dorp, 1966; Nugteren, Beerthuis and van Dorp, 1966), iris of pig (van Dorp, Jouvenaz and Struijk, 1967), rat stomach (Pace-Asciak, Coceani and Wolfe, 1967) rat epididymal fat pad (Shaw and Ramwell, 1968b), intestinal mucosa (van Dorp, 1966; Nugteren *et al.,* 1966; Vonkeman, 1966), brain (Kataoka, Ramwell and Jessup, 1967; Pace-Asciak, Coceani and Wolfe, 1967), human endometrial curettings (van Dorp, 1966), thymus, heart, liver, kidney and human decidua (van Dorp, 1966; Nugteren *et al.,* 1966; Vonkeman, 1966). Prostaglandin $E_2$ is formed when arachidonic acid is infused into frog perfused intestine (Kunze, 1970).

When dihomo-gamma-linolenic acid (all-cis-eicosa-8,11,14-trienoic acid), arachidonic acid (all-cis-eicosa-5,8,11,14-trienoic acid), and all-cis-eicosa-5,8,11,14,17-pentanoic acid are added to homogenates of sheep vesicular glands they are metabolized to prostaglandins $E_1$, $E_2$ and $E_3$ respectively (van Dorp *et al.,* 1964a, b; Bergström *et al.,* 1964a, b). However, arachidonic acid is converted by homogenates of guinea-pig lung to both prostaglandin $E_2$ and $F_{2\alpha}$ (Änggård and Samuelsson, 1965; Vane, 1971). Although metabolites of prostaglandins $E_2$ and $F_{2\alpha}$ are also formed there is no evidence that $E_2$ is converted to $F_{2\alpha}$ in the lung; guinea-pig liver is the only tissue in which there is evidence of conversion of $E_2$ to $F_{2\alpha}$ (Hamberg and Israelsson, 1970). 8,11,14-eicosatrienoic acid is converted to prostaglandin $E_1$ in the rat epididymal fat pad (Shaw and Ramwell, 1968b). The synthesis of prostaglandins $E_2$ and $F_{2\alpha}$ in cell free homogenates of guinea-pig lung is inhibited by anti-inflammatory drugs (Vane, 1971).

Prostaglandin synthetases are associated with the microsome fraction (van Dorp, 1967; Samuelsson, 1967; Wolfe, Coceani and Pace-Asciak, 1967). As shown in Fig. 1 prostaglandin biosynthesis may be initiated

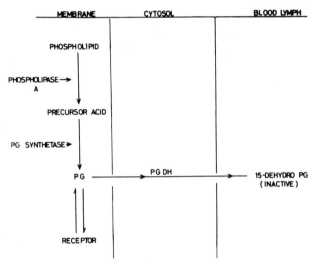

Fig. 1. Possible sequence of events in intracellular synthesis and inactivation of prostaglandins, PGDH = 15-hydroxyprostaglandin dehydrogenase. Modified from Änggård (1971).

and possibly controlled by hydrolysis of microsomal precursors esterified to phospholipids (Lands, Lee and Smith, 1971). Phospholipase A could be the enzyme which splits the precursor acids from the phospholipids (Kunze and Vogt, 1971) before the synthetases convert them rapidly into prostaglandins (Änggård, 1971).

### Removal from the circulation

When the prostaglandins have been synthesized by their tissue of origin they may act near their site of formation before they enter the circulation. Although prostaglandins are stable in blood (Ferreira and Vane, 1967) the half-life of prostaglandins in the circulation is short because of rapid removal by vascular beds, such as the pulmonary circulation. In one passage through the lungs 90-95% of prostaglandins $E_1$ and $E_2$ are removed from the blood in cat, dog and rabbit *in vivo* (Ferreira and Vane, 1967) and prostaglandins $E_1$, $E_2$ and $F_{2\alpha}$ are almost completely inactivated by the pulmonary circulation of cat, dog, rat and guinea-pig (Biron, 1968a; McGiff, Terragno, Strand, Lee, Lonigro and Ng, 1969; Horton and Jones, 1969; Piper and Vane, 1969a). Following intravenous injection of tritium labelled $PGE_1$ in healthy male subjects most of the radioactivity disappears from the blood within 10 minutes of injection (Granström, 1967) and the pulmonary circulation of man removes 90% of injected prostaglandin (Biron, 1968b). Prostaglandins $E_1$, $E_2$, $F_{2\alpha}$ and $A_2$ are enzymically inactivated during passage through the pulmonary circulation of guinea-pig isolated perfused lungs (Piper, Vane and Wyllie, 1970) but in the dog *in vivo* prostaglandins $A_1$ and $A_2$ pass through the lungs unchanged (McGiff *et al.*, 1969). The inactivation is probably due to the action of 15-hydroxyprostaglandin dehydrogenase and prostaglandin $\Delta^{13}$ reductase (see later). These enzymes inactivate prostaglandins at different rates (Änggård and Samuelsson, 1966). In guinea-pig isolated lungs prostaglandins $E_1$, $E_2$ and $F_{2\alpha}$ are 80-95% removed in one passage through the lungs but $A_2$ is only 60-75% removed (Piper *et al.*, 1970).

Similar removal mechanisms for prostaglandins exist in other parts of the body; more than 80% of prostaglandins $E_1$, $E_2$ and $F_{2\alpha}$ is removed in the liver and more than 60% of $E_1$ and $E_2$ in the hindquarters (Ferreira and Vane, 1967; Vane, 1969). Rat liver removes up to 95% of circulating prostaglandin $E_1$ in a single passage (Dawson, Jessup, McDonald-Gibson, Ramwell and Shaw, 1970).

After intravenous injection of tritium labelled prostaglandins $E_1$ and $F_{2\alpha}$ to mice, autoradiographic studies show that the label accumulates in the liver, kidneys, connective tissue and myometrium but that there is no significant uptake in the endometrium (Hansson and Samuelsson, 1965; Green, Hansson and Samuelsson, 1967). Subcutaneous administration of tritium labelled prostaglandin $E_1$ to rats leads to high concentrations of radioactivity in the liver and kidneys and lower concentrations in the lungs, pituitary gland, adrenal gland, ovaries and uterus (Samuelsson, 1964b).

## Breakdown

Prostaglandins are metabolized by enzymes in the tissues and converted to forms which usually have less biological activity than the parent compound. Guinea-pig lung and dog kidney convert 30-40% of prostaglandin $E_1$ to less polar metabolites in one circulation (Piper *et al.,* 1970; Nakano, 1970).

Several enzyme systems which metabolize prostaglandins have been isolated from tissue preparations *in vitro.*

(a) *15-hydroxyprostaglandin dehydrogenase.* This enzyme catalyses oxidation of prostaglandins at C-15 and was first isolated from homogenates of swine lung (Änggård and Samuelsson, 1966) but is also present in tissues of guinea-pig, rat and man. In swine it occurs in many tissues, the highest concentrations being found in the lung, spleen and kidney (the cortex contains three times more than the medulla) and lower concentrations in the stomach, testicle, small intestine, heart and adipose tissue (Larsson and Änggård, 1970). This enzyme has been purified and investigated for substrate specificity (Änggård and Samuelsson, 1966; Nakano, Änggård and Samuelsson, 1969a; Vonkeman, Nugteren and van Dorp, 1969; Shio, Ramwell, Anderson and Corey, 1970). In swine lung homogenates 15-hydroxyprostaglandin dehydrogenase converts prostaglandins to 15-keto compounds and is most active in converting $E_1$ and $E_2$. It is only about 60% as active in oxidizing prostaglandin $E_3$ and those of the F series and even less effective in converting those of the A series. 15-hydroxyprostaglandin dehydrogenase is stereospecific with regard to configuration of the molecule at C-15; constituents of the cyclopentane ring are not important but the length of the side-chain is (Nakano *et al.,* 1969a; Shio *et al.,* 1970).

(b) *Prostaglandin* $\Delta^{13}$ *reductase.* Prostaglandin $\Delta^{13}$ reductase catalyses reduction of $\Delta^{13}$ double bond of prostaglandins. The highest concentrations of this enzyme are found in the liver, spleen, small intestine and kidney of swine whilst fairly high concentrations occur in the adrenals, pancreas, adipose tissue, brain, lung and stomach (Larsson and Änggård, 1970).

(c) *β-oxidation.* Prostaglandins are also metabolized by $β$-oxidation of the carboxylic acid side chain and this metabolic pathway has been demonstrated in the mitochondria of rat liver (Hamberg, 1968) and in homogenates of rat lung and kidney (Nakano and Morsy, 1971). $β$-oxidation results in the formation of dinor- and tetranor-derivatives of prostaglandins. When enzymes for dehydrogenation and $β$-oxidation occur in the same tissue, dehydrogenation must precede $β$-oxidation because the dinor- and tetranor-derivatives are poor substrates for 15-hydroxyprostaglandin dehydrogenase (Nakano, Änggård and Samuelsson, 1969b).

(d) *ω-oxidation.* Enzymes catalysing ω-oxidation of the side chain of prostaglandins are found in human seminal plasma (Hamberg and Samuelsson, 1966), guinea-pig and human liver microsomes (Israelsson, Hamberg and Samuelsson, 1969). See Fig. 2.

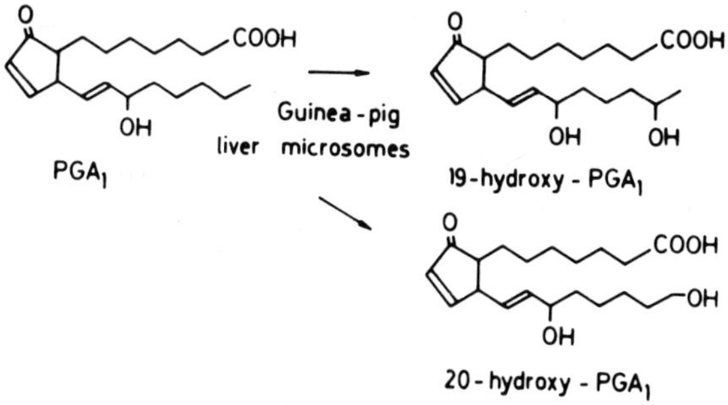

Fig. 2. ω-hydroxylation of $PGA_1$. Reproduced from Samuelsson *et al.* (1971) with permission of the authors and publisher.

(e) *Reduction of C-9 keto prostaglandins.* The particle-free fraction of guinea-pig liver contains enzymes which metabolize prostaglandin $E_2$ to seven metabolites, one of which is prostaglandin $F_{2\alpha}$. This is the first example of an E prostaglandin being converted into an F prostaglandin (Hamberg and Israelsson, 1970).

The metabolic pathways for breakdown of prostaglandins vary between *in vitro* systems from different species and also between different animals *in vivo*.

## In vitro metabolism

In the supernatant from homogenates of lung from guinea-pig and swine, prostaglandins are metabolized by oxidation of the C-15 hydroxyl group (by 15-hydroxyprostaglandin dehydrogenase) and by reduction of the $\Delta^{13}$ double bond (by prostaglandin $\Delta^{13}$ reductase) (Änggård and Samuelsson, 1964, 1965; Änggård, Gréen and Samuelsson, 1965; Änggård, 1971). In guinea-pig lung the metabolites are 15-keto-dihydro-prostaglandin $E_1$ and dihydro-prostaglandin $E_1$ (Änggård and Samuel-sson, 1964) but in swine lung prostaglandin $E_1$ is converted to 15-keto-prostaglandin $E_1$ (Änggård and Samuelsson, 1966), Fig. 3. Prostaglandin $E_2$ and $E_3$ are metabolized in these tissues by analogous reactions (Änggård *et al.*, 1965; Änggård and Samuelsson, 1965). One or both of these reactions takes place in lung tissue of sheep, rat and man and also in kidney and intestine of sheep and guinea-pig and in rat stomach (Änggård and Samuelsson, 1966; Pace-Asciak, Morawska and Wolfe, 1970). Prostaglandin $E_1$ is metabolized in a similar way in the supernatant of homogenates of spleen, kidney and liver of swine and in particle-free homogenates of guinea-pig liver. The metabolic pathway has recently been determined and is shown in Fig. 4 (Änggård, 1971; Hamberg, Israelsson and Samuelsson, 1971). Firstly, the C-15 hydroxyl

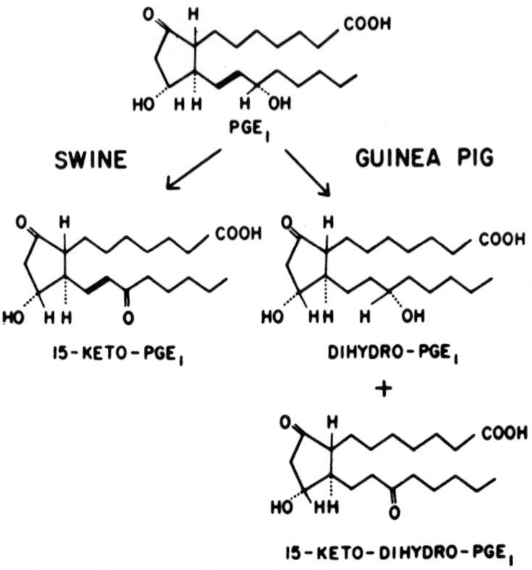

Fig. 3. Formation of metabolites of PGE₁ in guinea-pig and swine lung. Reproduced from Änggård (1971) with permission of the author and publisher.

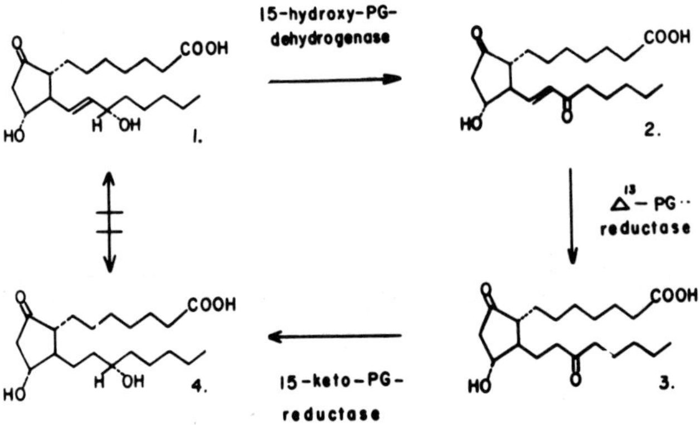

Fig. 4. The pathway for the initial steps in the metabolism of PGE₁ in the supernatant from spleen, kidney and liver from swine. PGE₁ = (1), 15-keto-PGE₁ = (2), 15-keto-dihydro PGE₁ = (3) and dihydro PGE₁ = (4). Reproduced from Änggård (1971) with permission of the author and publisher.

group is oxidized by 15-hydroxyprostaglandin dehydrogenase, then the 15-keto-prostaglandin $E_1$ so formed is reduced by $\Delta^{13}$-prostaglandin reductase to 15-keto-dihydro-prostaglandin $E_1$ and finally dihydro-prostaglandin $E_1$ is formed by a stereospecific reduction of the keto group, not by a direct reduction of the double bond in prostaglandin $E_1$. The enzyme catalysing the latter reaction is not identical with 15-hydroxyprostaglandin dehydrogenase.

When prostaglandins are incubated with mitochondria of rat liver they undergo $\beta$-oxidation and are degraded by one or two carbon units (Hamberg, 1968). High concentrations of prostaglandins $E_1$, $B_1$, $F_{1\alpha}$ and $F_{1\beta}$ are converted to their C-18 homologues but low concentrations of prostaglandin $E_1$ are converted to a mixture of C-16 and C-18 homologues. Prostaglandin $A_1$ and the prostaglandin metabolites 11 and 15-dihydroxy-9-ketoprostanoic acid and 11$\alpha$-hydroxy-9, 15 diketoprostanoic acid are metabolized to a mixture of C-16 and C-18 homologues but low concentrations of prostaglandin $A_1$ are converted to the C-16 homologue.

In the blood-perfused rat liver, prostaglandins $E_1$ and $F_{1\alpha}$ are rapidly removed from the blood and decarboxylated. The pharmacologically inactive products are excreted into the bile and venous effluent (Dawson, Ramwell and Shaw, 1968; Dawson *et al.*, 1970). Although not positively identified the metabolites appear to include dihydro-prostaglandin $E_1$ and 15-keto-dihydro-prostaglandin $E_1$.

When prostaglandin $A_1$ is incubated with microsomes of guinea-pig liver it undergoes $\omega$-hydroxylation and is converted to a mixture of 19-hydroxy-prostaglandin $A_1$ and 20-hydroxy-prostaglandin $A_1$. Prostaglandin $E_1$ and 11$\alpha$-hydroxy-9, 15 diketoprostanoic acid (a metabolite of prostaglandin $E_2$) are not metabolized by this enzyme system (Israelsson *et al.*, 1969).

Enzymes present in the supernatant of guinea-pig liver homogenates convert prostaglandin $E_2$ into seven metabolites (Hamberg and Israelsson, 1970). It is interesting that prostaglandin $F_{2\alpha}$ occurs among these metabolites as this is the only example of an E prostaglandin being converted to an F prostaglandin in a biological system. A small percentage of these metabolites arise by a non-enzymic reaction which may also occur under physiological conditions. When prostaglandin $E_1$ is incubated with human plasma and homogenates of human uterus and swine ovary, there is little metabolic degradation but prostaglandin $E_1$ is more effectively metabolized by homogenates of human placenta (Nakano, Montague and Darrow, 1971).

*In vivo metabolism*

When tritium-labelled prostaglandin $E_2$ is injected intravenously into male subjects, 50% of the radioactivity appears in the urine in the first 5 hr and less than 3% in the following 12 hr (Hamberg and Samuelsson, 1969a). The metabolite of prostaglandin $E_2$ recovered from the urine is 7$\alpha$-hydroxy-5, 11 diketo-tetranorprosta-1, 16-dioic acid (Samuelsson, Granström, Gréen and Hamberg, 1971). Four sets of reactions are involved in the metabolism of prostaglandin $E_2$ in man (Fig. 5). Firstly, prostaglandin $E_2$ undergoes dehydrogenation of the alcohol group in the side chain (by the action of 15-hydroxyprosta-

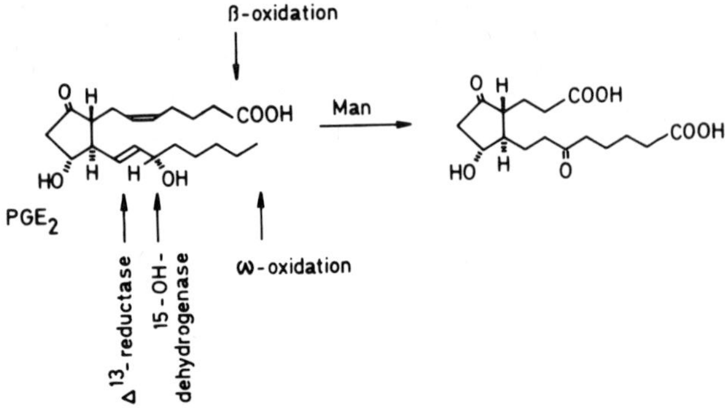

Fig. 5. Conversion of $PGE_2$ to 7α-hydroxy-5,11-diketotetranorprosta-1-16-dioic acid in man.

The reactions involved include those due to $\Delta^{13}$ prostaglandin reductase and 15-hydroxyprostaglandin dehydrogenase and also β-oxidation and ω-oxidation. Reproduced from Samuelsson *et al.* (1971) with permission of the authors and publisher.

glandin dehydrogenase) then reduction of the *trans* double bond (by prostaglandin $\Delta^{13}$ reductase) followed by two steps of β-oxidation and finally ω-oxidation. The order of the first two reactions is known but the sequence of β-oxidation and ω-oxidation has yet to be determined. Prostaglandin $E_2$ is initially rapidly converted to 11α-hydroxy-9, 15-diketoprost-5-enoic acid because this metabolite appears in the venous blood of one arm 1.5 min after intravenous injection of tritium-labelled prostaglandin $E_2$ into the other arm (Hamberg and Samuelsson, unpublished).

In similar experiments with tritium-labelled prostaglandin $F_{2\alpha}$ more than 90% of the radioactivity appears in the urine in the first 5 hr (Granström and Samuelsson, 1969a). Prostaglandin $F_{2\alpha}$ is mainly converted to a metabolite which corresponds to that of prostaglandin $E_2$ described above and is 5, 7-dihydroxy-11-ketotetranorprosta-1, 16-dioic acid. Two other metabolites have been identified as 5β, 7α, 11-trihydroxy-tetranorprosta-1, 16-dioic acid and 5β, 7α, 16-trihydroxy-11-keto-tetranorprostanoic acid. Prostaglandins $E_1$ and $F_{1\alpha}$ are converted to the same principal metabolites as prostaglandins $E_2$ and $F_{2\alpha}$ respectively (Samuelsson *et al.*, 1971; Granström and Samuelsson, 1971).

In the guinea-pig the main urinary metabolite of prostaglandin $E_2$ is 5β, 7α-dihydroxy-11-ketotetranorprostanoic acid (Hamberg and Samuelsson, 1969b). The steps in conversion of prostaglandin $E_2$ to this metabolite include oxidation of the secondary alcohol group in the side chain, reduction of the *trans* double bond, β-oxidation of the carboxyl side chain and reduction of the keto group in the 5-membered ring. Prostaglandin $F_{2\alpha}$ is metabolized by analogous reactions and the main urinary metabolite has been identified as 5β, 7α-dihydroxy-11-

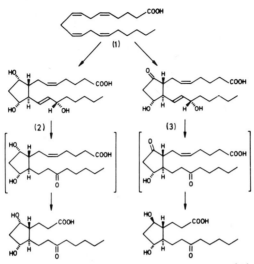

Fig. 6. Metabolism of prostaglandins in the guinea-pig. Arachidonic acid = (1), $PGF_{2\alpha}$ = (2), $PGE_2$ = (3). Reproduced from Samuelsson *et al.* (1971) with permission of the authors and publisher.

ketotetranorprostanoic acid (Granström and Samuelsson, 1969b). The metabolism of prostaglandins $E_2$ and $F_{2\alpha}$ in the guinea-pig *in vivo* is shown in Fig. 6.

The rat degrades prostaglandins by more complex metabolic pathways than either man or guinea-pig (Gréen, 1969). Prostaglandin $E_2$ is metabolized by three separate pathways. In one, prostaglandin $E_2$ is oxidized by 15-hydroxyprostaglandin dehydrogenase, reduced by $\Delta^{13}$ reductase, $\beta$-oxidized and the resulting metabolite is then further oxidized to the $\omega$-hydroxy and dicarboxylic acid metabolites. In a second pathway, prostaglandin $E_2$ is converted to the 5$\beta$-hydroxy derivative which is identical with the main urinary metabolite in the guinea-pig but the metabolic pathway is unknown. In a third pathway, prostaglandin $E_2$ undergoes initial $\beta$-oxidation to the C-16 derivative, then dehydration and the resulting metabolite is oxidized further to the $\omega$1- and $\omega$2-hydroxylated derivatives and dicarboxylic acid. Prostaglandin $F_{2\alpha}$ is converted into three metabolites by steps analogous to the first pathway for prostaglandin $E_2$ and, in addition, two further C-16 and C-18 derivatives are formed by $\beta$-oxidation (Samuelsson *et al.*, 1971).

In the rat, as in man and guinea-pig, the main prostaglandin metabolites appear in the urine but in experiments using radioactively-labelled prostaglandins carbon dioxide produced by decarboxylation can be detected in expired air (Miller and Krake, 1968) and other fragments of the parent prostaglandins are utilized in fatty acid and phospholipid biosynthesis (Dawson *et al.*, 1970).

Metabolism of prostaglandins results in curtailment of their activity because the metabolites usually have less pharmacological activity than the parent compound when tested in the various systems used for assaying prostaglandins. An exception is dihydro-prostaglandin $E_1$ which is more active than prostaglandin $E_1$ in depressing guinea-pig blood pressure (Änggård, 1966).

## Conclusions

Prostaglandins can be extracted from many tissues taken from animals of different species. These substances are also easily released by widely differing stimuli which have only cell distortion or damage in common (Piper and Vane, 1971). However, stimulation of release of prostaglandins can be equated with stimulation of synthesis of prostaglandins (Piper and Vane, 1971) and since prostaglandins are synthesized/released by manoeuvres such as agitation of chopped tissue it seems likely that prostaglandins are synthesized by homogenization of tissues during extraction procedures. If this is so, it explains why prostaglandins may be extracted from most of the non-fluid tissues examined and suggests that the amounts of prostaglandins obtained by homogenization in a watery medium may be erroneously high. It would also account for the apparent lack of regional distribution of prostaglandins, for example, in tissues of the central nervous system.

Synthesis of prostaglandins occurs enzymically from essential fatty acids which are possibly derived from phospholipids (Lands *et al.*, 1971). Prostaglandins are rapidly metabolized by several enzyme systems which are widely distributed throughout the cells of the body. Prostaglandins may be synthesized and metabolized by the same cell (Änggård, 1971) in which case, the 'release' of prostaglandins detected in various *in vivo* and *in vitro* systems could be an overflow of prostaglandins occurring when the metabolizing mechanism is saturated.

The enzymes synthesizing prostaglandins can be blocked by anti-inflammatory drugs (Vane, 1971) and it may be possible to modify the action of the metabolizing enzymes. These enzymes are more specific for some prostaglandins and their metabolites than others and since some of the prostaglandins have therapeutic actions this enzyme specificity is important. For instance, prostaglandins $E_1$ and $E_2$ have a bronchodilator action in man (Cuthbert, 1969, 1971) and it should be possible to produce an analogue which has the desired bronchodilator action but is not so rapidly metabolized as the parent compound.

Since they are so rapidly metabolized, prostaglandins are likely to act either intracellularly or close to their site of synthesis; the rapid removal of prostaglandins from the circulation makes it unlikely that they are circulating hormones (Vane, 1969). The exact physiological role of prostaglandins is still unknown but many possibilities exist and evidence is accumulating to suggest that they participate in defence reactions such as inflammation, pyrexia and pain (Vane, 1971; Collier, 1971). Prostaglandins may modulate the release of other agonists (Hedqvist, 1970; Piper and Walker, to be published) and modify blood flow in organs such as the lung and kidney (Liljestrand, 1967; Piper and Vane, 1971; McGiff *et al.*, 1970; Aitken and Vane, 1971; Herbaczynska-Cedro and Vane, 1972). Also the presence of high concentrations of prostaglandin $E_2$ and $F_{2\alpha}$ in human amniotic fluid during spontaneous abortion and the release of prostaglandin $F_{2\alpha}$ during labour (Karim, 1968; Karim and Devlin, 1967; Karim and Hillier, 1970) strongly suggests that one of their physiological actions is to cause the uterus to contract rhythmically and expel its contents.

## REFERENCES

Aitken, J. W. and Vane, J. R. (1971). Blockade of angiotensin-induced prostaglandin release from dog kidney by indomethacin. *Pharmacologist*, **13**, 564.

Alabaster, V. A. and Bakhle, Y. S. (1970). The release of biologically active substances from isolated lungs by 5-hydroxytryptamine and tryptamine. *British Journal of Pharmacology*, **40**, 582P.

Ambache, N. (1957). Properties of irin, a physiological constituent of the rabbit's iris. *Journal of Physiology*, **135**, 114.

Ambache, N., Brummer, H. C., Rose, J. G. and Whiting, J. (1966). Thin-layer chromatography of spasmogenic unsaturated hydroxy-acids from various tissues. *Journal of Physiology*, **185**, 77P.

Ambache, N., Kavanagh, L. and Whiting, J. (1965). Effect of mechanical stimulation on rabbits' eyes: release of active substances in anterior chamber perfusates. *Journal of Physiology*, **176**, 378.

Änggård, E. (1965). The isolation and determination of prostaglandins in lungs of sheep, guinea-pig, monkey and man. *Biochemical Pharmacology*, **14**, 1507.

Änggård, E. (1966). The biological activities of three metabolites of prostaglandin $E_1$. *Acta Physiologica Scandinavica*, **66**, 509.

Änggård, E. (1971). Studies on the analysis and metabolism of the prostaglandins. *Annals of the New York Academy of Sciences*, **180**, 200.

Änggård, E., Gréen, K. and Samuelsson, B. (1965). Synthesis of tritium-labelled prostaglandin $E_2$ and studies on its metabolism in guinea-pig lung. *Journal of Biological Chemistry*, **240**, 1932.

Änggård, E. and Samuelsson, B. (1964). Smooth muscle stimulating lipids in sheep iris. The identification of prostaglandin $F_{2\alpha}$. *Biochemical Pharmacology*, **13**, 281.

Änggård, E. and Samuelsson, B. (1965). Biosynthesis of prostaglandins from arachidonic acid in guinea-pig lung. *Journal of Biological Chemistry*, **240**, 3518.

Änggård, E. and Samuelsson, B. (1966). Purification and properties of a 15-hydroxyprostaglandin dehydrogenase from swine lung. *Arkiv för Kemi*, **25**, 293.

Bennett, A., Friedman, C. A. and Vane, J. R. (1967). Release of prostaglandin $E_1$ from the rat stomach. *Nature (London)*, **216**, 873.

Bennett, A., Murray, J. G. and Wyllie, J. H. (1968). Occurrence of prostaglandin $E_2$ in the human stomach, and a study of its effects on human isolated gastric muscle. *British Journal of Pharmacology and Chemotherapy*, **32**, 339.

Bergström, S., Carlson, L. A. and Weeks, J. R. (1968). The prostaglandins: A family of biologically active lipids. *Pharmacological Reviews*, **20**, 1.

Bergström, S., Danielsson, H., Klenberg, D. and Samuelsson, B. (1964a). The enzymatic conversion of essential fatty acids into prostaglandins. *Journal of Biological Chemistry*, **239**, PC 4006.

Bergström, S., Danielsson, H. and Samuelsson, B. (1964b). The enzymatic formation of prostaglandin $E_2$ from arachidonic acid. *Biochimica et Biophysica Acta*, **90**, 207.

Bergström, S., Dressler, F., Krabisch, L., Ryhage, R. and Sjövall, J. (1962). The isolation and structure of a smooth muscle stimulating factor in normal sheep and pig lungs. *Arkiv für Kemi*, **20**, 63.

Berry, E. M., Edmonds, J. F. and Wyllie, J. H. (1971). Release of prostaglandin $E_2$ and unidentified factors from ventilated lungs. *British Journal of Surgery*, **58**, 189.

Biron, P. (1968a). Vasoactive hormone metabolism by the pulmonary circulation. *Clinical Research*, **16**, 112.

Biron, P. (1968b). *La Presse,* Montreal, 21st December.

Bradley, P. B., Samuels, G. M. R. and Shaw, J. E. (1969). Correlation of prostaglandin release from the cerebral cortex of cats with the electrocorticogram, following stimulation of the reticular formation. *British Journal of Pharmacology*, **37**, 151.

Bygdeman, M. and Holmberg, O. (1966). Isolation and identification of prostaglandins from ram seminal plasma. *Acta Chemica Scandinavica*, **20**, 2308.

Bygdeman, M. and Samuelsson, B. (1966). Analyses of prostaglandins in human semen. *Clinica Chimica Acta*, **13**, 465.

Coceani, F. and Wolfe, L. S. (1965). Prostaglandins in brain and the release of prostaglandin-like compounds from the rat cerebellar cortex. *Canadian Journal of Physiology and Pharmacology*, **43**, 445.

Coceani, F., Pace-Asciak, C., Volta, F. and Wolfe, L. S. (1967a). Presenza e liberazione di prostaglandine dallo stomacho di ratto. *Bolletino della societa italiana di biologia sperimentale*, **43**, 76.

Coceani, F., Pace-Asciak, C., Volta, F. and Wolfe, L. S. (1967b). Effect of nerve stimulation on prostaglandin formation and release from the rat stomach. *American Journal of Physiology*, **213**, 1056.

Collier, H. O. J. (1971). Prostaglandins and aspirin. *Nature (London)*, **232**, 17.

Crowshaw, K. (1971). Prostaglandin biosynthesis from endogenous precursors in rabbit kidney. *Nature New Biology*, **231**, 240.

Crowshaw, K. and Szylk, J. Z. (1970). Distribution of prostaglandins in rabbit kidney. *Biochemical Journal*, **116**, 421.

Cuthbert, M. F. (1969). Effect on airways resistance of prostaglandin $E_1$ given by aerosol to healthy and asthmatic volunteers. *British Medical Journal*, **4**, 723.

Cuthbert, M. F. (1971). Bronchodilator activity of aerosols of prostaglandins $E_1$ and $E_2$ in asthmatic subjects. *Proceedings of the Royal Society of Medicine*, **64**, 15.

Davies, B. N., Horton, E. W. and Withrington, P. G. (1968). The occurence of prostaglandin $E_2$ in splenic venous blood of the dog following splenic nerve stimulation. *British Journal of Pharmacology and Chemotherapy*, **32**, 127.

Dawson, W., Jessup, S. J., McDonald-Gibson, W., Ramwell, P. W. and Shaw, J. E. (1970). Prostaglandin uptake and metabolism by the perfused rat liver. *British Journal of Pharmacology*, **39**, 585.

Dawson, W., Ramwell, P. W. and Shaw, J. E. (1968). Metabolism of prostaglandins by the rat isolated liver. *British Journal of Pharmacology*, **34**, 668P.

Dorp, D. A. van (1966). The biosynthesis of prostaglandins. *Memoirs of the Society for Endocrinology*, **14**, 39.

Dorp, D. A. van (1967). Aspects of the biosynthesis of prostaglandins. *Progress in Biochemical Pharmacology*, **3**, 71.

Dorp, D. A. van, Beerthuis, R. K., Nugteren, D. H. and Vonkeman, H. (1964a). The biosynthesis of prostaglandins. *Biochimica et Biophysica Acta*, **90**, 204.

Dorp, D. A. van, Beerthuis, R. K. Nugteren, D. H. and Vonkeman, H. (1964b). Enzymatic conversion of all-*cis*-polyunsaturated fatty acids into prostaglandins. *Nature (London)*, **203**, 839.

Dorp, D. A. van, Jouvenaz, G. H. and Struijk, C. B. (1967). The biosynthesis of prostaglandin in pig eye iris. *Biochimica et Biophysica Acta*, **137**, 396.

Eliasson, R. (1959). Studies on prostaglandin. Occurrence, formation and biological actions. *Acta Physiologica Scandinavica*, **46**, Suppl. 158, 1.

Euler, U. S. von (1934). Zur Kenntnis der pharmakologischen Wirkungen von Nativsekreten und Extrackten männlicher accessorischer Geschlechtsdrüsen. *Naunym-Schmiedebergs Archiv für experimentelle Pathologie und Pharmakologie*, **175**, 78.

Euler, U. S. von (1935). A depressor substance in the vesicular gland. *Journal of Physiology (London)*, **84**, 21P.

Euler, U. S. von (1937). On the specific vasodilating and plain muscle stimulating substances from accessory genital glands in man and certain animals (prostaglandin and vesiglandin). *Journal of Physiology (London)*, **88**, 213.

Euler, U. S. von and Hammarström, S. (1937). Über das Vorkommen des prostaglandins in Tierorganen. *Skandinavishes Archiv. für Physiologie*, **77**, 96.

Ferreira, S. H. and Vane, J. R. (1967). Prostaglandins: their disappearance from and release into the circulation. *Nature (London)*, **216**, 868.

Ferreira, S. H., Moncada, S. and Vane, J. R. (1971). Indomethacin and aspirin abolish prostaglandin release from the spleen. *Nature New Biology*, **231**, 237.

Ferreira, S. H. and Moncada, S. (1972). Inhibition of prostaglandin synthesis augments the effects of sympathetic nerve stimulation on the cat spleen. *British Journal of Pharmacology*, **43**, 419P.

Gilmore, N. (1968). Ph.D. Thesis, University of London.

Gilmore, N., Vane, J. R. and Wyllie, J. H. (1968). Prostaglandin released by the spleen. *Nature (London)*, **218**, 1135.

Gilmore, N., Vane, J. R. and Wyllie, J. H. (1969). Prostaglandin release by the spleen in response to infusion of particles. *Prostaglandins, Peptides and Amines* (Eds P. Mantegazza and E. W. Horton), p. 21. Academic Press.

Goldblatt, M. W. (1933). A depressor substance in seminal fluid. *Journal of the Society of Chemical Industry (London)*, **52**, 1056.

Goldblatt, M. W. (1935). Properties of human seminal plasma. *Journal of Physiology (London)*, **84**, 208.

Granström, E. (1967). On the metabolism of prostaglandin $E_1$ in man. *Progress in Biochemical Pharmacology*, **3**, 89.

Granström, E. and Samuelsson, B. (1969a). The structure of a urinary metabolite of prostaglandin $F_{2\alpha}$ in man. *Journal of the American Chemical Society*, **91**, 3398.

Granström, E. and Samuelsson, B. (1969b). The structure of the main urinary metabolite of prostaglandin $F_{2\alpha}$ in the guinea-pig. *European Journal of Biochemistry*, **10**, 411.

Granström, E. and Samuelsson, B. (1971). On the metabolism of prostaglandin $F_{2\alpha}$ in female subjects. *Journal of Biological Chemistry*, **246**, 5254.

Greaves, M. W., McDonald-Gibson, W. and Søndergaard, J. S. (1971). Recovery of prostaglandin-like fatty acids from human allergic contact eczema using a skin perfusion method. *British Journal of Pharmacology*, **41**, 416P.

Greaves, M. W., Søndergaard, J. and McDonald-Gibson, W. (1971). Recovery of prostaglandin in human cutaneous inflammation. *British Medical Journal*, **2**, 258.

Gréen, K. (1969). Structures of urinary metabolites of prostaglandin $F_{2\alpha}$ in the rat. *Acta Chemica Scandinavica*, **23**, 1453.

Gréen, K., Hansson, E. and Samuelsson, B. (1967). Synthesis of tritium labeled prostaglandin $F_{2\alpha}$ and studies of its distribution by autoradiography. *Progress in Biochemical Pharmacology*, **3**, 85.

Hall, W. J. (1966). Prostaglandins in human menstrual fluid and endometrial curettings. *Memoirs of the Society for Endocrinology*, **14**, 65.

Hamberg, M. (1968). Metabolism of prostaglandins in rat liver mitochondria. *European Journal of Biochemistry*, **6**, 135.

Hamberg, M. and Israelsson, U. (1970). Metabolism of prostaglandin $E_2$ in guinea-pig liver. I. Identification of seven metabolites. *J. of Biological Chemistry*, **245**, 5107.

Hamberg, M., Israelsson, U. and Samuelsson, B. (1971). Metabolism of prostaglandin $E_2$ in guinea-pig liver. *Annals of the New York Academy of Sciences*, **180**, 164.

Hamberg, M. and Samuelsson, B. (1966). Prostaglandins in human seminal plasma. *Journal of Biological Chemistry*, **241**, 257.

Hamberg, M. and Samuelsson, B. (1967). New groups of naturally occurring prostaglandins. *Nobel Symposium 2, Prostaglandins*, (Eds. S. Bergström and B. Samuelsson), p. 63, Almqvist and Wiksell, Stockholm.

Hamberg, M. and Samuelsson, B. (1969a). The structure of the major urinary metabolite of prostaglandin $E_2$ in man. *Journal of the American Chemical Society*, **91**, 2177.

Hamberg, M. and Samuelsson, B. (1969b). The structure of a urinary metabolite of prostaglandin $E_2$ in the guinea-pig. *Biochemical and Biophysical Research Communications*, **34**, 22.

Hansson, E. and Samuelsson, B. (1965). Autoradiographic distribution studies of [3]H-labeled prostaglandin $E_1$ in mice. *Biochimica et Biophysica Acta*, **106**, 379.

Hedqvist, P. (1970). Control by prostaglandin $E_2$ of sympathetic neurotransmission in the spleen. *Life Sciences*, **9**, 269.

Herbaczynska-Cedro, K. and Vane, J. R. (1972). An intra-renal role for prostaglandin production. *Proceedings of the Fifth International Congress on Pharmacology*. In press.

Hickler, R. B., Birbari, A. E., Qureshi, E. U. and Karnovsky, M. L. (1966). Purification and characterization of the vasodilator and antihypertensive lipid of rabbit renal medulla. *Transactions of the Association of American Physicians*, **79**, 278.

Higgs, G. A. and Youlten, L. J. F. (1972) Prostaglandin production by rabbit peritoneal leucocytes *in vitro. British Journal of Pharmacology,* **44,** 330P.

Holmes, S. W. (1970). The spontaneous release of prostaglandins into the cerebral ventricles of the dog and the effect of external factors on this release. *British Journal of Pharmacology,* **38,** 653.

Holmes, S. W. and Horton, E. W. (1968a). The identification of four prostaglandins in dog brain and their regional distribution in the central nervous system. *Journal of Physiology (London),* **195,** 731.

Holmes, S. W. and Horton, E. W. (1968b). Prostaglandins and the central nervous system. Prostaglandin Symposium of the Worcester Foundation (Eds P. W. Ramwell and J. E. Shaw), p. 21. Interscience, New York.

Hopkin, J. M., Horton, E. W., Whittaker, V. P. (1968). Prostaglandin content of particulate and supernatant fractions of rabbit brain homogenates. *Nature (London),* **217,** 71.

Horton, E. W. (1969). Hypotheses on physiological roles of prostaglandins. *Physiological Reviews,* **49,** 122.

Horton, E. W. and Jones, R. L. (1969). Prostaglandins $A_1$, $A_2$ and 19-hydroxy $A_1$; their actions on smooth muscle and their inactivation on passage through the pulmonary and hepatic portal vascular beds. *British Journal of Pharmacology,* **37,** 705.

Horton, E. W. and Main, I. H. M. (1967). Central nervous actions of the prostaglandins and their identification in the brain and spinal cord. Nobel Symposium 2, Prostaglandins (Eds S. Bergström and B. Samuelsson), p. 253. Almqvist and Wiksell, Stockholm.

Horton, E. W. and Thompson, C. J. (1964). Thin-layer chromatography and bioassay of prostaglandins in extracts of semen and tissues of the male reproductive tract. *British Journal of Pharmacology and Chemotherapy,* **22,** 183.

Horton, E., Jones, R., Thompson, C. and Poyser, N. (1971). Release of prostaglandins. *Annals of the New York Academy of Sciences,* **180,** 351.

Israelsson, U., Hamberg, M. and Samuelsson, B. (1969). Biosynthesis of 19-hydroxy-prostaglandin $A_1$. *European Journal of Biochemistry,* **11,** 390.

Karim, S. M. M. (1966). Isolation of prostaglandins in human amniotic fluid. *Journal of Obstetrics and Gynaecology of the British Commonwealth,* **73,** 903.

Karim, S. M. M. (1967). The identification of prostaglandins in human umbilical cord. *British Journal of Pharmacology and Chemotherapy,* **29,** 230.

Karim, S. M. M. (1968). Appearance of prostaglandin $F_{2\alpha}$ in human blood during labour. *British Medical Journal,* **4,** 618.

Karim, S. M. M. and Devlin, J. (1967). Prostaglandin content of amniotic fluid during pregnancy and labour. *Journal of Obstetrics and Gynaecology of the British Commonwealth,* **74,** 230.

Karim, S. M. M. and Hillier, K. (1970). Prostaglandins and spontaneous abortion. *Journal of Obstetrics and Gynaecology of the British Commonwealth,* **77,** 837.

Karim, S. M. M., Hillier, K. and Devlin, J. (1968). Distribution of prostaglandins $E_1$, $E_2$, $F_{1\alpha}$ and $F_{2\alpha}$ in some animal tissues. *Journal of Pharmacy and Pharmacology,* **20,** 749.

Karim, S. M. M., Sandler, M. and Williams, E. D. (1967). Distribution of prostaglandins in human tissues. *British Journal of Pharmacology and Chemotherapy,* **31,** 340.

Kataoka, K., Ramwell, P. W. and Jessup, S. (1967). Prostaglandins; localization in subcellar particles of rat cerebral cortex. *Science* (New York), **157,** 1187.

Kunze, H. (1970). Formation of $(1\text{-}^{14}C)$ prostaglandin $E_2$ and two prostaglandin metabolites from $(1\text{-}^{14}C)$ arachidonic acid during vascular perfusion of the frog intestine. *Biochimica et Biophysica Acta,* **202**, 180.

Kunze, H. and Vogt, W. (1971). Significance of phospholipase A for prostaglandin formation. *Annals of the New York Academy of Sciences,* **180**, 123.

Kurzrok, R. and Lieb, C. C. (1930). Biochemical studies of human semen. II. The action of semen on the human uterus. *Proceedings of the Society for Experimental Biology and Medicine,* **28**, 268.

Laity, J. L. H. (1969). The release of prostaglandin $E_1$ from the rat phrenic nerve diaphragm preparation. *British Journal of Pharmacology,* **37**, 698.

Lands, W., Lee, R. and Smith, W. (1971). Factors regulating the biosynthesis of various prostaglandins. *Annals of the New York Academy of Sciences,* **180**, 107.

Larsson, C. and Änggård, E. (1970). Distribution of prostaglandin metabolizing enzymes in tissues of the swine. *Acta Pharmacologica et Toxicologica,* **28**, supplement 1, 61.

Lewis, G. P. and Matthews, J. (1969). The cause of the vasodilatation accompanying free fatty acid release in rabbit adipose tissue. *Journal of Physiology (London),* **202**, 95P.

Liljestrand, G. (1967). Discussion remarks to Änggård and Samuelsson: The metabolism of prostaglandins in lung tissue. Nobel Symposium 2, Prostaglandins. (Ed. S. Bergström and B. Samuelsson), p. 107. Almqvist and Wiksell, Stockholm.

Lindsey, H. E. and Wyllie, J. H. (1970). Release of prostaglandins from embolized lungs. *British Journal of Surgery,* **57**, 738.

Maddox, I. S. and Sykes, J. A. C. (1972). Prostaglandin production by mouse tumours. *British Journal of Pharmacology.* In press.

McGiff, J. C., Terragno, N. A., Strand, J. C., Lee, J. B., Lonigro, A. J. and Ng, K. K. F. (1969). Selective passage of prostaglandins across the lung. *Nature (London),* **223**, 742.

McGiff, J. C., Crowshaw, K., Terragno, N. A., Lonigro, A. J., Strand, J. C., Williamson, M. A., Lee, J. B. and Ng, K. F. F. (1970). Prostaglandin-like substances appearing in canine renal venous blood during renal ischaemia. *Circulation Research,* **27**, 765.

Miller, W. L. and Krake, J. J. (1968). Metabolism of $C^{14}$-prostaglandin $E_1$ by rats: Exhaled $C^{14}O_2$ and urinary excretion of $C^{14}$ activity. *Federation Proceedings,* **27**, 241.

Nakano, J. (1970). Metabolism of prostaglandin $E_1$ in dog kidneys. *British Journal of Pharmacology,* **40**, 317.

Nakano, J., Änggård, E. and Samuelsson, B. (1969a). Substrate specificity and inhibition of 15-hydroxyprostaglandin dehydrogenase (PGDH). *Pharmacologist,* **11**, 238.

Nakano, J., Anggård, E. and Samuelsson, B. (1969b). 15-hydroxyprostanoate dehydrogenase. Prostaglandins as substrates and inhibitors. *European Journal of Biochemistry,* **11**, 386.

Nakano, J., Montague, B. and Darrow, B. (1971). Metabolism of prostaglandin $E_1$ in human plasma, uterus and placenta in swine ovary and rat testicle. *Biochemical Pharmacology,* **20**, 2512.

Nakano, J. and Morsy, N. H. (1971). Beta-oxidation of prostaglandins $E_1$ and $E_2$ in rat lung and kidney homogenates. *Clinical Research,* **19**, 142.

Nugteren, D. H., Beerthuis, R. K. and Dorp, D. A. van (1966). The enzymic conversion of *all-cis* 8, 11, 14 eicosatrienoic acid into prostaglandin $E_1$. *Recuil des travaux chimiques des Pays–Bas et de la Belguique,* **85**, 405.

Pace-Asciak, C., Coceani, F. and Wolfe, L. S. (1967). Comparison of the conversion of arachidonic acid into prostaglandins by some tissues. *Proceedings of the Canadian Federation of Biological Sciences,* **10**, 80.

Pace-Asciak, C., Morawska, K. and Wolfe, L. S. (1970). Metabolism of prostaglandin $F_{1\alpha}$ by the rat stomach. *Biochemica et Biophysica Acta,* **218**, 288.

Palmer, M. A., Piper, P. J. and Vane, J. R. (1970a). The release of rabbit aorta contracting substance (RCS) from chopped lung and its antagonism by anti-inflammatory drugs. *British Journal of Pharmacology,* **40**, 581P.

Palmer, M. A., Piper, P. J. and Vane, J. R. (1970b). Release of vasoactive substances from lungs by injection of particles. *British Journal of Pharmacology,* **40**, 547P.

Pickles, V. R., Hall, W. J., Best, F. A. and Smith, G. N. (1965). Prostaglandins in endometrium and menstrual fluid from normal and dysmenorrhoeic subjects. *Journal of Obstetrics and Gynaecology of the British Commonwealth,* **72**, 185.

Piper, P. J. and Vane, J. R. (1969a). The release of prostaglandins during anaphylaxis in guinea-pig isolated lungs. *Prostaglandins, Peptides and Amines* (Eds P. Mantegazza and E. W. Horton), p. 15. Academic Press, London.

Piper, P. J. and Vane, J. R. (1969b). Release of additional factors in anaphylaxis and its antagonism by anti-inflammatory drugs. *Nature (London),* **223**, 29.

Piper, P. J., Vane, J. R. and Wyllie, J. H. (1970). Inactivation of prostaglandins by the lungs. *Nature (London),* **225**, 600.

Piper, P. J. and Vane, J. R. (1971). The release of prostaglandins from lung and other tissues. *Annals of the New York Academy of Sciences,* **180**, 363.

Posner, J. (1970). The release of prostaglandin $E_1$ from bovine iris. *British Journal of Pharmacology,* **40**, 163P.

Poyser, N. L., Horton, E. W., Thompson, C. J. and Los, M. (1971). Identification of prostaglandin $F_{2\alpha}$ released by distension of guinea-pig uterus *in vitro. Nature (London),* **230**, 526.

Ramwell, P. W. and Shaw, J. E. (1966). Spontaneous and evoked release of prostaglandins from the cerebral cortex of anesthetised cats. *American Journal of Physiology,* **211**, 125.

Ramwell, P. W. and Shaw, J. E. (1970). Biological significance of the prostaglandins. *Recent Progress in Hormone Research,* **26**, 139.

Ramwell, P. W., Shaw, J. E., Douglas, W. W. and Poisner, A. M. (1966). Efflux of prostaglandin from adrenal glands stimulated with acetylcholine. *Nature (London),* **210**, 273.

Ramwell, P. W., Shaw, J. E. and Jessup, R. (1966). Spontaneous and evoked release of prostaglandins from frog spinal cord. *American Journal of Physiology,* **211**, 998.

Ramwell, P. W., Shaw, J. E. and Kucharski, J. (1965). Prostaglandin release from the rat phrenic nerve-diaphragm preparation. *Science (New York),* **149**, 1390.

Samuelsson, B. (1964a). Identification of a smooth muscle-stimulating factor in bovine brain. *Biochimica et Biophysica Acta,* **84**, 218.

Samuelsson, B. (1964b). Synthesis of tritium-labeled prostaglandin $E_1$ and studies on distribution and excretion in the rat. *Journal of Biological Chemistry,* **239**, 4091.

Samuelsson, B. (1967). Biosynthesis and metabolism of prostaglandins. *Progress in Biochemical Pharmacology,* **3**, 59.

Samuelsson, B. (1969). Biosynthesis and metabolism of prostaglandins. *Abstracts of the 4th International Congress of Pharmacology, Basle,* p. 11.

Samuelsson, B., Granström, E., Gréen, K. and Hamberg, M. (1971). Metabolism of prostaglandins. *Annals of the New York Academy of Sciences,* **180**, 138.

Shaw, J. E. and Ramwell, P. W. (1968a). Inhibition of gastric secretion in rats by prostaglandin $E_1$. Prostaglandin Symposium of the Worcester Foundation for Experimental Biology (Eds P. W. Ramwell and J. E. Shaw), p. 55. Interscience, New York.

Shaw, J. E. and Ramwell, P. W. (1968b). Release of prostaglandin from rat epididymal fat pad on nervous and hormonal stimulation. *Journal of Biological Chemistry,* **243**, 1498.

Shio, H., Ramwell, P. W., Andersen, N. H. and Corey, E. J. (1970). Sterospecificity of the prostaglandin 15-dehydrogenase from swine lung. *Experientia,* **26**, 355.

Smith, J. B. and Willis, A. L. (1970). Formation and release of prostaglandins by platelets in response to thrombin. *British Journal of Pharmacology,* **40**, 545P.

Strong, C. G., Boucher, R., Nowaczynski, W. and Genest, J. (1966). Renal vasodepressor lipid. *Proceedings of the Mayo Clinic,* **41**, 433.

Suzuki, T. and Vogt, W. (1965). Prostaglandins in einem Darmstoffpräparat aus Froschdarm. *Naunyn-Schmiedebergs Archiv für experimentelle Pathologie und Pharmakologie,* **252**, 68.

Vane, J. R. (1969). The release and fate of vasoactive hormones in the circulation. *British Journal of Pharmacology,* **35**, 209.

Vane, J. R. (1971). Inhibition of prostaglandin synthesis as a mechanism of action for aspirin-like drugs. *Nature New Biology,* **231**, 232.

Vogt, W. and Distelkotter, B. (1967). Release of prostaglandin from frog intestine. Nobel Symposium 2, Prostaglandins (Eds S. Bergström and B. Samuelsson), p. 237. Almqvist and Wiksell, Stockholm.

Vogt, W., Meyer, V., Kunze, H., Lufft, E. and Babilli, S. (1969). Entstehung von SRS-C in der durchströmten Meerschweinchenlunge durch Phospholipase A. Identifizierung mit Prostaglandin. *Naunyn-Schmiedebergs Archiv. für experimentelle Pathologie und Pharmakologie,* **262**, 124.

Vonkeman, H. (1966). De biosynthese van prostaglandines. *Chemisch Weekblad,* **62**, 361.

Vonkeman, H., Nugteren, D. H. and Dorp, D. A. van (1969). The action of prostaglandin 15-hydroxydehydrogenase on various prostaglandins. *Biochimica et Biophysica Acta,* **187**, 581.

Wallach, D. P. (1965). The enzymic conversion of arachidonic acid to prostaglandin $E_2$ with acetone powder preparations of bovine seminal vesicles. *Life Sciences,* **4**, 361.

Weinheimer, A. J. and Spraggins, R. L. (1969). The occurrence of two new prostaglandin derivatives (15-epi-PGA$_2$ and its acetate, methyl ester) in the gorgonian *Plexaura homonalla. Tetrahedron Letters,* **59**, 5185.

Williams, E. D., Karim, S. M. M. and Sandler, M. (1968). Prostaglandin secretion by medullary carcinoma of the thyroid. *Lancet,* **1**, 22.

Willis, A. L. (1969). Parallel assay of prostaglandin-like activity in rat inflammatory exudate by means of cascade superfusion. *Journal of Pharmacy and Pharmacology,* **21**, 126.

Willis, A. L. (1971). *Ph.D. Thesis,* University of London.

Wolfe, L. S., Coceani, F. and Pace-Asciak, C. (1967). Brain prostaglandins and studies of the action of prostaglandins on the isolated rat stomach. Nobel Symposium 2, Prostaglandins (Eds S. Bergström and B. Samuelsson), p. 265. Almqvist and Wiksell, Stockholm.

# CHAPTER IV

# Cyclic AMP and the Mechanism of Action of the Prostaglandins

K. J. Hittelman and R. W. Butcher

In the many biological systems in which the prostaglandins have been shown to have profound physiological effects, we remain relatively uninformed about their precise mechanism of action at the molecular level. We do know, however, that in several tissues the prostaglandins exert their action upon a biochemical system which controls the metabolism of one of the body's most important regulatory agents, a small, ubiquitous molecule known as cyclic adenosine-3',5'-monophosphate or cyclic AMP. Since cyclic AMP plays a crucial role in endocrinological regulation of many tissues, it would be well to review here briefly the metabolism and role of cyclic AMP in order to be able to discuss more easily some of the biochemical effects of the prostaglandins.

Cyclic AMP has been found throughout the animal kingdom as well as in a number of bacteria. Rall, Sutherland, and Berthet (1957) showed it to be involved in adrenaline and glucagon-stimulated glycogenolysis in mammalian liver. This role has now been further defined to the point that we now believe cyclic AMP to be the means of intracellular information transfer between the extracellular glycogenolytic hormones and those intracellular regulatory enzymes which when activated by cyclic AMP give rise to the overt glycogenolytic response of the liver cell. The discovery of cyclic AMP in biological systems and its implication as a courier of biochemical information have greatly improved our understanding of hormone/effector systems, and it is now known that a very large number of target tissues respond to their relevant hormones by increasing intracellular production of cyclic AMP (Robison, Butcher and Sutherland, 1971).

## 1. INTRACELLULAR CONCENTRATIONS OF CYCLIC AMP

Intracellular concentrations of cyclic AMP reflect the relative activities of at least two enzymes which function in opposition to each other (Fig. 1). The production of cyclic AMP is catalyzed by a hormone-sensitive enzyme called adenyl cyclase. In the reaction over which this

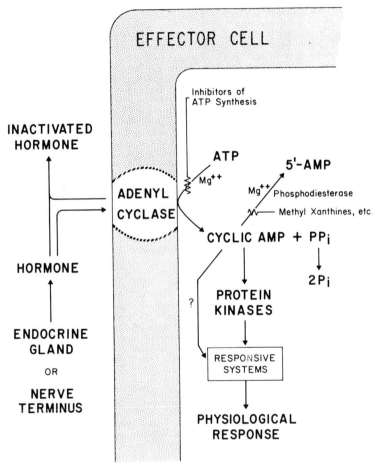

Fig. 1. The metabolism of cyclic AMP. The details of this figure are explained in the text. The protein kinases are members of a family of enzymes whose activity is dependent upon the presence of cyclic AMP. They are thought to be the first stage in the mechanism whereby cyclic AMP exerts its effects within the cell. Reproduced from Hittelman K. J. and Butcher, R. W. in *Effects of drugs on cellular control systems* (Eds B. R. Rabin and R. B. Freedman), Macmillan, London, 1971, with permission of the publisher.

enzyme presides, adenosine-5′-triphosphate (ATP) is cyclized to cyclic AMP (Rall and Sutherland, 1962).

With very few exceptions, adenyl cyclase is known to be an enzyme which resides in the plasma membrane of cells. This, of course, fits quite well with our belief that the enzyme serves as an information transducer between circulating hormones and the actual intracellular effector sites. It is also interesting to note that the enzyme is built into the cell membrane in such a way that it displays what we may call sidedness (Øye and Sutherland, 1966). This is illustrated by the observation that in most cells cyclic AMP is formed only at the inner surface of the cell, and hence cyclic AMP is produced only intracellularly (Fig. 2); for while cells can metabolize ATP at the outer surface of the cell membrane, the product is not cyclic AMP, but, rather, adenosine-5′-diphosphate (ADP).

Perhaps the most striking and functionally significant property of adenyl cyclase is that its catalytic activity is under a remarkable degree of control by hormones (Robison, *et al.,* 1971). That is, whereas in the absence of a hormone adenyl cyclase may only form cyclic AMP at a negligible rate, this rate may increase by as much as an order of magnitude or more in the presence of a relevant hormone. This property, of course, makes adenyl cyclase an outstanding candidate as a control point in the regulation of cyclic AMP metabolism.

Sharing the task with adenyl cyclase of regulating the intracellular concentration of cyclic AMP is a specific cyclic AMP phosphodiesterase (PDase) (Butcher and Sutherland, 1962). This enzyme hydrolyzes cyclic AMP to yield 5′-AMP. Like adenyl cyclase, phosphodiesterase enjoys an extremely wide phylogenetic distribution. However, in contrast to adenyl cyclase the PDase may exist in both soluble and membrane-bound forms in the same cell (DeRobertis, Arnaiz, Alberici, Butcher and Sutherland, 1967).

In some tissues, such as the adrenal cortex, it can be shown that administration of a relevant hormone (ACTH in this case) results in increased cyclic AMP production to the extent that intracellular concentrations may rise by as much as two to three orders of magnitude (Grahame-Smith, Butcher, Ney and Sutherland, 1967). This is as one might expect: Hormonal activation of adrenocortical adenyl cyclase by ACTH stimulates the cyclase to produce cyclic AMP at a rate far greater than the rate at which PDase can destroy it. Cyclic AMP consequently accumulates intracellularly and discharges its functions.

However, there are many data in the literature which suggest that in other tissues PDase is present in cells at far greater activity than is adenyl cyclase. If these observations accurately reflect the state of the intact cell (which they probably do not), they pose somewhat of a dilemma with respect to the regulation of intracellular concentrations of cyclic AMP, for we must find some way of explaining the ability of cyclic AMP to

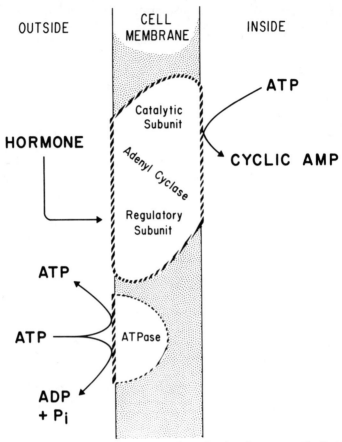

Fig. 2. Sidedness of the typical mammalian adenyl cyclase system. Cyclic AMP is produced on the inside of the plasma membrane, opposite the side at which the hormone binds. The regulatory subunit refers to that part of the cyclase system to which the hormone binds and through which it exerts its stimulatory effect upon the catalytic subunit. Further details are in the text. Reproduced from Butcher, R. W. in *Biochemical actions of Hormones* (Ed. G. Litwak), Academic Press, New York (in press), with permission of the publisher.

fulfill its function in these tissues under conditions where it would seem impossible for it to accumulate in significant enough amounts to exert its action. At present, we can propose the following possible explanations:

(1) Adenyl cyclase and phosphodiesterase may somehow be separated from each other within the cell. This kind of compartmentalization at a subcellular level is, of course, a widely recognized phenomenon for other opposing biochemical functions, such as the processes of fatty acid

synthesis and oxidation. Thus, a segregation of the enzymes producing and destroying cyclic AMP might permit sufficient accumulation of the nucleotide for it to serve its functions. Rall and Sattin (1970) presented some evidence for such a mechanism in brain tissues.

(2) Phosphodiesterase as well as adenyl cyclase may be under h rmonal control, but in a reciprocal manner. That is, agents or cconditions which increase adenyl cyclase activity may decrease PDase activity and *vice versa.* It is especially intriguing, for instance, to speculate on a possible role of cyclic AMP itself acting as a regulator of PDase activity. With such a mechanism, one can envisage cyclic AMP ensuring its own accumulation by directly affecting the enzyme which destroys it. Although there is presently no evidence directly supporting this position, it is known that the activity of PDase is affected by a number of other agents (Cheung, 1970). The relationships between these agents and a concomitant effect on adenyl cyclase remain to be elucidated.

(3) The explanation which is presently most acceptable is also one of the simplest. There is evidence that cyclic AMP-mediated events may be triggered by only small changes in intracellular concentrations of cyclic AMP. For instance, hormone-stimulated lipolysis, a cyclic AMP-dependent event, was shown to increase to a maximum of 13 times its basal rate while cyclic AMP levels only increased by slightly more than twice (Butcher, Robison, Hardman and Sutherland, 1968). Although cyclic AMP could be increased to much higher concentrations, no additional effects on lipolysis occurred. Thus, it is reasonable to suspect that a hormone-stimulated adenyl cyclase might be able to increase intracellular cyclic AMP concentrations sufficiently to trigger desired physiological effects, even in the presence of very high PDase activity.

The fact is, of course, that increases in intracellular cyclic AMP concentrations can be measured in intact cells stimulated by a relevant hormone. Thus, adenyl cyclase must be able to produce cyclic AMP at a rate greater than that at which PDase can destroy it. Among the things one would like to know to help resolve this question are the maximal activities of adenyl cyclase and PDase in intact cells, but these are very difficult data to obtain. One can, however, use published data on intact fat cells (Butcher and Baird, 1968) and with a few reasonable assumptions, maximal adenyl cyclase and PDase activities can be roughly estimated. Interestingly, it turns out that the maximal activities of these two enzymes may be about equal.

Figure 1 summarizes our current knowledge of the relationship between adenyl cyclase and PDase and illustrates the three primary possibilities for control of intracellular cyclic AMP concentrations: (1) Modulation of the activity of adenyl cyclase; (2) modulation of the activity of PDase; or (3) a concerted modulation of the activities of both of these enzymes simultaneously. We do not mean to imply that there may not be other means of controlling intracellular levels of cyclic AMP. There is, for instance, leakage of the nucleotide out of cells, and at least in certain unicellular organisms this appears to play a role in controlling intracellular cyclic nucleotide accumulations. Further, there may be other mechanisms of which we are at present unaware. Nevertheless, there is now an overwhelming body of evidence which suggests that one of the primary control points in the regulation of intracellular cyclic AMP concentrations is at the level of adenyl cyclase, and this control is usually found to result from hormonal stimulation of adenyl cyclase. This is sensible, too, from an energetic point of view, for the substrate for adenyl cyclase—ATP—is also the primary source of energy in living organisms. It would thus be disadvantageous to an organism to squander ATP in continuously generating cyclic AMP only to have it promptly degraded to 5′-AMP without using it for a regulatory function.

## 2. THE SECOND MESSENGER HYPOTHESIS

Although the biological role of cyclic AMP had only begun to be elucidated in 1957, a sufficient number of hormone/effector systems had been tested by 1965 to show that cyclic AMP plays a pivotal role in the mediation of a large number of hormonal responses (Robison, et al., 1971). It was on the basis of such frequent occurrence of cyclic AMP in these systems that Sutherland, Øye and Butcher (1965) formally proposed the 'Second Messenger Hypothesis'.

According to this hypothesis (Fig. 3), a circulating hormone or neurohormone is called a first messenger. This agent impinges upon a target cell at a specific receptor site which is intimately related to the adenyl cyclase system. As a result of the interaction between the hormone and the adenyl cyclase system, the catalytic activity of the enzyme is increased, thus increasing production of cyclic AMP and its intracellular concentration. In effect what has happened is that the extracellular form of information, the hormone, has been translated by adenyl cyclase at the cell membrane, resulting in an altered intracellular concentration of cyclic AMP (the second messenger). It is, in fact, the altered level of intracellular cyclic AMP that changes the metabolic behaviour of the cell so that it can be said to have 'responded to the hormone'. In some tissues, such a scheme of information transfer can be extended even further. For instance, thyroid, adrenal cortex, anterior pituitary, and gonads may respond to increased intracellular cyclic AMP concentrations by increasing in turn the rates at which they secrete their own hormones; and these hormones can thus be termed 'third messengers'.

How is it, one may ask, that a single, small, ubiquitous molecule like cyclic AMP can be responsible for evoking such a wide variety of specific

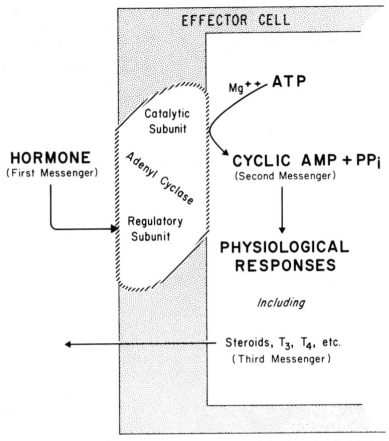

Fig. 3. The second messenger system. The details of this figure are explained in the text. Reproduced from Hittelman, K. J. and Butcher, R. W. in *Effects of drugs on cellular control systems* (Eds. B. R. Rabin and R. B. Freedman), Macmillan, London, 1971, with permission of the publisher.

physiological responses to hormones? The answer is that in great measure this apparent versatility is only illusory, and is really a reflection of the different enzyme profiles of different cells. Any specific cell type can respond to its relevant hormones only by using that metabolic machinery which it has available to it. Whereas an increased intracellular concentration of cyclic AMP in response to ACTH in adrenocortical cells results in increased steroidogenesis, ACTH cannot elicit the same response in fat cells (even though it increases cyclic AMP levels) because they do not have the sufficient enzyme complement necessary for steroid production. Further, although adipose tissue, cardiac muscle, and liver all respond to adrenaline by increasing their intracellular concentrations of cyclic AMP and all share several cyclic AMP-dependent processes, many of the pursuant biochemical and physiological changes which occur appear in one tissue but not in the others. Thus, the nature and specificity of the response of a cell to a relevant hormone are not determined by cyclic AMP itself, but, rather by the highly specific hormone-receptor interaction at adenyl cyclase, and by the enzymatic constitution of the cell.

## 3. PROSTAGLANDINS AND THE SECOND MESSENGER SYSTEM

The first indication that prostaglandins might exert some of their effects at the level of the second messenger system came in 1964 when Steinberg, Vaughan, Nestel, Strand and Bergström reported that prostaglandin $E_1$ ($PGE_1$) acted as an antagonist of both lipolysis and phosphorylase activation in rat epididymal fat cells stimulated by lipolytic hormones. Then, Orloff, Handler and Bergström (1965) showed that $PGE_1$ blocked the actions of vasopressin and theophylline (a phosphodiesterase inhibitor) on movements of water and ions in toad bladder. Since these processes observed to be affected by $PGE_1$ are regulated by cyclic AMP, these reports suggested that prostaglandins might act by altering intracellular levels of cyclic AMP.

The involvement of prostaglandins in cyclic AMP metabolism was demonstrated directly in 1967-1968 (Butcher and Sutherland, 1967; Butcher, Pike and Sutherland, 1967; Butcher and Baird, 1968) in a series of experiments which, though baffling at first, served to underscore the sometimes bewildering array of effects that the prostaglandins can have. In experiments on intact epididymal fat pads from rats it was observed that $PGE_1$ greatly inhibited adrenaline-induced cyclic AMP accumulation whereas $PGE_1$ alone caused an increase in cyclic AMP levels. These observations raised the possibility that the prostaglandin acted as an antagonist of cyclic AMP production in the presence of adrenaline, but as an agonist in its absence.

This puzzle was shortly resolved when experiments were performed on isolated, intact adipocytes derived from the epididymal fat pads. It was found that when isolated fat cells were incubated for 10 minutes with adrenaline and caffeine (another phosphodiesterase inhibitor), cyclic AMP levels increased about 10-fold. If, after maximum cyclic AMP levels were reached, $PGE_1$ was added, cyclic AMP levels were rapidly reduced back to low control values. Interestingly, $PGE_1$ was found not to have any effect on cyclic AMP levels in the absence of hormone stimulation. Thus, the original observation that $PGE_1$ could act as agonist or antagonist of cyclic AMP accumulation under appropriate conditions is explained by the cellular heterogeneity of the intact fat pad. In fact, in adipocytes $PGE_1$ has the effect of decreasing hormonally elevated cyclic AMP levels; in the stromovascular elements which comprise the non-adipocyte portion of the fat pad, $PGE_1$ effects an increase in cyclic AMP.

These studies on adipose tissue opened the way to general investigations on the effects of prostaglandins on the second messenger system. As shown in Table 1, prostaglandins have been demonstrated to affect cyclic AMP levels in a number of tissues. As we have seen, the response of adipose cells to prostaglandins is just the opposite of the way in which other tissues respond, and we will come back to this again later.

As there are several factors involved in the regulation of intracellular cyclic AMP levels, the direct observation that prostaglandins change these levels tells us little of *how* this change might be brought about. But what can be done toward this end, of course, is to test the effects of prostaglandins on the individual components of the second messenger system, particularly adenyl cyclase and phosphodiesterase. When this was done, it was found that in corpus luteum (Marsh, 1970), leukocytes and platelets (Robison, Arnold and Hartmann, 1969; Wolfe and Shulman,

Table 1

Effects of prostaglandins on intracellular cyclic AMP concentrations in various tissues[1]

| | Tissue and Effect | |
| Prostaglandin | ↑ cyclic AMP | ↓ cyclic AMP |
| --- | --- | --- |
| $E_1$ | thyroid<br>lung<br>spleen<br>platelets<br>diaphragm<br>foetal bone<br>adenohypophysis<br>adipose (stromovascular) | white adipocytes[2]<br>brown adipocytes[2] |
| $E_2$ | platelets<br>foetal bone | white adipocytes[2] |
| $F_{1\alpha}$ | | white adipocytes[2] |
| $A_1$ | | white adipocytes[2] |

[1] See Butcher (1970) and Robison *et al.* (1971) for references and further details.

[2] Prostaglandins decrease cyclic AMP levels only if the cells are hormonally stimulated. There is no effect on unstimulated cells.

1969; Scott, 1970; Moskowitz, Harwood, Reid and Krishna, 1971), lymphocytes (Novogrodsky and Katchalski, 1970), anterior pituitary (Zor, Kaneko, Schneider, McCann, Lowe, Bloom, Borland and Field, 1969) and thyroid (Zor, Kaneko, Lowe, Bloom and Field, 1969), prostaglandins increased the activity of adenyl cyclase. Thus, in several tissues where prostaglandins act to increase cyclic AMP, they probably do so by stimulating the production of cyclic AMP. As yet, no effects of prostaglandins have been observed on the PDase.

Fat cells appear to be quite different from other tissues in which prostaglandins affect cyclic AMP levels since in fat cells prostaglandins *decrease* the cyclic nucleotide concentration (Table 1). And while one might suspect the prostaglandins to act on fat cells by inhibiting adenyl cyclase, this has not been shown to be the case and the site of action of the prostaglandins in adipose tissue remains a mystery.

One of the major obstacles in elucidating the site of action of prostaglandins in fat cells is that these effects have not yet been elicited in cell-free systems. Although adrenaline and $\beta$-adrenoceptor blocking agents will, respectively, stimulate and inhibit adenyl cyclase in fat cell homogenates, $PGE_1$ is ineffective. Also, $PGE_1$ has not been shown to activate PDase, another action it might have which could explain its cyclic AMP-lowering activity.

Experiments have been carried out to determine whether prostaglandins could inhibit the effects of exogenous cyclic AMP on lipolysis. However, because there are so many unknowns under such experimental conditions, such as rates of penetration, diffusion, sequestration, and destruction of the exogenous cyclic AMP, and its ultimate intracellular distribution, it is very difficult to interpret such experiments.

One of the more attractive hypotheses for explaining the action of prostaglandins in fat cells comes from a study by Steinberg and Vaughan (1967) who demonstrated that $PGE_1$ inhibited lipolysis induced by the family of PDase inhibitors called methyl xanthines. Since there is presumably always an endogenous rate of cyclization of ATP occurring, accumulation of significant levels of cyclic AMP will occur in the presence of these inhibitors. When the cyclic AMP concentration attains a sufficient level, lipolysis will be triggered. Under such circumstances, lipolysis may be inhibited by prostaglandins in two ways: (1) Prostaglandins may interfere with the action of accumulated cyclic AMP, or (2) prostaglandins may inhibit the activity of adenyl cyclase. Obviously, only in the latter instance would one be able to explain both the inhibition of lipolysis as well as the observed decrease in cyclic AMP concentrations effected by $PGE_1$. Thus, it is tempting to speculate that in fat cells, $PGE_1$ exerts its antilipolytic effect by inhibiting adenyl cyclase.

Two other ideas about the actions of prostaglandins should be mentioned here. One is the proposal that the action of luteinizing hormone (LH) in stimulating steroidogenesis in mouse ovary may be mediated by prostaglandin (Kuehl, Humes, Tarnoff, Cirillo and Ham, 1970). This hypothesis is based on the observation that an inhibitor of prostaglandin-induced cyclic AMP formation in ovary also inhibited the action of LH. This may be a case, then, where adenyl cyclase responds to a hormone-induced change in the prostaglandin level, rather than responding directly to the hormone itself. We must await further studies for illumination of this peculiar system.

Shaw and Ramwell (1968) have presented data which indicate that prostaglandins constitute part of a feedback loop which regulates the formation of cyclic AMP. They suggest that in fat cells as adenyl cyclase activity and cyclic AMP concentration go up pursuant to hormonal stimulation, so too does the intracellular level of prostaglandin. As a result, a negative feedback is imposed on adenyl cyclase, limiting further formation of cyclic AMP. The experiments of Christ and Nugteren (1970) tend to support this hypothesis. As has been pointed out (Butcher, 1970), this hypothesis is attractive for fat cells, but the opposite effects of prostaglandins in non-adipose cell types would mean that these cells would be at the mercy of a positive feedback loop—a very unstable position. So this proposal, too, must be viewed with caution pending further investigation.

## 4. PROSTAGLANDINS AND CYCLIC AMP IN DISEASE

It is now generally believed that the function of some prostaglandins is to mediate defensive reactions, and perhaps to alter body temperature through their pyrogenic properties. However, virtually nothing is known at present about the effects of prostaglandins on the second messenger system in these or other pathophysiological states. Because of the crucial role played by cyclic AMP in the control of metabolism, and the striking effects prostaglandins can have on the second messenger system, it seems entirely reasonable to suspect that the prostaglandins may exert their actions in some acute inflammatory and chronic disease states through effects on levels of cyclic AMP. It would not be surprising, for example, to one day find that the primary cause of an endocrinopathy lay in an aberrant prostaglandin metabolism, with consequent over- or under-production of cyclic AMP and a resultant over- or under-production of hormone.

The recent scientific literature has presented two instances which hint that we may be very close to defining more accurately the role of prostaglandins in altering cyclic AMP metabolism and pursuant physiological events. The first case is that of the disease cholera. It has been shown that cholera toxin and prostaglandins both markedly stimulate transmucosal secretion of water and electrolytes in dog jejunum (Pierce, Carpenter, Elliott and Greenough, 1971). Furthermore, cholera toxin also dramatically increases the activity of intestinal adenyl cyclase (Sharp and Hynie, 1971). Since the movement of water and electrolytes across the intestinal mucosa is thought to be under the control of cyclic AMP, all of these observations point to the involvement of the second messenger system in the gastrointestinal sequelae of cholera. An attempt has been made to tie all these ends together with the suggestion that the action of cholera toxin is to stimulate the synthesis or release of prostaglandins (Bennett, 1971). Thus, the proposed sequence of events following administration of cholera toxin would be: cholera toxin → increased mucosal prostaglandin levels → stimulation of mucosal adenyl cyclase → increased intracellular cyclic AMP levels → increased water and electrolyte secretion. It must be stressed that this scheme is only hypothetical at present, but it is certainly open to confirmation or refutation in the laboratory.

The second instance in which prostaglandins may be implicated to be involved in pathophysiological alterations of cyclic AMP metabolism stems from investigations into the mechanism of action of aspirin and similar anti-inflammatory drugs. It has been shown that these drugs interfere with prostaglandin metabolism in spleen (Ferreira, Moncada and Vane, 1971), platelets (Smith and Willis, 1971) and lung (Vane, 1971). This is of considerable interest in relation to the second messenger system, of course, because prostaglandins are known to have marked effects on cyclic AMP metabolism in platelets and bronchiolar smooth muscle. Thus, we may soon find that many of the therapeutic actions of aspirin and related drugs are based on alterations induced in prostaglandin metabolism which in turn affect the function of the second messenger system.

At present, these inferences are purely speculative, of course. But they are amenable to rigorous testing, and such studies are no doubt under way in a number of laboratories. The appeal of the hypothesis that prostaglandins function as important control elements in cyclic AMP metabolism lies not so much in the fact that the hypothesis is readily open to scientific scrutiny as it does in its scope and simplicity. The broad occurrence of the prostaglandins is certainly matched by the ubiquity of the second messenger system, and such a unifying concept of prostaglandin action is quite attractive—especially when compared with the staggering and unlikely alternative of having to explain each of the many actions of the prostaglandins on the basis of individual mechanisms.

This work was supported by Grant AM-13904 from the National Institutes of Health.

# REFERENCES

Bennett, A. (1971). Cholera and prostaglandins. *Nature,* **231**, 536.

Butcher, R. W. (1970). Prostaglandins and cyclic AMP. Role of Cyclic AMP in Cell Function (Eds P. Greengard and E. Costa), p. 173. Raven Press, New York.

Butcher, R. W. and Baird, C. E. (1968). Effects of prostaglandins on adenosine $3',5'$-monophosphate levels in fat and other tissues. *Journal of Biological Chemistry,* **243**, 1713.

Butcher, R. W., Pike, J. E. and Sutherland, E. W. (1967). The effects of prostaglandin $E_1$ on adenosine $3',5'$-monophosphate levels in adipose tissue. Nobel Symposium 2, Prostaglandins (Eds S. Bergström and B. Samuelsson), p. 133. Interscience Publishers, New York.

Butcher, R. W., Robison, G. A., Hardman, J. G. and Sutherland, E. W. (1968). The role of cyclic AMP in hormone actions. *Advances in Enzyme Regulation,* **6**, 357.

Butcher, R. W. and Sutherland, E. W. (1962). Adenosine $3',5'$-phosphate in biological materials. I. Purification and properties of cyclic $3',5'$-nucleotide phosphodiesterase and use of this enzyme to characterize adenosine $3',5'$-phosphate in human urine. *Journal of Biological Chemistry,* **237**, 1244.

Butcher, R. W. and Sutherland, E. W. (1967). The effects of the catecholamines, adrenergic blocking agents, prostaglandin $E_1$, and insulin on cyclic AMP levels in the rat epididymal fat pad *in vitro. Annals of the New York Academy of Sciences,* **139**, 849.

Cheung, W. Y. (1970). Cyclic nucleotide phosphodiesterase. Role of Cyclic AMP in Cell Function (Eds P. Greengard and E. Costa), p. 51. Raven Press, New York.

Christ, E. J. and Nugteren, D. H. (1970). The biosynthesis and possible function of prostaglandins in adipose tissue. *Biochimica et Biophysica Acta,* **218**, 296.

DeRobertis, E., Arnaiz, G. R. DeL., Alberici, M., Butcher, R. W. and Sutherland, E. W. (1967). Subcellular distribution of adenyl cyclase and cyclic phosphodiesterase in rat brain cortex. *Journal of Biological Chemistry,* **242**, 3487.

Ferreira, S. H., Moncada, S. and Vane, J. R. (1971). Indomethacin and aspirin abolish prostaglandin release from the spleen. *Nature New Biology,* **231**, 237.

Grahame-Smith, D. G., Butcher, R. W., Ney, R. L. and Sutherland, E. W. (1967). Adenosine $3',5'$-monophosphate as the intracellular mediator of the action of adrenocorticotropic hormone on the adrenal cortex. *Journal of Biological Chemistry,* **242**, 5535.

Kuehl, F. A., Humes, J. L., Tarnoff, J., Cirillo, V. J. and Ham, E. A. (1970). Prostaglandin receptor site: Evidence for an essential role in the action of luteinizing hormone. *Science (New York),* **169**, 883.

Marsh, J. M. (1970). The stimulatory effect of prostaglandin $E_2$ on adenyl cyclase in bovine corpus luteum. *Federation of European Biochemical Societies Letters,* **7**, 283.

Moskowitz, J., Harwood, J. P., Reid, W. D. and Krishna, G. (1971). The interaction of norepinephrine and prostaglandin $E_1$ on the adenyl cylase system of human and rabbit blood platelets. *Biochimica et Biophysica Acta,* **230**, 279.

Novogrodsky, A. and Katchalski, E. (1970). Effect of phytohemagglutinin and prostaglandins on cyclic AMP synthesis in rat lymph node lymphocytes. *Biochimica et Biophysica Acta,* **215**, 291.

Orloff, J., Handler, J. S. and Bergström, S. (1965). Effect of prostaglandin (PGE₁) on the permeability response of the toad bladder to vasopressin, theophylline and adenosine 3′,5′-monophosphate. *Nature (London)*, **205**, 397.

Øye, I. and Sutherland, E. W. (1966). The effect of epinephrine and other agents on adenyl cyclase in the cell membrane of avian erythrocytes. *Biochimica et Biophysica Acta*, **127**, 347.

Pierce, N. F., Carpenter, C. C. J., Elliott, H. L. and Greenough, W. B. (1971). Effects of prostaglandins, theophylline, and cholera exotoxin upon transmucosal water and electrolyte movement in canine jejunum. *Gastroenterology*, **60**, 22.

Rall, T. W. and Sattin, A. (1970). Factors influencing the accumulation of cyclic AMP in brain tissue. Role of Cyclic AMP in Cell Function (Eds P. Greengard and E. Costa), p. 113. Raven Press, New York.

Rall, T. W. and Sutherland, E. W. (1962). Adenyl cyclase. II. The enzymatically catalyzed formation of adenosine 3′,5′-phosphate and inorganic pyrophosphate from adenosine triphosphate. *Journal of Biological Chemistry*, **237**, 1228.

Rall, T. W., Sutherland, E. W. and Berthet, J. (1957). The relationship of epinephrine and glucagon to liver phosphorylase. *Journal of Biological Chemistry*, **224**, 463.

Robison, G. A., Arnold, A. and Hartmann, R. C. (1969). Divergent effects of epinephrine and prostaglandin E₁ on the level of cyclic AMP in human blood platelets. *Pharmacological Research Communications*, **1**, 325.

Robison, G. A., Butcher, R. W. and Sutherland, E. W. (1971). Cyclic AMP. Academic Press, New York.

Scott, R. E. (1970). Effects of prostaglandins, epinephrine and NaF on human leukocyte, platelet and liver adenyl cyclase. *Blood*, **35**, 514.

Sharp, G. W. G. and Hynie, S. (1971). Stimulation of intestinal adenyl cyclase by cholera toxin. *Nature* (London), **229**, 266.

Shaw, J. E. and Ramwell, P. W. (1968). Release of prostaglandin from rat epididymal fat pad on nervous and hormonal stimulation. *Journal of Biological Chemistry*, **243**, 1498.

Smith, J. B. and Willis, A. L. (1971). Aspirin selectively inhibits prostaglandin production in human platelets. *Nature New Biology*, **231**, 235.

Steinberg, D. and Vaughan, M. (1967). *In vitro* and *in vivo* effects of prostaglandins on free fatty acid metabolism. Nobel Symposium 2, Prostaglandins (Eds S. Bergström and B. Samuelsson), p. 109. Interscience Publishers, New York.

Steinberg, D., Vaughan, M., Nestel, P. J., Strand, O. and Bergström, S. (1964). Effects of the prostaglandins on hormone-induced mobilization of free fatty acids. *Journal of Clinical Investigation*, **43**, 1553.

Sutherland, E. W., Øye, I. and Butcher, R. W. (1965). The action of epinephrine and the role of the adenyl cyclase system in hormone action. *Recent Progress in Hormone Research*, **21**, 623.

Vane, J. R. (1971). Inhibition of prostaglandin synthesis as a mechanism of action for aspirin-like drugs. *Nature New Biology*, **231**, 232.

Wolfe, S. M. and Shulman, N. R. (1969). Adenyl cyclase activity in human platelets. *Biochemical and Biophysical Research Communications*, **35**, 265.

Zor, U., Kaneko, T., Lowe, I. P., Bloom, G. and Field, J. B. (1969). Effect of thyroid-stimulating hormone and prostaglandins on thyroid adenyl cyclase activation and cyclic adenosine 3′,5′-monophosphate. *Journal of Biological Chemistry*, **244**, 5189.

Zor, U., Kaneko, T., Schneider, H. P. G., McCann, S. M., Lowe, I. P., Bloom, G., Borland, B. and Field, J. B. (1969). Stimulation of anterior pituitary adenyl cyclase activity and adenosine $3',5'$-cyclic phosphate by hypothalamic extract and prostaglandin $E_1$. *Proceedings of the National Academy of Sciences,* **63**, 918.

# CHAPTER V

# Pharmacology and Therapeutic Applications of Prostaglandins in the Human Reproductive System

Sultan M. M. Karim and Keith Hillier

High concentrations of prostaglandins are found in many organs of the reproductive system and their secretions. They were first discovered in human seminal fluid (von Euler, 1934, 1935; Goldblatt, 1933, 1935; Bergström and Samuelsson, 1962; Samuelsson, 1963; Hamberg and Samuelsson, 1966a, 1966b) and have since been shown to be present in menstrual fluid (Pickles, Hall, Best and Smith, 1965); amniotic fluid (Karim, 1966; Karim and Devlin, 1967; Karim and Hillier, 1970); blood of women during spontaneous abortion and term labour (Karim, 1968; Karim and Hillier, 1970) and umbilical cord and placental blood vessels (Karim, 1967; Hiller, 1970).

Prostaglandins also have pharmacological actions on the reproductive system including the female genital tract. Physiological roles ascribed to these substances in relation to human reproduction include a contribution to the control of vessel tone in the umbilical blood vessels during gestation and at birth (Karim, 1967; Hillier and Karim, 1968; Hillier, 1970); menstruation (Pickles et al., 1965); parturition and spontaneous abortion (Karim, 1966, 1968, 1969a, b, 1971b, d).

Studies carried out during the past two years with naturally-occurring prostaglandins indicate that they have clinical usefulness as abortifacients, for the induction of labour and as contraceptives.

## 1. NON-PREGNANT UTERUS

*In vitro* Studies

The effect of human semen and seminal fluid extracts on the isolated strips of non-pregnant human uterus is generally to decrease the amplitude and frequency of spontaneous contractions (Kurzrok and

Lieb, 1930; Cockrill, Miller and Kurzrok, 1935; Eliasson, 1959, 1966a, b; Bygdeman and Eliasson, 1963a, b; Eglinton, Raphael, Smith, Hall and Pickles, 1963; Pickles and Hall, 1963; Sandberg, Ingelman-Sundberg and Rydén, 1963a, b, 1965; von Euler and Eliasson, 1967; Bygdeman, 1964, 1967; Bygdeman, Hamberg and Samuelsson, 1966; Bygdeman and Hamberg, 1967). This inhibitory effect could be due to the greater proportion of prostaglandin E (PGE) compounds present in human semen.

Pure $PGE_1$, $PGE_2$ and $PGE_3$ all decrease the tone, frequency and amplitude of uterine strip contractions (Bygdeman, 1964, 1967; Bygdeman and Eliasson, 1963a, b, c; Pickles and Hall, 1963; Sandberg *et al.*, 1963a, b, 1965; Sandberg, Ingelman-Sundberg and Rydén, 1964; Eliasson, 1959), although some of these investigators have reported occasional stimulation or stimulation followed by inhibition with E compounds.

Prostaglandin A (PGA) and prostaglandin B (PGB) compounds and their 19-hydroxy derivatives, which are all present in human seminal fluid, also produce relaxation of the non-pregnant myometrial strips but are less active than the E compounds (Bygdeman, 1967; Bygdeman and Hamberg, 1967).

In contrast, the prostaglandin F$\alpha$ (PGF$\alpha$) compounds will only cause contraction of the non-pregnant strips and higher doses than those of E prostaglandins are required. $PGF_{2\alpha}$ is more active than $PGF_{1\alpha}$ (Bygdeman and Eliasson, 1963a, b, c; Bygdeman, 1964; Pickles and Hall, 1963; Sandberg *et al.*, 1965; Pickles, Hall, Clegg and Sullivan, 1966).

On the isolated non-pregnant cervix $PGE_2$ always causes a marked relaxation whilst $PGF_{2\alpha}$ produces a variable effect (Najak, Hillier and Karim, 1970).

### *In vivo* Studies

The effect of prostaglandins upon the non-pregnant uterus *in situ* is of considerable interest because of their possible implication in fertility control. Karim, Hillier, Somers and Trussell (1971b) studied the effect of prostaglandins on the non-pregnant uterus *in situ*. In two subjects, rapid intravenous injections of $PGE_2$, in doses of 20, 40 and 60 $\mu$g, were given at 20-minute intervals. With the two lower doses there was a marked increase in uterine activity without side effects; 60 $\mu$g caused, in addition, a transient increase in heart rate of 10 beats per minute. Intravenous injections of 100 $\mu$g. $PGF_{2\alpha}$ had no effect but, 250 $\mu$g caused a marked, though short-lived, increase in uterine activity. 500 $\mu$g produced additionally a mean increase in systolic and diastolic blood pressures of 24 mm Hg lasting approximately five minutes.

In four subjects, intramuscular and subcutaneous injections of 1-2 mg

$PGE_2$ caused an increase in uterine activity within less than five minutes of the injection and this lasted several hours. There was, however, no effect on the cardiovascular system; all women complained of pain at the site of injection. Intramuscular and subcutaneous injections of 10-20 mg $PGF_{2\alpha}$ caused stimulation of uterine activity starting within a few minutes of injection and lasting for 2-3 hours. With this dose, all patients complained of pain at the site of injection.

Continuous intravenous infusion of $PGE_2$, in amounts of 10, 20 or 40 $\mu$g per minute for 60 minutes, caused an increase in uterine activity in the three women studied. This started within 2-5 minutes of the onset of infusion and continued for up to 60 minutes after stopping the infusion. There were no effects upon the electrocardiogram, heart rate, systolic and diastolic pressures. One of the three women was post-menopausal, another at mid-cycle and the third in the late secretory phase of the cycle. Intravenous infusions of 100, 200 and 300 $\mu$g per minute $PGF_{2\alpha}$ were given to three women for 60 minutes. Two were in the late secretory phase and one at day 7 of the cycle. Stimulation of uterine activity was recorded in all cases starting 5 minutes before the onset of infusion and continuing for at least one hour after stopping the infusion. There was no effect on the cardiovascular system but one woman passed a loose stool after stopping the infusion and there was uterine bleeding in two women in the late secretory phase of the cycle.

Roth-Brandel, Bygdeman and Wiqvist (1970b) have also carried out studies on the non-pregnant myometrium *in situ.* Their material included 19 gynaecologically normal volunteers at different stages of the menstrual cycle. Increasing doses of $PGE_1$ from 5-100 $\mu$g and $PGF_{2\alpha}$ from 20-200 $\mu$g were given at 30-60 minute intervals. At the end of the experiment one international unit of vasopressin was given as an additional check of the phase of the cycle. The threshold dose of $PGE_1$ was from 20-50 $\mu$g and a marked elevation in tone ensued, particularly with the higher doses of 50-100 $\mu$g. The elevated tone decreased to normal levels over a 30-40 minute period. $PGF_{2\alpha}$ had approximately the same effect as $PGE_1$ but the threshold dose was in the region of 50 $\mu$g. They found, however, that some degree of tachyphylaxis developed towards the end of the experiment and as $PGF_{2\alpha}$ was generally injected at this time, it is possible that the threshold dose for this substance might have been lower than 50 $\mu$g.

From these studies it appears that the non-pregnant uterus is more sensitive than the mid-pregnant uterus in its response to $PGF_{2\alpha}$ (Bygdeman, Kwon, Mukherjee, Roth-Brandel and Wiqvist, 1970; Wiqvist, Bygdeman, Kwon, Mukherjee and Roth-Brandel, 1968), although the former is certainly less sensitive than the term uterus as, at that time, 5 $\mu$g per minute of $PGF_{2\alpha}$ generally produces stimulation of uterine activity (Karim, Trussell, Patel and Hillier, 1968).

There was no cyclic variation in the sensitivity of the uterus to prostaglandins but some differences in the patterns of response were seen. For example, Roth-Brandel *et al* (1970b) observed that 100 μg of $PGE_1$ increased the tone at both the 8th and 13th day of the cycle; whilst on the 8th day there was no increase in amplitude or frequency of contractions, on the 13th day there was a marked increase in both parameters. The work of Roth-Brandel *et al* (1970b) and Karim *et al.* (1971b) has proven that the response of the uterus *in situ* to prostaglandins is only stimulation, unlike that *in vitro* when inhibition of uterine activity with E prostaglandins is seen. Roth-Brandel *et al.* (1970b), however, commented on the fact that with 50-100 μg $PGE_1$, four of their cases exhibited an inhibition of activity for 40-60 seconds prior to the stimulatory effect. This could have coincided with changes in arterial blood pressure. Other cases did not exhibit this inhibition.

It has been claimed that oxytocin and vasopressin may increase the sensitivity of the uterus to prostaglandins (Eliasson, 1966a, b; Eliasson and Posse, 1960). Embrey (1971) and Hillier and Embrey (unpublished) have also suggested that prostaglandins might sensitize the uterus to oxytocin or vice versa. Roth-Brandel *et al.* (1970b) injected 50 μg $PGE_1$ prior to, and during, the infusion of oxytocin and vasopressin in four women at day 12, 17, 19 and 27. They observed that during the oxytocin and vasopressin-induced stimulation, single intravenous injections of prostaglandin produced less effect, suggesting that a synergistic action did not occur. However, the authors commented that tachyphylaxis may occur and this could be a partial explanation. A similar tachyphylactic phenomenon has also been described with the intrauterine route of administration (Embrey and Hillier, 1971).

The observed effect of prostaglandins on the non-pregnant uterus *in vivo* cannot support the hypothesis of a physiological role for these compounds in promoting sperm migration by inhibiting uterine contractility in the period following ejaculation, as has been suggested by Eliasson (1966a) and Eliasson and Posse (1960). However, experimental conditions were not identical and, therefore, conclusions should be drawn cautiously.

More recently, Karim (1971d) has shown that intravaginal administration of 2-5 mg $PGE_2$ or 20-50 mg $PGF_{2\alpha}$ increased activity of the intact non-pregnant human uterus at all stages of the cycle. The uterus appears to be particularly sensitive before the onset of menstrual bleeding (Fig. 1).

## Prostaglandins and Menstruation

Pickles (1957) reported the presence of a smooth muscle stimulant in menstrual fluid and called the active fraction the 'menstrual stimulant'.

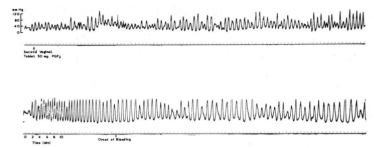

Fig. 1. Records of uterine activity in a 20-year-old subject on the 6th day after first missed period. Record started 4 hr after intravaginal administration of 50 mg $PGF_{2\alpha}$. Reproduced from Karim (1971d) with permission of the publishers.

Later work showed that this was a complex mixture of several substances all of lipid origin (Clitheroe, 1961; Clitheroe and Pickles, 1961; Pickles and Ward, 1965). Two main components were identified as $PGF_{2\alpha}$ and $PGE_2$ with the former predominating (Eglinton *et al.* 1963). 'Two others are most probably $PGF_{1\alpha}$ and $PGE_1$' (Pickles, 1967).

Prostaglandins are also present in the endometrium and, prostaglandin-like substances have been shown to be present in circulating blood during menstruation (Pickles *et al.,* 1965). The possibility exists, therefore, that prostaglandins play a role in the process of menstruation perhaps by increasing uterine contractility.

Karim (1971a, d) administered doses of $PGE_2$ and $PGF_{2\alpha}$ intravaginally to 12 women who had passed their expected date of menstruation by 2-7 days; in 11, menstruation was induced and the menstrual bleeding was always preceded by a marked increase in uterine activity (Fig. 1).

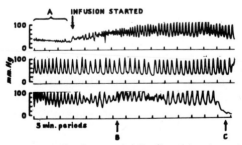

Fig. 2. Continuous record of prostaglandin $F_{2\alpha}$ induced uterine activity in a woman at 18 weeks. Intravenous infusion 50 μg/min.
A = Part of control period spontaneous activity.
B = Sitting up to pass urine.
C = Intact sac expelled.
Reproduced from Karim and Filshie (1970a) with permission of the publishers.

It is becoming apparent that prostaglandins may play a role as fertility regulating agents either as early abortifacients or in a luteolytic and menses-inducing role. Future work must establish whether the drug is best administered before the expected date of menstruation or whether it should be given if the period is missed and a pregnancy test is positive. If it can be established with certainty that the earlier the pregnancy the more sensitive and susceptible is the uterus and ovum to prostaglandins, then it may be advantageous to adminster them even before a pregnancy test has been proven positive. It is certain that this use of these compounds may give rise to some ethical problems. The results, so far, have generated a cautious optimism and much excitement since they may provide an alternative to present methods of contraception and abortion, providing side effects of nausea, diarrhoea and uterine pain can be minimized by formulation modification and different routes of administration.

Dysmenorrhoea and the associated pain is far from being understood and there is some evidence implicating $PGF_{2\alpha}$. It has been shown (Pickles *et al.*, 1965) that the amount of $PGF_{2\alpha}$ in menstrual fluid is higher in women with dysmenorrhoea than in normal women; present work has shown that long-term infusion of high doses of $PGF_{2\alpha}$ in a number of patients resulted in many instances of menstrual-like pain (Hillier unpublished observations; Wiqvist *et al.* unpublished observations; quoted from Roth-Brandel *et al.*, 1970b) and possibly in menstrual bleeding (Karim, 1971a; Karim *et al.*, 1971b; Hillier, unpublished observations). It is now clear that E prostaglandins will also stimulate the non-pregnant uterus and can produce dysmenorrhoeic-type pains. The 'menstrual stimulants' of Pickles *et al.* (1965) should probably now be adjudged to consist of E prostaglandins in addition to $PGF_{2\alpha}$.

## 2. EARLY PREGNANT UTERUS

*In vitro* Studies

In contrast to the inhibitory effect on strips of non-pregnant human uterus, seminal fluid and total seminal fluid extracts generally produce stimulation of strips from the pregnant uterus at 12-20 weeks. In 2 out of 10 strips, however, some inhibition was evident (Bygdeman, 1964, 1967; Bygdeman and Eliasson, 1963a, b, c, d).

The effect of pure prostaglandin $E_1$ on uterine strips from early pregnancy is complex. In half the uteri studied, $PGE_1$ stimulated the uterus initially but higher doses inhibited the motility.

Prostaglandin $F_{1\alpha}$ contracted pregnant uterine strips and this was 30 times more active than on non-pregnant strips (Bygdeman, 1964). With higher doses there was further stimulation and unlike E compounds no inhibition was recorded with $PGF_{1\alpha}$ (Bygdeman, Hamberg and Samuelsson, 1966). Prostaglandin $F_{2\alpha}$ is also a more potent stimulant of the pregnant than the non-pregnant uterine strips.

## *In vivo* Studies

### *The use of prostaglandins as abortifacients:*

Investigations thus far carried out on the intact human uterus, have basically attempted to clarify whether the prostaglandins are of potential clinical usefulness in obstetrics and gynaecology. This has been only partially answered by the work reviewed below but nevertheless important information has been obtained to further this aim.

There is now ample evidence to suggest that the administration of prostaglandin $E_1$, $E_2$, $F_{1\alpha}$ and $F_{2\alpha}$ cause an increase in activity in the non-pregnant human uterus at all stages of the menstrual cycle and in the pregnant uterus throughout gestation (Karim *et al.,* 1968; Karim, Trussell, Hillier and Patel, 1969; Karim, Hillier, Trussell, Patel and Tamusange, 1970; Karim, 1969a, b, 1970, 1971a, d; Karim and Filshie, 1970a, b; Karim and Filshie, 1972; Bygdeman and Wiqvist, 1970; Roth-Brandel, Bygdeman and Wiqvist, 1970a, b; Embrey, 1969, 1970a, b).

It is still necessary to know exactly how the sensitivity of the uterus to prostaglandins alters during gestation; whether the doses required and the side effects produced are compatible with an acceptable therapeutic ratio; how the efficacy and side effects vary with the route of administration and how the efficacy and safety compare with present methods of inducing abortion.

### *(i) The Intravenous Route*

In 1968, Bygdeman, Kwon, Mukherjee and Wiqvist and Wiqvist *et al.* administered short-term intravenous infusion of $PGE_1$ and $PGE_2$ in eight patients at 16 to 22 weeks gestation and in seven patients near term. At the lower end of the dose range used (0.6-8 $\mu$g per minute), in mid-trimester patients, there was a 'preferential increase in tone, whereas at term the increase in amplitude and frequency was greater'. However, with higher doses both tone and amplitude of contractions increased at both mid-trimester and term and in the latter 'the unphysiological elevation of tone frequently occurred with doses little higher than those required to increase amplitude and frequency of contraction'. The threshold dose in the mid-trimester patients was slightly lower than at term and they equated the response of 4 $\mu$g per minute $PGE_1$ and $PGE_2$ to that of 50 mU per minute oxytocin in mid-pregnancy. This led them to suggest that $PGE_1$ and $PGE_2$ were less active than oxytocin on the uterus in mid-pregnancy (as 50 mU oxytocin is approximately equal to 0.1 $\mu$g) and at term this difference may be even higher. They also suggested that the pattern of activity produced by oxytocin was more regular than that produced with prostaglandin. The only side effects observed were vomiting and this occurred with $PGE_2$ at a dose of 8 $\mu$g per minute.

The most clinically complete results have, in the main, been obtained by using continuous slow infusions of prostaglandins. Prostaglandins $E_1$, $E_2$ and $F_{2\alpha}$ have been used for the induction of therapeutic abortion and in the management of missed abortion (Karim and Filshie, 1970a, b, 1972; Roth-Brandel, Bygdeman, Wiqvist and Bergström, 1970c; Wiqvist and Bygdeman, 1970a; Embrey, 1970a, Karim, 1970, 1971a, d).

Karim and Filshie (1970a, b) established the regime of slow infusion at a constant rate throughout the induction of abortion (Fig. 2). They have reported in detail the successful induction of abortion in 50 out of 52 cases receiving 5 $\mu$g per minute of $PGE_2$ and in 14 of 15 cases receiving 50 $\mu$g per minute of $PGF_{2\alpha}$. The gestational age for both series varied between 9 and 22 weeks and the induction/abortion interval for the successful cases between 6-27½ hours (mean 12.5 hours) with $PGF_{2\alpha}$ and from 4½-54½ hours (mean 15 hours 50 minutes) with $PGE_2$. In both series only seven of the patients were first trimester, the remainder being second trimester. With these dose levels, 3 of the 15 patients receiving $PGF_{2\alpha}$ experienced vomiting and 7 diarrhoea, whilst 13 of the 52 receiving $PGE_2$ had vomiting or nausea and 4 had diarrhoea. Side effects were adequately contained with suitable treatment.

Karim and Filshie (1972) have reported the largest series of induction of abortion with the intravenous infusion of 5 $\mu$g per minute $PGE_2$. The case material consisted of 139 women in the first and second trimester of pregnancy. Abortion occurred in 130 women and was complete in 105. Of the 25 women in whom partial products of conception were retained, 19 were in the first trimester of pregnancy. The data is summarized in Table 1 and the relative distribution of the induction/abortion interval with gestational age is shown in Fig. 3.

Karim and Filshie (1972) have also shown that infusion of 5 $\mu$g per minute $PGE_2$ for several hours does not have any effect on blood clotting mechanisms, cell morphology, cell count or fibrinogen degradation products. In the same series it was also shown that $PGE_2$ has no antidiuretic effect in the dose used. According to these authors there have not been any serious adverse effects when $PGE_2$ is infused for the termination of pregnancy. Side effects encountered include nausea and vomiting in 50 patients and diarrhoea in 9 patients. The side effect causing some concern was the development of redness over the course of the vein from the site of the cannula. Some patients complained of pain

Table 1

Summary of Therapeutic Abortion with Prostaglandin E₂ in 139 women

| Parity | No. of Cases | Maturity | Average Induction/Abortion Interval |
|---|---|---|---|
| 0 | 55 (3 failed†) | 9-22 weeks | 19 hours 30 min |
| 1 | 19 (1 failed†) | 8-19 weeks | 15 hours |
| 2 | 24 (1 failed†) (1 discontinued) | 5-19 weeks | 17 hours |
| 3 | 13 | 6-24 weeks | 15 hours |
| 4 | 15 (3 failed†) | 11-20 weeks | 14 hours 45 min |
| 5 | 10 | 6-20 weeks | 19 hours 30 min |
| 7 | 1 | 18 weeks | 7 hours 30 min |
| 8 | 1 | 13 weeks | 9 hours 45 min |
| 10 | 1 | 16 weeks | 27 hours |

† No abortion within 48 hours. Infusion rate 5 μg/min PGE₂.
Data from Karim and Filshie, 1972.

in the forearm. The redness developed into phlebitis in one patient, who had an infusion for over 24 hours. The phlebitis rapidly subsided spontaneously after the infusion was discontinued. In most patients a mild pyrexia was recorded (less than 1°C) which subsided after abortion. In 17 patients the pyrexia exceeded 1°C. Headache developed in 4 women which responded to mild analgesics such as paracetamol. One patient complained of a transient blurring of vision but no apparent

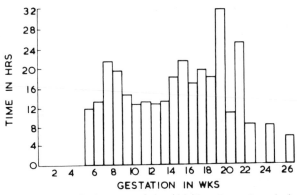

Fig. 3. Relationship between induction abortion interval and duration of pregnancy in 130 cases of pregnancy terminated with intravenous infusion of PGE₂. Height of the columns represents the mean abortion time for the patients studied at that gestational age.

cause was determined. Blood loss after the abortion was less than 200 ml in all except 4 women but only one woman required a blood transfusion of two pints.

Embrey (1970a) had a similar success rate inducing nine abortions successfully out of 11 patients using $PGE_1$ and $PGE_2$ at 9-28 weeks pregnancy. The average induction/abortion interval in this series was 17½ hours with a range of 10-27 hours. The dose used by Embrey, in the range 2-5 μg per minute, was generally lower and the duration shorter than that used by Karim and Filshie (1970a, b, 1972). With this dose level, Embrey noticed no undesirable side effects.

The Swedish workers, Wiqvist and Bygdeman (1970a, b) suggested that in the early weeks of pregnancy the uterus and ovum may be particularly susceptible to the action of prostaglandins compared with the mid-trimester. In their first series, 8 women were infused with $PGF_{2\alpha}$ at 6 to 12 weeks and 4 women at 13-16 weeks gestation. The dose range was increased step-wise between 13-300 μg per minute until a slight or moderate menstrual-like pain occurred. The infusion time was up to 7 hours on the first day and 7 hours on the second day. In 6 of the 7 women at 6-8 weeks, bleeding started within 3-7 hours of the start of the first day's infusion and the conceptus was partially or completely expelled after the first day's infusion. Abortion was accomplished in 3 out of the 5 remaining cases; bleeding started in 4 of these within 3-31 hours but in one of the failures no bleeding occurred. Diarrhoea or vomiting occurred in 5 of the patients at an infusion rate of 50-160 μg per minute but this readily disappeared upon reducing the infusion rate.

It was the suggestion of the authors that the vascular system between the small ovum and the uterine wall is susceptible to contractions in early pregnancy, but that the amniotic sac and placenta, later in pregnancy, are less susceptible. In the former case, the initiating mechanism may be traumatic in origin and/or may be caused by impaired corpora lutea activity. However, maintenance of the infusion for 1-2 days will probably interrupt pregnancy at any stage of gestation.

In a second series of 22 early pregnant women at 8 weeks gestation or less, $PGF_{2\alpha}$ was given by intravenous infusion for 7.6 hours. There was partial or complete expulsion of the conceptus in 20 patients. In contrast, when $PGF_{2\alpha}$ was administered in the 9th-12th week of pregnancy, only 6 out of 19 women were terminated, despite using an infusion time of 13.6 hours; in 28 patients in the 13th-20th week of gestation, abortion was only induced in 4 patients. From this study it would, therefore, appear that the greatest degree of success and the shortest induction/abortion interval is obtained during the early stages of gestation.

The frequency of side effects were directly related to the dose of $PGF_{2\alpha}$ administered. At a dose rate of 50 μg per minute, 12% had nausea or diarrhoea and at 75 µg per minute, 30% had nausea and/or diarrhoea. They suggested that the dose range which induced effective uterine contractions was very similar to the dose producing generalised side effects. Karim and Filshie (1970a, b) experienced a higher rate of side effects when a dose of 50 µg per minute $PGF_{2\alpha}$ was administered; over 40% had diarrhoea.

Hillier and Embrey (1972) administered increasing doses of $PGE_2$ (2.5-20 µg per minute) and $PGF_{2\alpha}$ (5-200 µg per minute) for periods of up to 24 hours; 4 out of 9 patients receiving $PGE_2$ and 5 out of 10 receiving $PGF_{2\alpha}$, failed to abort. Side effects were similar to those reported by Karim and Filshie (1970a, b) but the incidence was greater.

Blood samples taken prior to the infusion, at the optimum dose and 12 hours after infusion, failed to show any significant changes in blood urea nitrogen, SGOT, alkaline phosphatase, total bilirubin, blood glucose, haematocrit, haemoglobin, platelet count, serum sodium, potassium and chloride. Neither albuminuria nor glycosuria developed. During the infusion there was no significant change in the plasma level of progesterone but in the post abortion sample, the levels had fallen to normal post-partum values. Similar findings have been reported by Karim and Filshie, 1972. In 6 of 11 patients examined, a mild neutrophil leucocytosis was seen with a corresponding relative fall in the lymphocyte count.

Six cases infused with $PGE_2$ and 5 with $PGF_{2\alpha}$ exhibited a local irritation and inflammation in the infusion arm; this was slight with $PGF_{2\alpha}$ but was severe in 2 cases with $PGE_2$. It was not diminished with hydrocortisone or an anti-histamine given systemically. Intra-ocular pressure, measured with a Schiötz tonometer, in 3 cases receiving $PGE_2$ and 3 receiving $PGF_{2\alpha}$ showed no alteration other than diurnal variation (Hillier and Embrey, 1972).

In some cases it has been shown that relatively low doses of prostaglandins given for short periods of time may result in abortion. For instance, Embrey (1970a) infused 2 patients at 9 and 10 weeks respectively with 2-3 µg per minute of $PGE_2$. The total infusion time in one case was 2¼ hours and in the other, 6 hours. The former patient failed to abort but the latter went on to abort after 24 hours. Another case at 28 weeks, infused with 2-4 µg of $PGE_2$ for 12 hours, went on to abort after 27 hours.

The high abortion success rate with moderate dosage infusion found by Karim and Filshie (1970a, b) and Embrey (1970a) contrasts markedly with the low rate of success reported by Wiqvist and Bygdeman (1970a, b). In order to achieve a high success rate the latter workers found it necessary to employ a mean infusion rate of 100 µg per minute of $PGF_{2\alpha}$.

The effect upon the uterine response of varying the route of administration of prostaglandins has been studied (Bygdeman *et al.,* 1970; Roth-Brandel *et al.,* 1970a; Karim *et al.,* 1971b; Wiqvist and Bygdeman, 1970b; Wiqvist, *et al.,* 1968). They have shown, in the mid-trimester, that single intravenous injections predominantly increase the tone of the uterus. Wiqvist *et al.* (1968) obtained a threshold dose for $PGE_1$ and $PGE_2$ of about 20-100 $\mu$g and a duration of effect from 18-40 minutes. No side effects were observed below 75 $\mu$g, but above this transient nausea and in one case an increase in pulse rate occurred. These results were confirmed by Roth-Brandel *et al.* (1970b) who showed that, at 10-20 weeks gestation, 100 $\mu$g of $PGE_1$ produced a marked increase in tone and this was of the same order as that produced by three international units of oxytocin. However, the time taken for the increase in tone, produced by prostaglandin, to decay to one half of its maximum elevated value was twice that of oxytocin. The time taken for the prostaglandin response to return to its basal level was 40-50 minutes.

The elevation in tone with $PGE_1$ was greater than oxytocin in the first and second trimester but the difference was only significant in the first trimester. No patients vomited but those receiving prostaglandins experienced a sensation of irritation in the throat and a feeling of warmness.

The effect of single intravenous injections of $PGF_{1\alpha}$ and $PGF_{2\alpha}$ is very similar to that of E compounds, although the former are less active; the mid-trimester threshold for $PGF_{1\alpha}$ being 200-500 $\mu$g and for $PGF_{2\alpha}$ around 100 $\mu$g. Thus, in mid-pregnancy, $PGF_{2\alpha}$ is about 8 times and $PGF_{1\alpha}$ 30-40 times less active than $PGE_1$ (Bygdeman *et al.,* 1970). These authors also suggested that $PGF_{2\alpha}$ was more active on the mid-trimester uterus than on the term uterus although only one injection of 100 $\mu$g was given to a full term patient.

The response manifested was a rapid elevation of uterine tone followed by a gradual return to the normal resting level. During the phase of relaxation contractions of increasing amplitude were superimposed upon the diminishing tone. The magnitude of the tone elevation as well as the duration of the response were dose dependent. Doses of $PGF_{1\alpha}$, up to 750 $\mu$g, produced no subjective side effects and had no influence on pulse rate or blood pressure. 500 $\mu$g of $PGF_{2\alpha}$, or above, however, caused subjective side effects in terms of chest discomfort and occasionally vomiting. No alteration in blood pressure was noted although in 5 out of 7 cases, a slight increase in pulse rate was noted. In contrast, Karim, Somers and Hillier (1971) have shown that 500 $\mu$g of $PGF_{2\alpha}$ given as a single intravenous injection produces an appreciable increase in arterial blood pressure lasting several minutes. Overall the effect of single intravenous injections of prostaglandins is relatively short-lived.

*(ii) The Intramuscular Route*

Prostaglandins are active when administered by the intramuscular route (Wiqvist *et al.,* 1968; Karim *et al.,* 1971b). A relative comparison of the intravenous or intramuscular routes shows that with the latter the onset of the response is delayed and is prolonged compared with the former. However, the side effects with the intramuscular route are concomitantly less, thus larger doses can be administered and this route has been used successfully for the attempted induction of abortion.

If the dose of $PGE_2$ administered intramuscularly is sufficiently large (1-2 mg) then the response of the uterus can be almost instantaneous, albeit this was shown on the non-pregnant uterus (Karim *et al.,* 1971b).

*(iii) Subcutaneous Route*

The effect of prostaglandins when given by the subcutaneous route has been little studied. Karim *et al.* (1971b) showed that subcutaneous injections of 10 mg of $PGF_{2\alpha}$ or 2 mg of $PGE_2$ given at mid-pregnancy, resulted in an almost immediate increase in the tone, frequency and amplitude of contraction; the duration of effect was from 2-3 hours (Fig. 4). With a total of six injections at 3-hourly intervals, it was possible to terminate two of four pregnancies at 14-18 weeks gestation. In the remaining two women, pregnancy was subsequently terminated with infusions of $PGE_2$ at a rate of 5 $\mu$g per minute. All patients experienced pain at the site of injection.

Roth-Brandel *et al.* (1970c) injected subcutaneous doses of 5 $\mu$g $PGF_{2\alpha}$ in four women at 13-18 weeks gestation; 5-6 injections per day were given every third hour for two days. Following this regime only one out of four women aborted. The stimulating effect of each injection usually lasted 1-2 hours. Subjective side effects of nausea and diarrhoea were noted in some of the patients on high doses but no details were given. No comment was made on pain at the site of injection.

Both the subcutaneous and the intramuscular injections are extremely painful and, at present, do not seem to be suitable routes of administration (Karim *et al.,* 1971b). However, with increased knowledge of the distribution of prostaglandins in tissue and the possible development of slow-release compounds or different vehicles for the injection, these may become suitable in the future.

*(iv) The Intra-amniotic Route*

Prostaglandins injected into the amniotic sac in three women at a dose of only 75 $\mu$g $PGE_1$ (Wiqvist *et al.,* 1968) had no effect on the uterus. Karim and Sharma (1971c) however, have shown that with intra-amniotic injection of 5 $\mu$g $PGE_2$ or 25 $\mu$g $PGF_{2\alpha}$ it is often possible to terminate a second trimester pregnancy with a single injection.

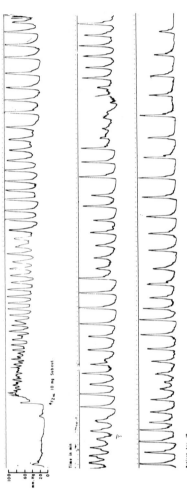

Fig. 4. Continuous record of the effect of a subcutaneous injection of 10 mg prostaglandin $F_{2\alpha}$ on the intact pregnant human uterus at 14 weeks. Reproduced from Karim, Hillier, Somers and Trussell (1971), with permission of the publishers.

## (v) The Intravaginal Route

In order to reduce the discomfort and patient care needed with continuous intravenous infusions and to try to overcome some of the side effects of intravenously administered prostaglandins, local application of the drug into the vagina has been used for the induction of abortion, labour and menstruation. Karim (1971d) has reported induction of abortion in 45 women using either $PGE_2$ or $PGF_{2\alpha}$ as impregnated lactose tablets or in the form of pessaries. In the study, 30 women received $PGE_2$ at 7-23 weeks gestation using a dose regime of 20 mg every 2½ hours, whilst 15 women at 9-22 weeks gestation received 50 mg of $PGF_{2\alpha}$ at 2½ hour intervals. The average induction/abortion interval using $PGE_2$ was 12½ hours and $PGF_{2\alpha}$, 14¾ hours. The increase in intrauterine pressure manifested itself during the first 15-30 minutes of the first instillation of the drug (Fig. 5) and thereupon the pattern

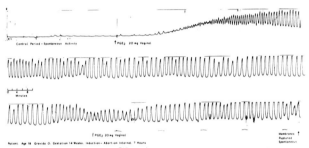

Fig. 5. Continuous record of the effect of intravaginal administration of prostaglandin $E_2$ on the pregnant uterus at 14 weeks. Reproduced from Karim and Sharma (1971a) with the permission of the publishers.

of response was very similar to that of an intravenous infusion (Karim and Sharma, 1971a). Table 2 shows composite results in 60 cases from Karim and Sharma (1971a and unpublished observations). The rate of absorption of $PGE_2$ and $PGF_{2\alpha}$ into the circulation from the vagina is not clear but Sandberg, Ingelman-Sundberg, Rydén and Joelsson (1968) showed that considerable but slow absorption of labelled $PGE_1$ from the vagina in the non-pregnant women takes place. Ten to 25% of the radioactivity was recovered in the urine within 24-32 hours. However, systemic absorption needs to take place before the drug can act upon the uterus, suggesting that the intravaginal route would suffer from no less side effects than the intravenous route, although it would be more acceptable and practical than the latter. However, the incidence of diarrhoea and vomiting seems to be considerably less with the vaginal route (Karim and Sharma, 1971a). Wiqvist *et al.* (1968) showed no effect upon the uterine contractility with vaginal instillation of 200 to 1000 $\mu$g of $PGE_1$. This was probably due to the low dose administered.

Table 2

Intravaginal administration of prostaglandins $E_2$ and $F_{2\alpha}$ for termination of pregnancy in 60 women.

| Parity | Prostaglandin | Gestation (Weeks) | No. of Women | Average Abortion Time |
|--------|---------------|-------------------|--------------|-----------------------|
| 0-9 | $PGE_2$ | 6-22 | 40 (1 failure†) | 17 hours |
| 0-7 | $PGF_{2\alpha}$ | 7-21 | 20 (3 failures†) | 19½ hours |

†No abortion

Lactose tablets containing $PGE_2$ 20 mg or $PGF_{2\alpha}$ 50 mg were administered every 2-2½ hours until abortion took place.

In six women abortion was incomplete and required evacuation of retained products of conception.

Data from Karim and Sharma (1971a) and unpublished observations.

### (vi) The Intrauterine (extra-amniotic) Route

Studies have been carried out whereby prostaglandins have been introduced directly into the uterine cavity via a small tube passed per vaginum between the amniotic membranes and the uterine wall. These studies arbitrarily found that instillations of the drug were required at intervals of approximately 1-2 hours in order to maintain a satisfactory level of uterine activity (Embrey and Hillier, 1971; Wiqvist and Bygdeman, 1970b).

Wiqvist and Bygdeman (1970b) studied 12 cases at 5-10 weeks gestation and one at 13 weeks. They instilled between 200-1000 $\mu$g $PGF_{2\alpha}$ in 9 cases and 25-75 $\mu$g of $PGE_2$ in three cases at 1-2 hourly intervals. Apart from the 13-week pregnancy the conceptus was completely or partially expelled. The interval between the first and last injections was between 2.5 and 9.3 hours, although the actual induction/abortion interval is not stated. In the only second trimester case, the interval between the first and last injection was 36 hours and, although dilatation of the cervix occurred, the conceptus was not expelled. According to these authors, side effects were virtually nil.

The study of Embrey and Hillier (1971) included 13 patients given $PGE_2$. Three of these were at 6-7 weeks gestation and the remainder, mid-trimester. In addition, two patients at 10 and 14 weeks received $PGF_{2\alpha}$. The dose administered was approximately 50-200 $\mu$g $PGE_2$ or 250-750 $\mu$g $PGF_{2\alpha}$ at 1-2 hourly intervals. Twelve of the 13 cases receiving $PGE_2$ aborted and the mean induction/abortion interval was 18 hours. The mean total dose of $PGE_2$ administered was 1177 $\mu$g. One patient at 17 weeks gestation, failed to abort after receiving intrauterine $PGE_2$ for 36 hours. Two other patients received a total of 3500 and 3800 $\mu$g of $PGF_{2\alpha}$ in divided doses. Ten of the 14 successful cases were complete whilst 4 were incomplete and the retained placenta or fragments were removed by evacuation. A further series of 15 mid-trimester patients (Embrey and Hillier, unpublished) in whom a Foley catheter was inserted and inflated to 35-40 ml and a similar regime for drug administration, successfully aborted but the induction/abortion interval was not reduced. However, the introduction of a Foley catheter increased the convenience of the procedure as thin Polythene catheters tend to be expelled by strong uterine contractions. It is noteworthy that Wiqvist and Bygdeman required only 1/10th of the usual total intravenous dose, whilst Embrey and Hillier required approximately 1/3rd of the total intravenous dose used in an earlier series at the same centre. The greater incidence of side effects observed by Embrey and Hillier (12 patients vomited and 1 patient had a loose stool) might reflect the higher doses used. The 2 patients receiving $PGF_{2\alpha}$ were symptom-free. (Table 3 shows results of intrauterine prostaglandins in 50 patients.)

Table 3

Induction of therapeutic abortion with intrauterine prostaglandins

| Prostaglandin | Patient | Successful Abortion | Failed Abortion | Mean Induction/Abortion Interval |
|---|---|---|---|---|
| $E_2$ | Primiparous | 19 | 1 | 22.3 hours |
| $E_2$ | Multiparous | 10 | 1 | 13.9 hours |
| $F_{2\alpha}$ | Primiparous | 12 | 1 | 21.4 hours |
| $F_{2\alpha}$ | Multiparous | 6 | – | 16.9 hours |
| | All primiparous | 31 | 2 | 22.0 hours |
| | All multiparous | 16 | 1 | 15.4 hours |

Complete abortions 39.
Incomplete abortions 11.
Results from Embrey and Hillier (unpublished observations).

In 8 of 14 cases, in which uterine activity was recorded, an almost immediate increase in uterine tone of 20-60 mm of mercury occurred. Gradually the hypertonus waned giving way to larger and usually frequent contractions (Fig. 6). In the remaining 6 cases there was little or virtually no increase in resting tone and the effect was essentially to produce a progressive increase in frequency and amplitude of

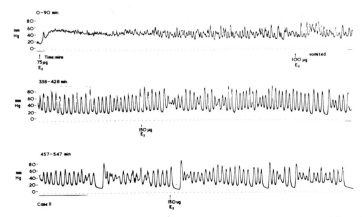

Fig. 6. Record of intrauterine pressure in a primiparous patient at 18 weeks' gestation. Doses of prostaglandin 75-150 μg were administered at approximately hourly intervals. Reproduced from Embrey and Hillier (1971) with permission of the publishers.

contraction. These two types of response did not appear to depend upon the gestation period but possibly represent a variable rate of absorption from different sites in the uterus. It is interesting to note that doses subsequent to those initially producing a marked hypertonus, did not continue to do so and it thus appears that a type of tachyphylaxis or tolerance to prostaglandins may develop. A similar observation has been made in non-pregnant women when a decrease in uterine sensitivity was observed upon repeated single intravenous injections at hourly intervals (Roth-Brandel *et al.,* 1970b). Uterine muscle fatigue or inertia may also play a part in this phenomenon.

Wiqvist and Bygdeman (1970a) showed that the uterus in the first trimester is more sensitive to intravenous $PGF_{2\alpha}$ than the second and therefore, abortion is much more easily induced during the first trimester. It is not yet clear, however, whether this is true for intrauterine and intravaginal routes of application (Embrey and Hillier, 1971; Karim, 1971a). Comparison of Wiqvist and Bygdeman's intrauterine results with those of Embrey and Hillier is difficult as the former workers used mainly $PGF_{2\alpha}$ and studied chiefly first trimester cases whilst the latter studied mainly the effect of $PGE_2$ on second trimester patients.

### (vii) The Oral Route

Oral administration of $PGE_2$ and $PGF_{2\alpha}$ has been found to be effective for the induction of labour at term. However, 10 times higher concentrations are required to stimulate the uterus in early pregnancy and at these dose levels, severe diarrhoea and vomiting occur (Karim, 1971d; Karim and Sharma, 1971b). For this reason it is unlikely that oral administration, in its present form will be acceptable for the termination of early pregnancy.

A W.H.O. sponsored conference held in Stockholm showed that, up to 8th March, 1971, a world total of 200 abortions had been induced with intravenous infusion of $PGF_{2\alpha}$ of which approximately 105 were complete. Prostaglandin $E_2$ was infused in 333 women and approximately 211 complete abortions were achieved. Intrauterine administration of $PGE_2$ and $PGF_{2\alpha}$ had been used for the induction of abortion in 60 cases of which 48 were complete. Sixty women, mainly in the mid-trimester, had been induced using the intravaginal route and 56 of these were complete. (W.H.O. Conference on Prostaglandins in Fertility Control, 1971).

The maximum acceptable intravenous dose of $PGF_{2\alpha}$ was subject to individual variation but generally was less than 100 $\mu$g per minute. Obvious side effects were vomiting and diarrhoea and local tissue reaction at the site of injection leading to venous erythema. With $PGE_2$ infusion the effective dose was 5 $\mu$g per minute and at this rate of infusion the incidence of diarrhoea was about 5%. Nausea, vomiting and venous erythema were evident.

The main problem that presents itself at this time with intravenous prostaglandins for the induction of abortion is the small difference in the dose required to stimulate uterine activity and that which produces side effects. This problem is mainly confined to the intravenous route and it is probable that the intrauterine, intravaginal and intra-amniotic routes of administration will furnish better therapeutic ratios. Side effects may be reduced by improvement in the drug formulation and drug delivery system. Some of the synthetic analogues now being tested may also prove to have a greater therapeutic ratio.

However, the alternative to a prostaglandin-induced abortion is either a surgical or intra-amniotic saline or glucose termination in mid-pregnancy. With greater experience, it is possible that prostaglandins will prove preferable to other methods of terminating pregnancy.

## 3. PREGNANT UTERUS AT TERM

*In vitro* Studies

Bygdeman (1964) studied the effect of total extracts of human semen on myometrial strips from one full term uterus. A dose of 0.025 to 0.05 units of seminal fluid extract stimulated spontaneous motility. The stimulation was, however, not linearly related to increasing doses of the extract. Prostaglandin $E_1$ in a concentration of 0.01 to 0.3 $\mu$g was without any effect.

The only other *in vitro* investigation on the effect of prostaglandins on term uterus was reported by Embrey and Morrison (1968). These authors studied the effects of prostaglandins $E_1$, $E_2$, $F_{1\alpha}$ and $F_{2\alpha}$ on 54 myometrial strips obtained from 29 uteri. Both $PGE_1$ and $PGE_2$ stimulated the upper segment of the uterus to contract. The strips from the lower segment were markedly less responsive to E prostaglandins. Prostaglandins $F_{1\alpha}$ and $F_{2\alpha}$ also stimulated the strips from upper segments whereas on the lower segment strips the stimulation was followed by inhibition.

## *In vivo* Studies—*Induction of Labour with Intravenous Infusions*

*F Compounds.* Karim (1969a) studied the effect of the continuous infusion of $PGF_{2\alpha}$ on the uterus in pregnant women at, or near, term. Initial studies were carried out in women with intrauterine foetal death and the infusion was at the rate of 0.05 $\mu$g/kg per minute. This usually produced uterine contractions after a latent period of 15-20 minutes and the pattern of uterine activity was found to be similar to that of normal spontaneous labour with complete relaxation between contractions without tendency to summation. The tone of the uterus did not increase. In the first series of 10 patients (Karim, 1968; Karim *et al.,* 1968) labour was successfully induced in all and this was followed by vaginal deliveries in 9 women with an average induction delivery interval of 6¾ hours. In the tenth case the foetus was delivered by Caesarean section for cephalo-pelvic disproportion. There were no side effects which could be ascribed to prostaglandin infusion and the babies were born in good condition. The third stage was normal in all cases. The above studies have since been extended to cover 100 women with successful inductions in 93 cases. The induction delivery interval has varied from 2¼ hours to 52 hours using infusion rates of 0.05-0.2 $\mu$g/kg per minute. In a separate study, it has been shown that $PGF_{2\alpha}$ infused at the rate of 4 $\mu$g/kg per minute in male and non-pregnant female volunteers is without any apparent effect on the cardiovascular system. However, 1 $\mu$g/kg per minute infusion does stimulate the gastrointestinal tract smooth muscle.

Embrey (1969) infused $PGF_{1\alpha}$ in one patient and $PGF_{2\alpha}$ in 5 patients at term. The infusion rate varied between 2 and 8 $\mu$g per minute but the duration of infusion was from 18-80 minutes. In spite of this brief duration of infusion, an increase in amplitude and frequency of contractions was demonstrated and labour was successfully induced in 3 women. There was no effect on the tone of the uterus and contractions began '15 to 30 minutes after infusion, and continued long afterwards, diminishing only slowly'. The maximum total dose infused in any patient was 200 $\mu$g. Of the remaining three cases, 'labour ensued within 48 hours in two'.

Roth-Brandel and Adams (1970) infused $PGF_{2\alpha}$ in 8 women. Each patient received $PGF_{2\alpha}$ at three different dose levels between 3.0 to 22.5 $\mu$g per minute for a total of 3 hours. With stepwise increase in doses these authors found that $PGF_{2\alpha}$ increased the frequency and amplitude of contractions but the increase in amplitude was small compared to the marked increase in frequency.

*E Compounds.* The effect of $PGE_1$ in four women at term was studied by Bygdeman, Kwon and Wiqvist (1967). The drug was given by continuous infusion at rates varying from 0.6 to 8 $\mu$g per minute. In term patients $PGE_1$, after a latent period of 15 minutes, stimulated the uterus to contract. The effect slowly disappeared after stopping the infusion. From a further study in seven patients, Bygdeman *et al.* (1968) concluded that with an infusion of $PGE_1$ and $PGE_2$ at rates of 4-8 $\mu$g per minute at term, 'the effect on amplitude and frequency of contractions was more dominant but unphysiological elevation of tone frequently occurred'. 'The latter reaction renders the E prostaglandins less suitable for induction of labour.' However, from the records of uterine activity and tables of results presented by these authors, there does not seem to be real evidence of frequent unphysiological elevation of uterine tones even at the rate of infusion of up to 8 $\mu$g per minute (Karim *et al.*, 1969).

Karim (1969a, b) and Karim *et al.* (1970) first reported on the use of $PGE_2$ for the induction of labour. These authors found that $PGE_2$ is about 10 times more active than $PGF_{2\alpha}$ in its uterine stimulating action at term. Thus, in a series of 50 cases, infusion of $PGE_2$ at the rate of 0.5 $\mu$g per minute induced uterine activity in all women after a latent period of 5 to 30 minutes. As with $PGF_{2\alpha}$ the prostaglandin-induced uterine activity was similar to that of normal spontaneous labour. Labour was successfully induced in all cases although in some cases the prostaglandin infusion had to be repeated on the following day. Two women were delivered by Caesarean section, one for foetal distress and another for cephalo-pelvic disproportion. Karim and associates have extended these studies and have induced labour with intravenous infusions of 0.5-2.0 $\mu$g per minute $PGE_1$ in over 500 women with a high success rate (Karim and Trussell, 1971; Karim, 1971d).

Embrey (1969) infused $PGE_2$ in eight patients and $PGE_1$ in one patient at the rate of 2-8 $\mu$g per minute. In spite of the very brief duration of infusion (maximum 75 minutes) labour was successfully induced in 7 of these women. Embrey considered the threshold dose to be of the order of 2 $\mu$g per minute (4 times higher than reported by Karim and associates) and 'in the range 2-6 $\mu$g per minute well marked oxytocic effects were observed in all patients'. The effect was essentially to increase both the frequency and amplitude of contractions. In one instance there was a transient increase in tone with 8 $\mu$g per minute which quickly disappeared when the infusion rate was reduced. 'No hypertonus was seen in any of the other tests.'

In a more recent publication, Embrey (1971) has reported the use of $PGE_1$ and $PGE_2$ for the induction of labour in 25 women at term. These include 9 cases previously reported and discussed above (Embrey, 1969). Of the additional 14 cases, 9 received infusion of 1 $\mu$g per minute (cf 2-8 $\mu$g per minute in earlier series) and in all labour was successfully induced. Four of the remaining five women were given 2 $\mu$g per minute and one, 3 $\mu$g per minute. From these studies and those of Karim and associates, it would appear that when infusion rates higher than 2 $\mu$g per minute $PGE_2$ are used, this may represent overdosage.

Another study on the use of $PGE_2$ for the induction of labour was reported by Beazley, Dewhurst and Gillespie (1970). $PGE_2$ was used in 40 patients between 29 and 42 weeks gestation and vaginal deliveries occurred in 37 women. In one patient labour was induced and the cervix dilated to 6 cm but the baby was delivered by Caesarean section for foetal distress. There were only 2 cases where $PGE_2$ in the dose used failed to adequately stimulate the uterus.

These authors commented that 'in our experience the effective dose of $PGE_2$ required to induce labour varied from patient to patient and we have demonstrated at least fourfold difference in the infusion rates required for patients near term'. They add that to initiate uterine contractions with $PGE_2$, it is more effective to commence infusion at 10 ng/kg per minute; (0.5 $\mu$g per minute for a 50 kg woman) and to double the infusion rate hourly up to 40-50 ng/kg per minute. These authors also reported transient uterine hypertonus in one case when $PGE_2$ was infused at the rate of 40 ng/kg per minute.

Roth-Brandel and Adams (1970) infused $PGE_2$ at a constant rate of 0.7 $\mu$g per minute in 13 women during a maximum period of 10 hours. Seven of these patients had 'normal vaginal deliveries as a result of prostaglandin stimulation'. One patient exhibited 'signs' of uterine hyperactivity which required termination of the infusion after 8 hours and 40 minutes. The membranes ruptured 90 minutes later and 'at the same time foetal bradycardia was noted and an immediate Caesarean section was performed'. The remaining 5 women were not given a further infusion of prostaglandin but labour was successfully induced in all cases with oxytocin the following day. It might be relevant to mention that in 3 of these 5 women who were 37-38 weeks pregnant, infusion of $PGE_2$ had resulted in some dilatation of the cervix.

In one woman, in the 39th week of pregnancy, $PGE_2$ was given at 0.7 $\mu$g per minute for 410 minutes and was interrupted due to 'irregular contraction complexes with periods of pathological tone elevation' (Roth-Brandel and Adams, 1970). Karim *et al.* (1970) have shown that such irregular contraction complexes and transient hypertonus are not an uncommon feature of normal spontaneous labour (see Karim, 1972). Table 4 shows a summary of the results from 500 women at, or near, term induced with $PGE_2$ and $PGF_{2\alpha}$ and Fig. 7 shows a typical trace from an induced labour at term.

Table 4

Summary of induction of labour with prostaglandins $E_2$ and $F_{2\alpha}$ in 500 women at or near term

| *Gravida* | *Prostaglandin* | *No. of Cases* | *Average Induction/Delivery Interval in hours* | *†Successful Induction* |
|---|---|---|---|---|
| 1 | $PGE_2$ | 56 | 12 | 55 |
| 2-13 | $PGE_2$ | 344 | 7½ | 342 |
| 1 | $PGF_{2\alpha}$ | 14 | 17 | 9 |
| 2-12 | $PGF_{2\alpha}$ | 86 | 10½ | 84 |

†Criteria for successful inductions:
 Stimulation of uterine activity followed by cervical dilatation.

$PGE_2$: 17 caesarean section:
        2 for failed induction; 13 for cephalopelvic disproportion; 2 for foetal distress.

$PGF_{2\alpha}$: 2 caesarean section.
        7 failed inductions (subsequently induced successfully with $PGE_2$).

Infusion rate: $PGE_2$: 0.5-2.0 μg per minute.
              $PGF_{2\alpha}$: 5.0-10.0 μg per minute.

Data from Karim (1971d); Karim and Trussell (1971).

## Double Blind Trials of Prostaglandins and Oxytocin for the Induction of Labour

Several double blind trials of prostaglandins and oxytocin for the induction of labour are in progress. In a trial reported by Karim (1971d) a total of 300 healthy normal women with normal pregnancies of 36-42 weeks of gestation and without any apparent complications were included. They were divided into three equal treatment groups of 100 women receiving $PGE_2$, $PGF_{2\alpha}$ or oxytocin.

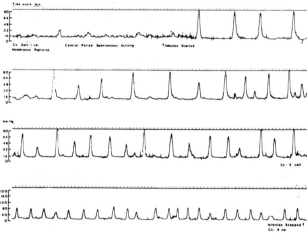

Fig. 7. Effect of an intravenous infusion of 0.006 μg/kg/min of prostaglandin $E_2$ on uterine activity at 36 weeks' gestation. Membranes had ruptured spontaneously 48 h previously. A normal vaginal delivery occurred 4 h 20 min after stopping the infusion. Induction delivery interval 7 h 30 min. Reproduced from Karim, Hillier, Trussell, Patel and Tamusange (1970) with the permission of the publishers.

The dose schedule for the administration of drugs is shown in Table 5.

The rate of infusion and therefore the administered dose was increased to the next higher level if, during the stipulated time interval of a given dose, adequate labour had not been induced. If the maximum dose had been reached, it was maintained until adequate labour had been induced, but not exceeding the 4 hours limit stipulated. The total duration of infusion was 12½ hours. Using the above protocol the successful inductions in the $PGF_{2\alpha}$, $PGE_2$ and oxytocin group were 67%,

Table 5

| Drug | Amount | Duration of Infusion |
|------|--------|---------------------|
| $PGF_{2\alpha}$ | 2.5 μg/min | 30 min |
| | 5.0 μg/min | 8.0 hours |
| | 10.0 μg/min | 4.0 hours |
| $PGE_2$ | 0.3 μg/min | 30 min |
| | 0.6 μg/min | 8.0 hours |
| | 1.2 μg/min | 4.0 hours |
| Oxytocin | 2mU/min | 30 min |
| | 4mU/min | 8.0 hours |
| | 8mU/min | 4.0 hours |

96% and 56% respectively. In all cases uterine activity was continuously recorded from a catheter introduced into the amniotic cavity.

Another double blind trial using $PGE_2$ and oxytocin for the induction of labour has been reported by Beazley and Gillespie (1971). There were 146 patients in each group. The dose of $PGE_2$ infused was between 0.21 to 6.7 $\mu$g per minute and of oxytocin 2.1-67.0 mU per minute. In spite of these high infusion rates, induction was successful in only 73% patients in each group. The reasons for the different results in the above two double blind trials may be related to the different dose schedule and criteria for successful induction followed by the two groups. Beazley *et al.* (1970) reported a successful induction rate of 95% using a much lower $PGE_2$ infusion rate. In a more recent study in which rapid infusion schedules were used for the induction of labour at term in 30 patients with intact membranes, Craft, Cullum, May, Noble and Thomas (1971) found $PGE_2$ to be considerably more effective than oxytocin in producing full cervical dilatation.

The results of other double blind studies, when available, may establish whether prostaglandins have clear advantages over oxytocin for the induction of labour.

## Oral and Vaginal Route of Administration

Following oral administration, $PGE_2$ and $PGF_{2\alpha}$ are absorbed into the circulation in quantities sufficient to produce a stimulant effect on the pregnant uterus at or near term (Karim, 1971c). Karim and Sharma (1971b) have used $PGE_2$ and $PGF_{2\alpha}$ given by mouth every 2 hours for the induction of labour. The dose of $PGE_2$ for adequate uterine contractions was 0.5-2.0 mg every 2 hours and that of $PGF_{2\alpha}$ 5-20 mg. The results of the first study involving 100 patients are shown in Table 6.

There have been no side effects with the dose schedule used. Karim and Sharma (1971a) have also used $PGE_2$ and $PGF_{2\alpha}$ administered intravaginally for the induction of labour. As with the oral route, the effect of each dose (0.5-2.0 mg $PGE_2$ and 5-10 mg $PGF_{2\alpha}$) lasts for 2½ hours and with repeated administration it is possible to induce labour.

## 4. INTRAUTERINE DEATH OF THE FOETUS

Intrauterine death of the foetus is usually followed by spontaneous contractions of the uterus and expulsion of its contents within a relatively short time. Retention of the products of conception, including the dead foetus, may, however, occur at any stage of pregnancy. This condition is termed missed abortion if the foetal death occurs before the 28th week of pregnancy or missed labour if the death occurs after the 28th week. Medical induction of labour is usually the treatment of

Table 6

Oral Administration of Prostaglandin $E_2$ for the Induction of Labour at Term

| Gravida | No. of Women | Average Induction/Delivery Interval | Average No. of Doses |
|---------|--------------|-------------------------------------|----------------------|
| Primigravida | 36 | 16½ hours (for 34 vaginal deliveries) | 7 |
| 2-9 | 64 | 9¾ hours (for 61 vaginal deliveries) | 4 |

Prostaglandin $E_2$ administered by mouth in a dose range of 0.5-2.0 mg every 2 hours. Three cases of Caesarean section for disproportion. In 2 cases $PGE_2$ failed to stimulate the uterus.

Data from Karim and Sharma (1970b) and unpublished results.

choice in these conditions and high concentrations of oxytocin have been infused with varying success.

### Missed Labour

In the series of induction of labour in 35 patients reported by Karim (1968) and Karim *et al.* (1969), there were seven cases of missed labour. $PGF_{2\alpha}$ infused at a rate of 3-5 µg per minute was effective in inducing labour and vaginal delivery occurred in every case within 24 hours. $PGE_2$ has also been shown to be effective for the induction of labour in cases of intrauterine foetal death in the third trimester. $PGE_2$ infusion at the rate of 0.52 µg per minute was successfully used for the induction of labour in 31 out of 33 such cases, with an average induction/delivery interval of 11½ hours (Karim, 1971d; Karim and Trussell, 1971). Results of 15 cases are shown in Table 7.

Filshie (1971) treated seven cases of missed labour with infusion of $PGE_2$. All delivered vaginally.

### Missed Abortion and Hydatidiform Mole

Karim (1971d) and Filshie (1971) used intravenous $PGE_2$ for the management of missed abortion and hydatidiform mole. Karim (1971d) infused 5 µg per minute in six cases at 19-24 weeks gestation. Foetal death had occurred 4-12 weeks beforehand. The case of hydatidiform mole was estimated to be at 20 weeks gestation. The induction/abortion interval varied from 2½ to 14 hours. Filshie (1971) also successfully

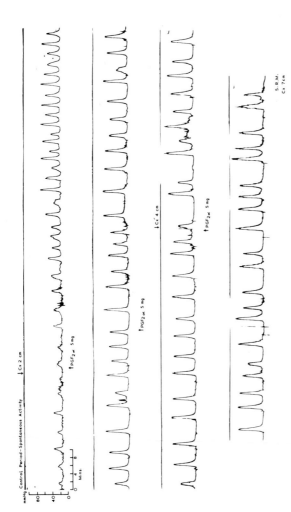

Fig. 8. Continuous record of the effect of orally administered prostaglandin $F_{2\alpha}$ on pregnant human uterus at term. $PGF_{2\alpha}$ 5 mg given by mouth every 2 hours until the patient was in established labour. Patient's age 24, gravida 2, gestation 40 weeks, induction delivery interval 9 hours. Reproduced from Karim and Sharma (1971b) with the permission of the publishers.

Table 7

Results of Treatment in 15 Cases of Missed Labour with Prostaglandin $E_2$ Infusion

| Case No. | Age | Parity | Gravida | Estimated Gestation (Weeks) At Death | Estimated Gestation (Weeks) At Delivery | Duration of Intrauterine Death (Weeks) | Infusion Rate (μg/minute) | Infusion Time (Hours) | Infusion/Delivery Interval (Hours) |
|---|---|---|---|---|---|---|---|---|---|
| 8 | 30 | 6 | 8 | 34 | 44 | 10 | 0.5 | 9 | 9 |
| 9 | 36 | 4 | 4 | 30 | 42 | 12 | 0.5 | 3½ | 3½ |
| 10 | 30 | 5 | 7 | 36 | 42 | 6 | 0.5 | 14 | 14 |
| 11 | 24 | 1 | 1 | 28 | 36 | 8 | 1.0 | 18 | 29½* |
| 12 | 24 | 2 | 2 | 38 | 42 | 4 | 0.5 | 7 | 7 |
| 13 | 38 | 6 | 8 | 40 | 44 | 4 | 0.5 | 11½ | 11½ |
| 14 | 26 | 2 | 2 | 34 | 42 | 8 | 2.0 | 6½ | 6½ |
| 15 | 32 | 9 | 9 | 38 | 42 | 4 | 0.5 | 4 | 5½ |
| 16 | 19 | 3 | 3 | 32 | 38 | 6 | 1.0 | 12 | 23 |
| 17 | 31 | 3 | 4 | 40 | 44 | 4 | 1.0 | 14 | C.S.† |
| 18 | 25 | 6 | 6 | 30 | 39 | 9 | 2.0 | 13¾ | 14 |
| 19 | 20 | 1 | 1 | 30 | 36 | 6 | 1.0 | 8 | 8 |
| 20 | 20 | 1 | 1 | 38 | 46 | 8 | 2.0 | 8½ | 12 |
| 21 | 24 | 2 | 3 | 38 | 42 | 4 | 0.5 | 10 | 13½ |
| 22 | 22 | 1 | 1 | 34 | 40 | 6 | 0.5 | 13 | 13 |

*Infused over two days.

†Caesarean Section for failed induction. $PGE_2$ infusion rate 0.5-2.0 μg/minute.

Data from Karim (1970).

treated five cases of missed abortion and one of hydatidiform mole with an infusion of 5 $\mu$g per minute of $PGE_2$ with a range of induction/ delivery interval of 1½ to 19 hours.

From these limited studies prostaglandins appear to be certainly more effective than oxytocin infusion for the treatment of missed abortion, missed labour and hydatidiform mole.

## REFERENCES

Beazley, J. M., Dewhurst, C. J. and Gillespie, A. (1970). Induction of labour with prostaglandin $E_2$. *Journal of Obstetrics and Gynaecology of the British Commonwealth*, **77**, 193.

Beazley, J. M. and Gillespie, A. (1971). Double blind trial of prostaglandin $E_2$ and oxytocin in induction of labour. *Lancet,* i, 152.

Bergström, S. and Samuelsson, B. (1962). Isolation of prostaglandin $E_1$ from human seminal plasma. *Journal of Biological Chemistry,* **237**, PC 3005.

Bygdeman, M. (1964). The effect of different prostaglandins on the human myometrium *in vitro. Acta Physiologica Scandinavica,* **63**, Suppl. 242, 1.

Bygdeman, M. (1967). Studies of the effects of prostaglandins in seminal plasma on human myometrium *in vitro.* Nobel Symposium 2, Prostaglandins (Eds S. Bergström and B. Samuelsson), p. 71. Almqvist and Wiksell, Stockholm.

Bygdeman, M. and Eliasson, R. (1963a). The effect of prostaglandin from human seminal fluid on the motility of the non-pregnant human uterus *in vitro. Acta Physiologica Scandinavica,* **59**, 43.

Bygdeman, M. and Eliasson, R. (1963b). Potassium and the reactivity pattern of the isolated human myometrium to prostaglandin from human seminal fluid. *Experientia,* **19**, 180.

Bygdeman, M. and Eliasson, R. (1963c). Potassium and the reaction pattern of the human myometrium to prostaglandin *in vitro. International Journal of Fertility,* **8**, 869.

Bygdeman, M. and Eliasson, R. (1963d). A comparative study on the effect of different prostaglandin compounds on the motility of the isolated human myometrium. *Medna exp.,* **9**, 409.

Bygdeman, M. and Hamberg, M. (1967). The effect of eight new prostaglandins on human myometrium. *Acta Physiologica Scandinavica,* **69**, 320-326.

Bygdeman, M., Hamberg, M. and Samuelsson, B. (1966). The content of different prostaglandins in human seminal fluid and their threshold doses on the human myometrium. *Memoirs of the Society for Endocrinology,* **14**, 49.

Bygdeman, M., Kwon, S. U., Mukherjee, T., Roth-Brandel, U. and Wiqvist, N. (1970). The effect of the prostaglandin F compounds on the contractility of the pregnant uterus. *American Journal of Obstetrics and Gynecology,* **106**, 567.

Bygdeman, M., Kwon, S. U., Mukherjee, T. and Wiqvist, N. (1968). Effect of intravenous infusion of prostaglandins $E_1$ and $E_2$ on motility of the pregnant human uterus. *American Journal of Obstetrics and Gynecology,* **102**, 317.

Bygdeman, M., Kwon, S. U. and Wiqvist, N. (1967). The effect of prostaglandin E$_1$ on human pregnant myometrium *in vivo*. Nobel Symposium 2, Prostaglandins (Eds S. Bergström and B. Samuelsson), p. 93. Almqvist and Wiksell, Stockholm.

Bygdeman, M. and Wiqvist, N. (1971). Early abortion in the human. *Annals of the New York Academy of Sciences,* **180,** 473.

Cockrill, J. R., Miller, E. G. and Kurzrok, R. (1935). The substance in human seminal fluid affecting uterine muscle. *American Journal of Physiology,* **112,** 577.

Clitheroe, H. J. (1961). The separation of three plain-muscle stimulants present in the human endometrium. *Journal of Physiology, Lond.,* **155,** 62.

Clitheroe, H. J. and Pickles, V. R. (1961). The separation of the smooth muscle stimulants in menstrual fluid. *Journal of Physiology, London,* **156,** 255.

Craft, I. L., Cullum, A. R., May, D. T. L., Noble, A. D. and Thomas, D. J. (1971). Prostaglandin E$_2$ compared with oxytocin for induction of labour. *British Medical Journal,* **3,** 276.

Eglinton, G., Raphael, R. A., Smith, G. N., Hall, W. J. and Pickles, V. R. (1963). The isolation and identification of two smooth muscle stimulants from menstrual fluid. *Nature, London,* **200,** 960, 993.

Eliasson, E. (1959). Studies on prostaglandin. Occurrence, formation and biological actions. *Acta Physiologica Scandinavica,* **46,** Suppl. 158, 1.

Eliasson, R. (1966a). Effect of posterior pituitary hormones on the myometrial response to prostaglandin. *Acta Physiologica Scandinavica,* **66,** 249.

Eliasson, R. (1966b). The effect of different prostaglandins on the motility of the human myometrium. *Memoirs of the Society for Endocrinology,* **14,** 77.

Eliasson, R. and Posse, N. (1960). The effect of prostaglandin on the non-pregnant human uterus *in vivo. Acta Obstetricia Gynecologica Scandinavica,* **39,** 112.

Embrey, M. P. (1969). The effect of prostaglandins on the human pregnant uterus. *Journal of Obstetrics and Gynaecology, British Commonwealth,* **76,** 783.

Embrey, M. P. (1970a). Induction of labour with prostaglandins E$_1$ and E$_2$. *British Medical Journal,* **2,** 256.

Embrey, M. P. (1970b). Induction of abortion by prostaglandins E$_1$ and E$_2$. *British Medical Journal,* **2,** 258.

Embrey, M. P. (1971). PGE compounds for induction of labour and abortion. *Annals of the New York Academy of Sciences,* **180,** 518.

Embrey, M. P. and Hillier, K. (1971). Therapeutic abortion by intrauterine instillation of prostaglandins. *British Medical Journal,* **1,** 588.

Embrey, M. P. and Morrison, D. L. (1968). The effect of prostaglandins on human pregnant myometrium *in vitro. Journal of Obstetrics and Gynaecology, British Commonwealth,* **75,** 829.

Euler, U. S. von (1934). Zur Kenntnis der Pharmakologischen Wirkungen von Nativsekreten and Extrackten männlicher accessorischer Geschlechtsdrüsen. *Arch. exp. Path. Pharmak.,* **175,** 78.

Euler, U. S. von (1935). A depressor substance in the vesicular gland. *Journal of Physiology, London,* **84,** 21P.

Euler, U. S. von and Eliasson, R. (1967). *Prostaglandins. Medicinal Chemistry Monographs,* Vol. 8, Academic Press, New York/London.

Filshie, G. M. (1971). The use of prostaglandin E$_2$ in the management of intrauterine death, missed abortion and hydatidiform mole. *Journal of Obstetrics and Gynaecology, British Commonwealth,* **78,** 87.

Goldblatt, M. W. (1933). A depressor substance in seminal fluid. *Journal of the Society for Chemistry and Industry, London,* **52**, 1056.

Goldblatt, M. W. (1935). Properties of human seminal plasma. *Journal of Physiology, London,* **84**, 208.

Hamberg, M. and Samuelsson, B. (1966a). Novel biological transformations of 8,11,14-eicosatrienoic acid. *Journal of the American Chemical Society,* **88**, 2349.

Hamberg, M. and Samuelsson, B. (1966b). Prostaglandins in human seminal plasma. *Journal of Biological Chemistry,* **241**, 257.

Hillier, K. (1970). Occurrence and actions of some prostaglandins in human umbilical and placental blood vessels. Ph.D. Thesis, University of London.

Hillier, K. and Embrey, M. P. (1972). High dose intravenous administration of $PGE_2$ and $PGF_{2\alpha}$ for the termination of mid-trimester pregnancies. *Journal of Obstetrics and Gynaecology, British Commonwealth,* **79**, 14.

Hillier, K. and Karim, S. M. M. (1968). Effects of prostaglandins, $E_1$, $E_2$, $F_{1\alpha}$ and $F_{2\alpha}$ on isolated human umbilical and placental blood vessels. *Journal of Obstetrics and Gynaecology, British Commonwealth,* **75**, 667.

Karim, S. M. M. (1966). Identification of prostaglandins in human amniotic fluid. *Journal of Obstetrics and Gynaecology, British Commonwealth,* **73**, 903.

Karim, S. M. M. (1967). The identification of prostaglandins in human umbilical cord. *British Journal of Pharmacology and Chemotherapy,* **29**, 230.

Karim, S. M. M. (1968). Appearance of prostaglandin $F_{2\alpha}$ in human blood during labour. *British Medical Journal,* **4**, 618.

Karim, S. M. M. (1969a). The role of prostaglandin $F_{2\alpha}$ in parturition. Prostaglandins, Peptides and Amines (Eds P. Mantegazza and E. W. Horton), p. 65. Academic Press, London.

Karim, S. M. M. (1969b). Effect of some prostaglandins on the pregnant human myometrium *in vivo*. Abstracts, 4th International Congress on Pharmacology, p. 337, Karger, Basel and New York.

Karim, S. M. M. (1970). The use of prostaglandin $E_2$ in the management of missed abortion, missed labour and hydatidiform mole. *British Medical Journal,* **3**, 196.

Karim, S. M. M. (1971a). Once-a-month vaginal administration of prostaglandin $E_2$ and $F_{2\alpha}$ for fertility control. *Contraception,* **3**, (3), 173.

Karim, S. M. M. (1971b). The role of prostaglandins in human parturition. *Proceedings of the Royal Society for Medicine,* **64**, 10.

Karim, S. M. M. (1971c). Effects of oral administration of prostaglandins $E_2$ and $F_2$ on the human uterus. *Journal of Obstetrics and Gynaecology, British Commonwealth,* **78**, 289.

Karim, S. M. M. (1971d). Action of prostaglandin in the pregnant woman. *Annals of the New York Academy of Sciences,* **180**, 483.

Karim, S. M. M. (1972). Prostaglandins and Reproduction: Physiological Roles and Clinical Uses of Prostaglandins in relation to human reproduction. In: Prostaglandins: Progress in Research (Ed. S. M. M. Karim), p. 71. Medical and Technical Press, Oxford and Lancaster.

Karim, S. M. M. and Devlin, J. (1967). Prostaglandin content of amniotic fluid during pregnancy and labour. *Journal of Obstetrics and Gynaecology, British Commonwealth,* **74**, 230.

Karim, S. M. M. and Filshie, G. M. (1970a). Therapeutic abortion using prostaglandin $F_{2\alpha}$. *Lancet,* **i**, 157.

Karim, S. M. M. and Filshie, G. M. (1970b). Use of prostaglandin $E_2$ for therapeutic abortion. *British Medical Journal*, 3, 198.

Karim, S. M. M. and Filshie, G. M. (1972). A study in the use of prostaglandin $E_2$ for therapeutic abortion. *Journal of Obstetrics and Gynaecology, British Commonwealth*, 79, 1.

Karim, S. M. M. and Hillier, K. (1970). Prostaglandins and spontaneous abortion. *Journal of Obstetrics and Gynaecology, British Commonwealth*, 77, 837.

Karim, S. M. M., Hillier, K., Somers, K. and Trussell, R. R. (1971b). The effect of prostaglandins $E_2$ and $F_{2\alpha}$ administered by different routes on uterine activity and the cardiovascular system in pregnant and non-pregnant women. *Journal of Obstetrics and Gynaecology, British Commonwealth*, 78, 172.

Karim, S. M. M., Hillier, K., Trussell, R. R., Patel, R. C. and Tamusange, S. (1970). Induction of labour with prostaglandin $E_2$. *Journal of Obstetrics and Gynaecology, British Commonwealth*, 77, 200.

Karim, S. M. M. and Sharma, S. (1971a). Therapeutic abortion and induction of labour by the intravaginal administration of prostaglandins $E_2$ and $F_{2\alpha}$. Journal of Obstetrics and Gynaecology, British Commonwealth, 78, 294.

Karim, S. M. M. and Sharma, S. D. (1971b). Oral administration of prostaglandins $E_2$ and $F_{2\alpha}$ for the induction of labour. *British Medical Journal*, 1, 260.

Karim, S. M. M. and Sharma, S. D. (1971c). Second trimester abortion with single intra-amniotic injection of prostaglandins $E_2$ and $F_{2\alpha}$. *Lancet*, 2, 47.

Karim, S. M. M., Somers, K. and Hillier, K. (1970). Cardiovascular actions of $PGF_{2\alpha}$ in man. *European Journal of Pharmacology*, 5, 117.

Karim, S. M. M. and Trussell, R. R. (1971). The use of prostaglandins in obstetrics. *The East African Medical Journal*, 48, 1.

Karim, S. M. M., Trussell, R. R., Patel, R. C. and Hillier, K. (1968). Response of pregnant human uterus to prostaglandin $F_{2\alpha}$-induction of labour. *British Medical Journal*, 4, 621.

Karim, S. M. M., Trussell, R. R., Hillier, K. and Patel, R. C. (1969). Induction of labour with prostaglandins $F_{2\alpha}$. *Journal of Obstetrics and Gynaecology, British Commonwealth*, 76, 769.

Kurzrok, R. and Lieb, C. C. (1930). Biochemical studies of human semen, II. The action of semen on the human uterus. *Proceedings of the Society for Experimental Biology and Medicine (New York)*, 28, 268.

Najak, Z., Hillier, K. and Karim, S. M. M. (1970). The action of prostaglandins on the human isolated non-pregnant cervix. *Journal of Obstetrics and Gynaecology, British Commonwealth*, 77, 701.

Pickles, V. R. (1957). A plain muscle stimulant in the menstrual fluid. *Nature, London*, 180, 1198.

Pickles, V. R. (1967). The prostaglandins. *Biological Reviews*, 42, 614.

Pickles, V. R. and Hall, W. J. (1963). Some physiological properties of the menstrual stimulant substances $A_1$ and $A_2$. *Journal of Reproduction and Fertility*, 6, 315.

Pickles, V. R., Hall, W. J., Best, F. A. and Smith, G. N. (1965). Prostaglandins in endometrium and menstrual fluid from normal and dysmenorrhoeic subjects. *Journal of Obstetrics and Gynaecology, British Commonwealth*, 72, 185.

Pickles, V. R., Hall, W. J., Clegg, P. C. and Sullivan, T. J. (1966). Some experiments on the mechanism of action of prostaglandins on the guinea-pig and rat myometrium. *Memoirs of the Society for Endocrinology*, 14, 89.

Pickles, V. R. and Ward, P. F. V. (1965). Menstrual stimulant component B, and possible prostaglandin precursors in the endometrium. *Journal of Physiology, London,* 178, 38P.

Roth-Brandel, U. and Adams, M. (1970). An evaluation of the possible use of prostaglandin $E_1$, $E_2$ and $F_{2\alpha}$ for induction of labour. *Acta Obstetricia Gynecologica Scandinavica,* 49, Supp., 5, 9.

Roth-Brandel, U., Bygdeman, M. and Wiqvist, N. (1970a). A comparative study of the influence of prostaglandin $E_1$, oxytocin and ergometrin on the pregnant human uterus. *Acta Obstetricia et Gynecologica Scandinavica,* 49, Suppl. 5, 1.

Roth-Brandel, U., Bygdeman, M. and Wiqvist, N. (1970b). Effect of intravenous administration of prostaglandin $E_2$ and $F_{2\alpha}$ on the contractility of non-pregnant human uterus *in vivo. Acta Obstetricia et Gynecologica Scandinavica,* 49, Suppl., 5, 19.

Roth-Brandel, U., Bygdeman, M., Wiqvist, N. and Bergström, S. (1970c). Prostaglandins for induction of therapeutic abortion. *Lancet,* 1, 190.

Samuelsson, B. (1963). Isolation and identification of prostaglandins from human seminal plasma. *Journal of Biological Chemistry,* 238, 3229.

Sandberg, F., Ingelman-Sundberg, A. and Rydén, G. (1963a). The effect of prostaglandin $E_1$ on the human uterus and the fallopian tubes *in vitro. Acta Obstetricia et Gynecologica Scandinavica,* 42, 269.

Sandberg, F., Ingelman-Sundberg, A. and Rydén, G. (1963b). The effect of purified prostaglandin $E_1$ on the human uterus and tubes. *International Journal of Fertility,* 8, 869.

Sandberg, F., Ingelman-Sundberg, A. and Rydén, G. (1964). The effect of prostaglandin $E_2$ and $E_3$ on the human uterus and fallopian tubes *in vitro. Acta Obstetricia et Gynecologica Scandinavica,* 43, 95.

Sandberg, F., Ingelman-Sundberg, A. and Rydén, G. (1965). The effect of prostaglandin $F_{1\alpha}$, $F_{1\beta}$, $F_{2\alpha}$ and $F_{2\beta}$ on the human uterus and the fallopian tubes *in vitro. Acta Obstetricia et Gynecologica Scandinavica,* 44, 585.

Sandberg, F., Ingelman-Sundberg, G., Rydén, G. and Joelsson, l. (1968). The absorption of tritium labelled prostaglandin $E_2$ from the vagina of non-pregnant women. *Acta Obstetricia et Gynecologica Scandinavica,* 47, 22.

World Health Organisation Conference. Prostaglandins in Fertility Control (Ed. K. Hillier). Research and Training Centre on Human Reproduction, Karolinska Institutet, Stockholm, March 8-10, 1971.

Wiqvist, N. and Bygdeman, (1970a). Induction of therapeutic abortion with intravenous prostaglandin $F_{2\alpha}$ *Lancet,* 1, 889.

Wiqvist, N. and Bygdeman, M. (1970b). Therapeutic abortion by local administration of prostaglandin. *Lancet,* 2, 716.

Wiqvist, N., Bygdeman, M., Kwon, S. U., Mukherjee, T. and Roth-Brandel, U. (1968). Effect of prostaglandin $E_2$ on the mid-pregnant human uterus. *American Journal of Obstetrics and Gynecology,* 102, 327.

# CHAPTER VI

# Vasoactive and Anti-hypertensive Effects of Prostaglandins and other Renomedullary Lipids

E. E. Muirhead

The normal kidney appears to exert a protective action toward hypertension (Braun-Menendez, Fasciolo, Leloir, Munoz and Taquini, 1946), recently termed the antihypertensive function of the kidney (Page and McCubbin, 1968). The specific nature of this function has not been elucidated. An earlier view that the kidney neutralizes pressor substances (renin [Braun-Menendez *et al.*, 1946], renotrophin [Braun-Menendez, 1958]) failed to materialize. To some (Ledingham, 1971; Borst and Borst de Geus, 1963; Guyton, Coleman, Bower and Harris, 1970) the kidney exerts its main antihypertensive effect by regulating external sodium and water balance and preventing fluid loads. According to this view, fluid loads cause expansion of the extracellular and intravascular volumes, thus increasing the cardiac output and by this means raising the arterial pressure. Under these conditions general autoregulation, possibly via myogenic reflexes of resistance vessels (Bayliss, 1902), may subsequently sustain the hypertensive state by increasing the peripheral vascular resistance. The vasoconstriction and concomitant decrease in venous return may lower the cardiac output to normal but at the expense of the hypertensive state. These haemodynamic views were well discussed recently by Ferrario, Page and McCubbin (1970). Others (Grollman, 1959; Grollman, Muirhead and Vanatta, 1949; Muirhead, Brown, Germain and Leach, 1970a, b; Green, Lucas and Floyer, 1970) support a more specific antihypertensive renal function, possibly of an endocrine nature, in the absence or reduction of which hypertensive mechanisms may be set in motion. Such a thesis would explain the absence of hypertension under conditions wherein the cardiac output is markedly elevated, as in anaemias, A-V fistulae and marked hyperthyroidism.

It is the purpose of this chapter to examine this controversy in terms of the renal medulla and its vasoactive and antihypertensive lipids.

## 1. ANTIHYPERTENSIVE FUNCTION OF THE WHOLE KIDNEY

In a modern sense, the Goldblatt experiment (Goldblatt, Lynch, Hanzal and Summerville, 1934) focused attention on the anti-hypertensive function of the kidney. Goldblatt and associates noted that constriction of one renal artery of the dog was associated with a modest and transient hypertension which became pronounced and sustained when the opposite renal artery was also constricted. Later, Goldblatt (1938) pointed out that the removal of the kidney opposite the renal artery constriction was also associated with a sustained elevation of the arterial pressure (now termed a one-kidney Goldblatt hypertension). The latter observation was confirmed for the dog by Blalock and Levy (1937), Fasciolo, Houssay and Taquini (1938) and Katz, Mendlowitz and Friedman (1938), and for the rabbit by Pickering and Prinzmetal (1938). Fasciolo coined the term 'the protective action of the normal kidney toward hypertension' to describe this phenomenon. When the rat was used in the Gollblatt experiment (Wilson and Byrom, 1939), it was noted that constriction of one renal artery often caused a sustained hypertensive state (termed a two-kidney Goldblatt hypertension). This was in part explained by vascular damage in the kidney opposite the arterial constriction. Byrom and Dodson (1949) made the important observation that removal of the clip constricting the renal artery of the rat at any time caused a prompt recession of the arterial pressure to baseline levels. Man with renovascular hypertension appeared to behave similarly to the rat (Maxwell and Prozan, 1962).

When additional hypertension-inducing experimental manipulations were developed, such as DOCA-salt (Selye, 1942), kidney wrap by either cellophane or a figure-of-eight suture (Page, 1939; Grollman, 1944), adrenal regeneration (Skelton, 1959) and salt-loading (Tobian, Ishii and Duke, 1969), it was observed that reduction of the renal mass by removal of one kidney potentiated the hypertensive state. Indeed, hypertension could be induced, under certain conditions, by a marked reduction of the renal mass as following uninephrectomy plus removal of the poles of the remaining kidney (Chanutin and Ferris, 1932). Thus, by the 1940's, it seemed that the presence of a normal renal mass blunted the hypertensive state while the reduction of the renal mass potentiated it.

Binephrectomy plus the intake of sodium causes hypertension (Braun-Menendez and von Euler, 1947; Leonards and Heisler, 1951; Orbison, Christian and Peters, 1952; Houck, 1954; Kolff, Page and Corcoran, 1954; Floyer, 1955; Ledingham and Pelling, 1970; Muirhead,

Jones and Graham, 1953; Muirhead, Stirman and Jones, 1959; Grollman *et al.,* 1949) and in the dog cardiovascular injury (Muirhead, Turner and Grollman, 1951; Kolff and Fischer, 1952) (termed renoprival hypertension). This hypertensive state is rapidly reverted by either perfusion of isolated normal kidneys (Kolff and Page, 1954; Kolff, Page and Corcoran, 1954) or whole kidney transplantation (Muirhead, Stirman, Lesch and Jones, 1956) despite maintenance of the sodium and water loads. Moreover, ureterocaval anastomosis (Grollman *et al.,* 1949; Floyer, 1955; Green *et al.,* 1970; Muirhead, Jones and Stirman, 1960a) and ureteroenteral anastomosis (Grollman *et al.,* 1949) prevent hypertension despite the same level of excretory renal insufficiency and the same fluid loads as following binephrectomy. Bilateral ureteral ligation, on the other hand, under the same conditions as ureterocaval anastomosis does not prevent the acute hypertensive state (see below). These observations suggested that sodium and fluid loads alone were not responsible for renoprival hypertension but rather that the absence of a unique non-excretory renal function made possible the influence toward hypertension of the sodium and fluid loads.

Perfusion of the intact donor kidney under hypertensive pressure not only reverts promptly sodium-loaded renoprival hypertension but reverts promptly also one kidney DOCA-salt (Gomez, Hoobler and Blaquier, 1960), Goldblatt (Tobian, Schonning and Seefeldt, 1964) and perinephritic (Kolff, 1958) types of hypertension. In some cases renal transplantation in man yields similar results (Ducrot, Jungers, Funck-Brentano, Perrin, Crosnier and Hamburger, 1960).

In summary, observations from various laboratories indicate that well perfused intact renal tissue opposes the hypertensive state as induced in experimental animals. Conversely, the reduction of the renal mass augments different types of experimental hypertension. The addition of well perfused intact renal tissue reverts several types of hypertension including that of man. Currently, a major question at issue concerns whether these antihypertensive influences of renal tissue are mediated by regulation of external sodium and water balance or whether there is a non-excretory antihypertensive renal function which, when deficient, allows hypertension-inducing mechanisms to operate.

The considerations below dealing with the renal medulla favour the non-excretory deficiency concept.

## 2. ANTIHYPERTENSIVE FUNCTION OF THE RENAL MEDULLA

The concept that the medulla of the kidney performs an antihypertensive function is based on five experimental models.

*Model No. 1* (Muirhead *et al.,* 1960a; Muirhead, 1962): Figure 1 summarizes results with this model which first suggested that the renal

RENAL ANTIHYPERTENSIVE FUNCTION AND SALINE LOAD

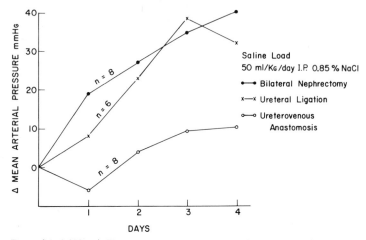

Fig. 1. (Model No. 1). Three groups of dogs yielded these data. Each received each day a high sodium load (about 7.5 mEq/kg) as saline intraperitoneally. One group had binephrectomy, one ureteral ligation plus contralateral nephrectomy, and one ureterovenous anastomosis plus contralateral nephrectomy. Ureteral ligation gave rise to the same level of hypertension as binephrectomy, while ureterovenous anastomosis protected against the hypertensive state. Modified from Muirhead *et al.* (1960a).

medulla might act as a structure performing an antihypertensive function.

Three manipulations were conducted on the dog and after each one the animal was given a high saline load intraperitoneally (50 ml/kg/day containing 7.5 mEq Na/kg/day). The three manipulations were: (a) bilateral nephrectomy; (b) ureteral ligation and contralateral nephrectomy; and (c) ureterovenous anastomosis and contralateral nephrectomy. Ureteral ligation, under these circumstances, gave rise to the same level of hypertension as binephrectomy while ureterovenous anastomosis protected against the hypertensive state. As indicated in Figure 2, bilateral ureteral ligation, under similar conditions, was also associated with a similar magnitude of hypertension. The point emphasized was that ureteral ligation was associated with extensive damage to the renal medulla and especially the papilla (Muirhead, Vanatta and Grollman, 1950) while ureterovenous anastomosis was attended by an intact and hypertrophied medulla. It was suggested that destruction of the renal medulla might be related to the sensitivity of the blood pressure to the saline load.

*Model No. 2* (Muirhead, Stirman and Jones, 1960b): This model was based on manipulations described diagrammatically in Figure 3. The left

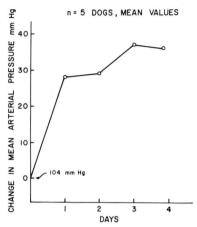

Fig. 2. Depicted are the changes in mean arterial pressure of the dog over four days time following bilateral ureteral ligation and a regimen consisting daily of saline intravenously (2.5 mEq Na/kg) and a diet containing about 3 gm of casein per kg. Hypertension was not averted by these manoeuvers whereas it was significantly blunted by unilateral ureterovenous anastomosis and contralateral nephrectomy as shown in figure 1 (Muirhead, unpublished).

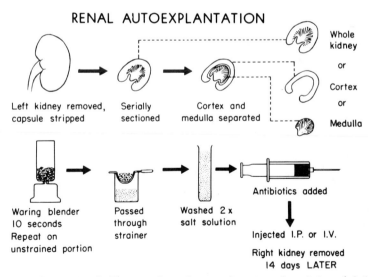

Fig. 3. (Model No. 2). The procedure of autoexplantation of renal tissue (whole kidney, cortex or medulla) as small particles is depicted diagrammatically.

kidney of the dog was removed and either whole kidney, dissected cortex or dissected medulla was fragmented in a small blender for a few seconds, washed, combined with an antibiotic mixture and injected back into the animal (medulla intravenously and whole kidney, cortex and medulla intraperitoneally). Fourteen days later the right kidney was removed, thus creating the renoprival state, and the animal was subjected to a hypertension-inducing regimen consisting of a saline load and dietary protein.

As indicated in Figure 4, the autotransplants of whole kidney and

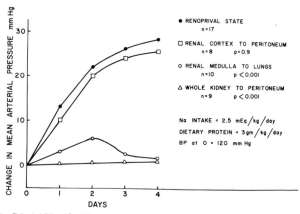

Fig. 4. (Model No. 2). The prevention of renoprival hypertension of the dog by fragmented whole kidney and renomedullary autotransplants is demonstrated. Modified from Muirhead *et al.* (1960b) by permission of the publisher.

medulla protected against renoprival hypertension while autotransplants of cortex did not. Thus, renomedullary tissue appeared to exert an antihypertensive action under these circumstances.

*Model No. 3* (Muirhead, Brown, Germain and Leach, 1970a, b): The third model dealt with a therapeutic rather than a preventive approach to the hypertensive state.

A one-kidney Goldblatt type hypertension was established in rats at the 'benign' level (tail arterial pressure 170 mm Hg). Then, either histocompatible fragmented renal cortex or histocompatible fragmented renal medulla was injected subcutaneously. Fourteen days later these transplants were removed.

While cortical tissue was *in situ*, the arterial pressure continued to rise (Figure 5). Conversely, while medullary tissue was present the arterial pressure dropped significantly and remained depressed as long as these transplants were present. Upon removal of the renomedullary transplants

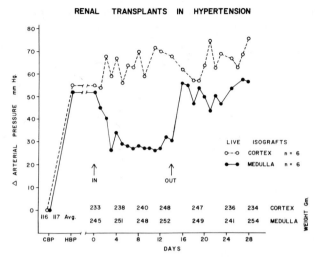

Fig. 5 (Model No. 3). Reversion of renovascular hypertension of the rat by transplanted fragmented histocompatible renal medulla is demonstrated. Renal cortex transplanted in an identical way failed to change the hypertensive state. Reproduced from Muirhead *et al.* (1970b) by permission of the publisher.

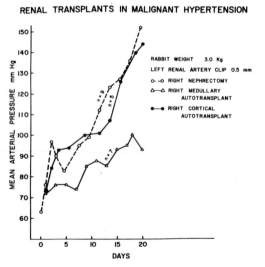

Fig. 6. (Model No. 4). Autotransplanted fragmented renal medulla prevented a lethal form of accelerated (malignant) renovascular hypertension of the white rabbit whereas autotransplanted fragmented renal cortex did not. Reproduced from Muirhead *et al.* (1972a) by permission of the publisher.

the pressure returned to the pre-transplant hypertensive level. This effect of renomedullary tissue depended on live cells since dead renomedullary transplants did not change the arterial pressure.

*Model No. 4* (Muirhead, Brooks, Pitcock and Stephenson, 1972a; Muirhead and Brooks, 1970): In the fourth model accelerated (malignant) hypertension of the rabbit was prevented by renomedullary tissue.

The stage was set for the accelerated hypertension by constricting the left renal artery with a rigid, narrow clip having a fixed gap (Brooks and Muirhead, 1971). When the right kidney was removed the mean arterial pressure rose to lethal levels (140-160 mm Hg) within three weeks. Autotransplanted fragmented renal medulla averted the lethal hypertension (Figure 6) while autotransplanted fragmented renal cortex did not. When the renomedullary transplants protective toward this hypertensive state were removed, the arterial pressure rose sharply and the animals died (Figure 7).

*Model No. 5* (Muirhead and Brooks, 1971; Muirhead, Brooks, Pitcock, Stephenson and Brosius, 1972b): This model demonstrated protection by renomedullary tissue against an extreme sodium-loading hyper-

RENOMEDULLARY  TRANSPLANTS  IN  HYPERTENSION

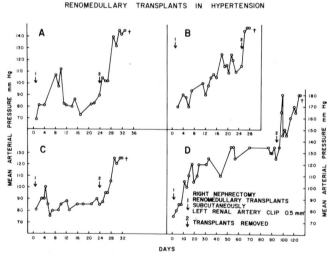

Fig. 7. (Model No. 4). The left renal artery of the white rabbit was constricted by the same narrow clip used for the experiments of Figure 6 and the medulla of the right kidney was autotransplanted subcutaneously. Protection against accelerated (malignant) hypertension was afforded for 22-24 days in three animals and for 90 days in one animal. At these times, the renomedullary transplants were removed. In each case, following ablation of the transplants, the arterial pressure rose sharply and the animal died. Reproduced from Muirhead *et al.* (1972a) by permission of the publisher.

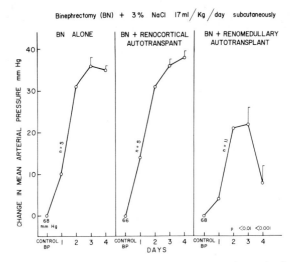

Fig. 8. (Model No. 5). In the panel on the extreme left is shown the development of renoprival hypertension of the white rabbit due to extreme sodium loading (about 9 mEq Na/kg/day). The middle panel demonstrates failure of renocortical autotransplants to prevent this hypertensive state. The last panel demonstrates the blunting and reversion of this type of hypertension by renomedullary autotransplants. Mean values are given plus the standard error of the mean for days 3 and 4. The p values refer to differences between the renomedullary group and the other groups for days 3 and 4. Reproduced from Muirhead and Brooks (1971) and Muirhead *et al.* (1972b) with permission of the publisher.

tension. There were three groups: group 1 had binephrectomy alone, group 2 had binephrectomy plus autotransplantation of renal cortex and group 3 had binephrectomy plus autotransplantation of renal medulla. The transplantation was performed 10 to 14 days before the second nephrectomy. Each group received daily subcutaneously 17 ml/kg of 3% sodium chloride (about 9 mEq Na/kg/day). The mean arterial pressure of groups 1 and 2 rose to +35 and +38 mm Hg, respectively, by the fourth day (Figure 8). The mean arterial pressure of group 3 lagged in elevation during the first two days, leveled off on the third day and returned to near baseline by the fourth day. The differences between this group and the first two groups were highly significant.

It appeared that the renoprival hypertension due to sodium loading was not solely due to haemodynamic changes, as contended by Ledingham (1971), Guyton *et al.* (1970) and others (Borst *et al.,* 1963; Merrill, Giordano and Heetderks, 1961; Dustan and Page, 1964; Ducrot, Kleinknecht, Jungers, Vantelon, Auvert, Zingraff and Funck-Brentano,

1970) but resulted from haemodynamic and possibly other changes attendant on the sodium excess but made permissible by the absence of renomedullary factors. This interpretation is in keeping with the observations of Green *et al.* (1970).

In summary, five experimental models involving three species (dog, rat and rabbit) support the view that the renal medulla acts as an antihypertensive organ, likely in an endocrine-like fashion. These models indicate an antihypertensive renomedullary action toward three types of hypertension, namely renoprival due to either a salt-protein regimen in the dog or extreme salt loading of the rabbit, 'benign' hypertension of the rat and 'malignant' hypertension of the rabbit. This antihypertensive effect of renomedullary tissue against a variety of hypertensive states seems to indicate a fundamental role of this structure in modifying the hypertensive state while also suggesting that a deficiency of the function involved may play a role in the pathogenesis of certain hypertensive states. Why the renal medulla modifies the hypertensive state in an extra-renal site and not within the Goldblatt kidney remains obscure. Some constraining influence on the renal medulla by the Goldblatt mechanism appears indicated but its nature (vascular, neural, biochemical, etc.) remains unknown.

## 3. VASODEPRESSOR LIPID (VDL) OF THE RENAL MEDULLA

As soon as the results of model No. 2 (described above) became apparent, crude extracts of dog renal medulla were prepared and these were tested for antihypertensive activity (Muirhead, Jones and Stirman, 1960c). The crude renomedullary extracts injected intravenously prevented renoprival hypertension of the dog due to the saline-dietary protein regimen and caused a prompt and sustained vasodepressor effect in hypertensive animals. Subsequent to this report, Lee, Hickler, Saravis and Thorn (1963) observed that similar extracts of rabbit renal medulla caused a prompt and marked vasodepressor effect in the prepared rat (under pentabarbitone anaesthesia, pentolinium-treated and with the vagi cut). Pursuing these results, Hickler, Lauler, Saravis, Vagnucci, Steiner and Thorn (1964) and Lee, Covino, Takman and Smith (1965) identified the principle as a lipid and suggested a relationship to prostaglandins. The extracted prostaglandin-like substance, which Lee *et al.* termed 'medullin', was identified as $PGA_2$ (at that time termed $PGE_2$-217) (Lee, Gougoutas, Takman, Daniels, Grostic, Pike, Hinman and Muirhead, 1966). $PGA_2$ or 'medullin' is unique in having a weak stimulating effect on gastrointestinal and genitourinary smooth muscle.

Later work clarified the nature of VDL. About 85% of the extracted renomedullary VDL consists of $PGE_2$, the remainder is made up almost entirely of $PGA_2$ (Daniels, Hinman, Leach and Muirhead, 1967). It is likely that this amount of $PGA_2$ is converted from $PGE_2$ during the extraction. However, it remains possible that small amounts of $PGA_2$ are available in the natural state.

VDL or prostaglandin identified as of the E series has been derived from the kidney of the dog, rabbit, pig, cat, rat, guinea pig and man (Daniels, 1971).

In summary, the indication that the renal medulla, as a tissue, possessed the ability to prevent renoprival hypertension led to tests of extracts of renal medulla for antihypertensive and vasoactive properties. As a consequence of such tests a vasodepressor lipid (VDL) was discovered in renomedullary extracts. The active depressor principle was subsequently identified as prostaglandin, mainly $PGE_2$.

## 4. THE RENOMEDULLARY PROSTAGLANDINS

It is customary to consider the 'renomedullary prostaglandins' as those compounds of this group which are extractable from renal medulla. Van Dorp (1971), however, demonstrated that the extractable prostaglandin is produced after the tissue is removed from the body, possibly during early autolysis. When the renal medulla was quickly homogenized little prostaglandin was extracted. These findings suggested that renomedullary prostaglandins, as those elsewhere (Pace-Asciak, Morawska, Coceani and Wolfe, 1968), are synthesized as they are needed. Nissen and Bojesen (1969) demonstrated a high concentration of the precursor of prostaglandin, arachidonic acid, within the medulla and especially the papilla. A deficiency of this essential fatty acid lowered the yield of $PGE_2$ from the renal medulla (van Dorp, 1971) stengthening the view that prostaglandins are synthesized *in situ* within renomedullary cells. Prostaglandins have not been derived from renal cortex. Moreover, the synthetase enzyme system for prostaglandin can be derived from medullary tissue (van Dorp, 1971).

The renomedullary prostaglandins are $PGE_2$, $PGA_2$ and $PGF_{2\alpha}$ (Figure 9) (Daniels *et al.,* 1967; Lee, Crowshaw, Takman, Attrep and Gougoutas, 1967; Crowshaw, McGiff, Strand, Lonigro and Terragno, 1970). As noted already, the prostaglandin most readily extractable from the renal medulla is $PGE_2$. Of these prostaglandins $PGE_2$ and $PGA_2$ are vasodepressor, apparently as a result of direct action on resistance vessels. In some species, $PGF_{2\alpha}$ elevates the arterial pressure possibly by constricting capacitance vessels (veins) and increasing the cardiac output while, in others, it lowers the arterial pressure.

In summary, three prostaglandins have been extracted from renal medulla. These are $PGE_2$, $PGA_2$ and $PGF_{2\alpha}$. Prostaglandins have not been extracted from renal cortex. The synthetase enzyme system for prostaglandins and the precursor of these prostaglandins, arachidonic

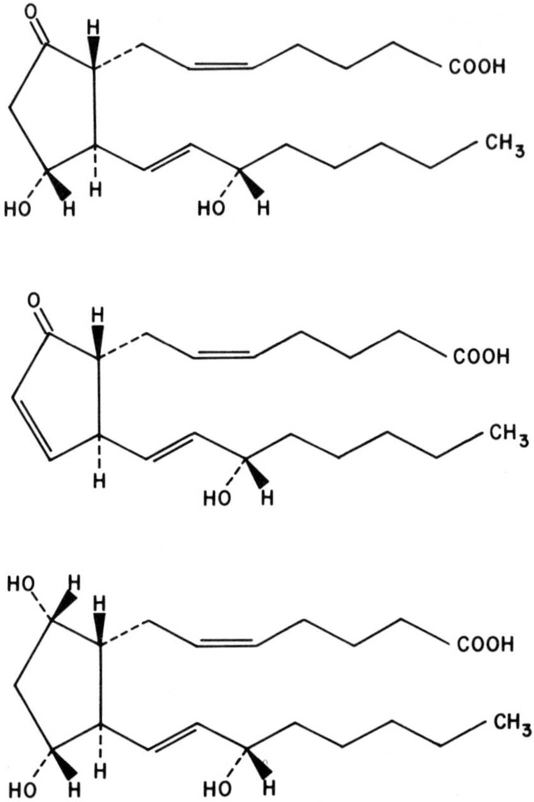

Fig. 9. These are the renomedullary prostaglandins.

acid, are present in renomedullary tissue. PGE$_2$ is the major renomedullary prostaglandin in terms of yield following extraction. It remains to be demonstrated whether PGA$_2$ is a natural product of renal medulla or results from the conversion of PGE$_2$ by dehydration of position 11 during the extraction procedure. PGE$_2$ and PGA$_2$ are vasodepressor agents while PGF$_{2\alpha}$ is depressor in some species and pressor in others.

## 5. CELLULAR SOURCE OF RENOMEDULLARY PROSTAGLANDINS

Indications are that the renomedullary interstitial cells are concerned with the synthesis of the renomedullary prostaglandins. The support for this view has been derived from histological examination, centrifugation and extraction.

The renomedullary interstitial cells (Figures 10 and 11) are located mainly within the interstitium of the inner medulla and between the vasa rectae, loops of Henle and the collecting ducts (Osvaldo and Latta, 1966; Muehrcke, Mandal and Volini, 1970; Tobian *et al.*, 1969). They form a ladder-like arrangement and have prominent cytoplasmic processes which orient themselves near the blood vessels and Henle's loop. Within the cytoplasm of these cells, including the processes, are prominent numbers of lipid vesicles. The lipid vesicles are membrane limited and on occasions appear to be within cisterns lined by ribosomal-like particles. The cells also have mitochondria and other organelles, a prominent Golgi apparatus, perinuclear and other cisterns and smooth and rough-lined endoplasmic reticulum.

Nissen (1968) and Nissen and Bojesen (1969) demonstrated the presence of simple saturated and unsaturated lipids within the lipid vesicles of the interstitial cells. The lipid droplets were then isolated by sucrose gradient centrifugation and were found to contain mainly triglycerides, cholesterol esters and free long chain fatty acids. The precursor of the renomedullary prostaglandins, arachidonic acid, was plentiful within the vesicles. These studies indicated a relationship of the

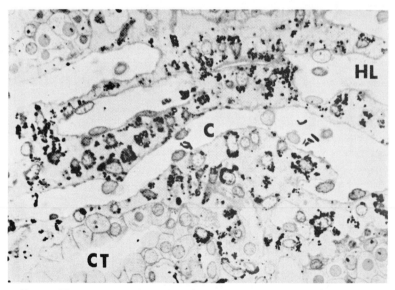

Fig. 10. The interstitial cells of the rat's renal medulla are shown when a semi-thin section (0.5 $\mu$) was stained with methylene blue-Azur II. The cytoplasmic vesicles containing lipids stain as dark granules. Note the extensions of cytoplasm as processes and location near a capillary (C), Henle's loop (HL) and a collecting duct (CT). Reproduced from Muehrcke *et al.* (1970) by permission of the authors and publisher.

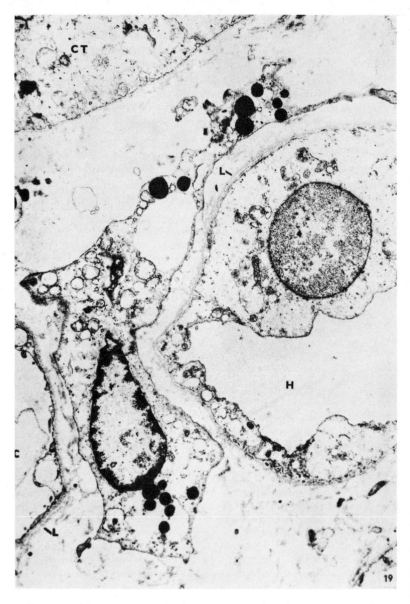

Fig. 11. An electronmicrograph of an interstitial cell of the renal papilla is shown. Note the elongated process, the prominent osmiophilic (lipid-containing) vesicles, two large cisterns, rough and smooth endoplasmic reticulum. The cell is interposed between Henle's loop (H) and a capillary (C). Reproduced from Osvaldo and Latta (1966) by permission of the authors and publisher.

lipid vesicles of the interstitial cells to the renomedullary prostaglandins. Bohman and Maunsbach (1969) also isolated the lipid vesicles of the interstitial cells and determined the presence of VDL, most likely $PGE_2$, within them.

In summary, it appears that the interstitial cells of the renal medulla are the cellular source of renomedullary prostaglandins. The prostaglandins appear to be within lipid vesicles in the cytoplasm of these cells which have processes in close contact with the vasa rectae and Henle's loop.

## 6. CARDIOVASCULAR EFFECTS OF RENOMEDULLARY PROSTAGLANDINS

The smooth muscle active principle in seminal fluid, discovered by von Euler (1934) and Goldblatt (1933) and termed 'prostaglandin' by von Euler (1935), was shown very early to be vasoactive. The intravenous injection of an extract of sheep vesicular gland into the cat caused a fall in arterial pressure but not if the animal was first eviscerated (von Euler, 1939). When prostaglandins were isolated and structurally characterized by Bergström and Sjövall (1957), the effects of the pure compounds on the cardiovascular system were studied in man and dog by Bergström, Duner, von Euler, Pernow and Sjövall (1959a) and Bergström, Eliasson, von Euler and Sjövall (1959b) and in the cat (Änggård and Bergström, 1963) and rabbit (Bergström and von Euler, 1963). Much of the earlier work resulted from the use of $PGE_1$. More recently, observations following the infusion of $PGE_2$ and $PGA_2$ became available.

Prostaglandins of the E and A series are powerful vasodilators when injected either intravenously or intraarterially (Horton, 1969). The dilator effect has been detected in most vascular beds. It is considered due to a direct action on vascular smooth muscle since relaxation of vascular strips from different viscera can be observed *in vitro* (Strong and Bohr, 1968).

The specific mechanism by which prostaglandins induce their smooth muscle activity remains controversial. The cell receptor thesis is usually invoked, i.e., that there are specific cellular receptor sites which, upon sufficient saturation, initiate the response through depolarization of the cell membrane (Khairallah, Page and Türker, 1967). Whether the mechanism is tied to the ouabain sensitive $Na^+ - K^+$ transport, the intracellular calcium pool or some other mechanism remains unsettled (Sunahara and Kadar, 1968; Strong and Bohr, 1968).

The direct action thesis has been subject to some challenge (see below under 'Prolonged Depressor Effect of PGE and PGA').

$PGE_1$ (Bergström *et al.,* 1959a; Steinberg, Vaughan, Nestel and Bergström, 1963) and $PGA_2$ (Lee, 1967) when injected intravenously in man as an infusion causes an increase in heart rate at a lower dose and a lowering of the arterial pressure plus the tachycardia at a higher dose. The tachycardia seems due to sympathetic activity since it is prevented by blocking sympathetic $\beta$ receptors while the blood pressure depression remains unaltered (Carlson and Oro, 1966; McCurdy and Nakano, 1966). $PGE_1$ and $PGE_2$ lower the arterial pressure of the dog (Steinberg *et al.*, 1963; Carlson and Oro, 1966; McCurdy and Nakano, 1966), cat (Horton and Main, 1963) and rabbit (Bergström *et al.*, 1959b) in a similar manner. It seems that an infusion high in the thoracic aorta is more depressor than an infusion low in the aorta and into veins (Carlson and Oro, 1966) (Figure 12).

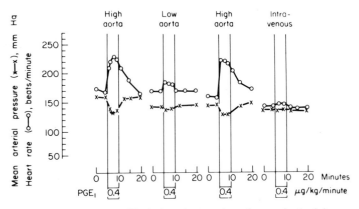

Fig. 12. The infusion of $PGE_1$ high in the aorta into the anesthetized dog caused a more profound vasodepression than the infusion low in the aorta or intravenously. Reproduced from Carlson and Oro (1966) by permission of the authors and publisher.

Injections of $PGF_{2\alpha}$ vary in different species. It elevates the arterial pressure of the dog and rat (Ducharme and Weeks, 1967; Ducharme, Weeks and Montgomery, 1968) but lowers it in the rabbit (Horton and Main, 1965) and cat (Änggård and Bergström, 1963). In the dog, the pressor effect was interpreted as due to venous constriction and a corresponding increase in cardiac output (Ducharme and Weeks, 1967; Ducharme *et al.*, 1968).

### Dose response to $PGE_2$ and $PGA_2$

As studied in the prepared animal, $PGA_2$ gave rise to a greater depressor effect in the dog than $PGE_2$ and a lesser effect in the rat (Weeks, personal communication). The effective depressor dose of $PGA_2$ in the rat was much lower than of $PGE_2$. These results were derived by the intravenous route and created problems in comparing the action of the two compounds.

The acute depressor effect is apparently dependent on the 15 OH radical (Änggård and Samuelsson, 1964, 1965; and Änggård, 1971) and is potentiated by the *trans*-double bond (Fried, Lin, Mehra, Koo and Dalvern, 1971). Upon one passage through the lungs, it is estimated that 90-95% of $PGE_2$ is converted to the 15 keto compound through the

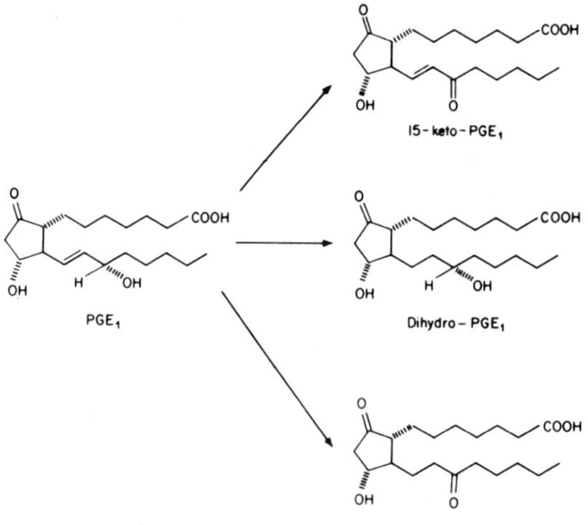

Fig. 13. This figure depicts the breakdown of $PGE_1$ by two enzyme systems described by Änggård and Samuelsson (1964) in lung and kidney tissue. The same breakdown is considered to involve $PGE_2$. 15-hydroxyprostaglandin dehydrogenase converts the 15 hydroxy to 15 keto whereupon the prostaglandin loses its vasodepressor effect. The second enzyme catalyzes the reduction of the *trans*-double bond at 13-14 position and converts the prostaglandin to the dihydro form. Reproduced from Daniels (1971) by permission of the author and publisher.

action of a specific dehydrogenase in pulmonary tissue (Ferreira and Vane, 1967; Biron, 1968). The 15 keto compound does not cause acute vasodepression (Figure 13). Conversely, conversion of $PGA_2$ to the 15 keto form is slow (McGiff, Tenagro, Strand, Lee, Lonigro and Ng, 1969). Thus, $PGA_2$ tends to circulate as a depressor prostaglandin longer than $PGE_2$. The 15 keto compound appears in the urine and is assumed to represent an end-stage metabolite. However, it remains to be demonstrated with certainty that the 15 keto conversion prevents all types of biological activity.

*Prolonged depressor effect of PGE and PGA*

Kannegiesser and Lee (1971) compared and contrasted the responses of E and A prostaglandins following their injection into the thoracic aorta in the anaesthetized cat. Results within the E series ($E_1$ and $E_2$) as well as those within the A series ($A_1$ and $A_2$) were comparable. Differences occurred between the E and A series.

Within pentolinium-treated animals the injection of the A compounds caused a gradual decrease in blood pressure followed by a slow return to the pre-injection level over 6 to 7 minutes. The E compounds, on the other hand, caused a prompt drop in arterial pressure followed by the same slow return. The drop in pressure afforded by the E compounds was significantly greater. Ganglion blockage augmented the early drop in pressure induced by A prostaglandins. As a consequence of this experience, these workers take issue with the concept that considers the depressor effect of prostaglandins E and A as solely due to a direct arteriolar dilatation; i.e., one due to a direct drug-smooth muscle receptor interaction. The early rapid fall in pressure by the E prostaglandins could be explained as a direct vasodilator effect but the sustained effect could not, since these compounds are inactivated by the lungs when the 15 hydroxy becomes the 15 keto compound. On the other hand, the lack of a prompt drop in pressure following the injection of A prostaglandins suggested little immediate vasodilatation while the prolonged effect could have been due to the long-lasting circulation of the 15 hydroxy form because of the slow conversion of this compound to the 15 keto form by the lungs. It was suggested that the vasodilatation produced by A prostaglandins and the prolonged effect of E prostaglandins might be mediated by an indirect mechanism, such as modification of the prostaglandin molecule giving it a different activity and the secondary release of other vasoactive compounds. In this connection, the Carlson and Oro (1966) observation of a more pronounced and prolonged depressor effect when $PGE_1$ was infused high in the thoracic aorta suggested, among various possibilities, a local effect such as an influence on baroreceptor activity. Moreover, the studies of Beck, Pollard, Harbo and Silver (1968) led them to postulate a 'third type' vasodilator system mediated via sympathetic nerves and giving rise to a sustained vasodepression. Evidence in support of mediation of this effect by prostaglandin of the E series was reported by these workers.

The depressor effect of $PGE_2$ has been studied in the spontaneously hypertensive rat (SH rat of the Okamoto and Aoki strain) following pentobarbitone anaesthesia, bilateral vagotomy and pentolinium treatment by Leach, Armstrong, Germain and Muirhead, 1971. $PGE_2$ evoked a more pronounced depressor effect while $PGA_2$ had greater sensitivity, evoking an effect at lower doses (Figure 14). Higher doses of $PGA_2$ appeared to make the animal temporarily insensitive to $PGA_2$ (tachyphylactic) while remaining very sensitive to $PGE_2$. Thus, $PGE_2$ in this system also differed in activity from $PGA_2$ and may have acted through different receptors on the same vascular bed, influenced a

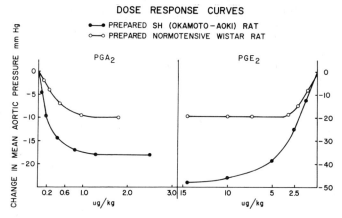

Fig. 14. The acute vasodepressor effect to increasing intravenous doses of $PGA_2$ and $PGE_2$ were compared in prepared SH and normotensive Wistar rats (anaesthetized, pentolium-treated and with vagi cut). Note that the scale for $PGE_2$ is twice the magnitude of that for $PGA_2$. $PGA_2$ caused a depressor effect at a lower dose but the depressor effect was less pronounced. The SH rat responded with a greater drop in arterial pressure. Reproduced from Leach *et al.* (1971) with permission of the publisher.

different vascular bed or operated through a different system such as an indirect system as suggested by Kannegiesser and Lee (1971) and Carlson and Oro (1966).

The SH rat, under pentobarbitone anaesthesia and intact vagi and ganglia, was injected intravenously with serially doubled low doses of $PGA_2$ until a pronounced acute depressor effect was attained (Leach *et al.*, 1971). This depressor dose was repeated two additional times at ten-minute intervals. Under these circumstances a unique phenomenon was observed (Figure 15). The mean arterial pressure slowly dropped (from 160-210 mm Hg to 125-160 mm Hg) as did the pulse rate. The entire phenomenon transpired over one half to one hour when a total dose averaging 4.85 µg/kg was injected. When the animal had the vagi cut and ganglionic blockade ahead of time, this phenomenon did not occur; rather the transient acute depressor effect lasting 5 to 7 minutes occurred. Cutting the vagi while the pressure was depressed, presumably under the influence of $PGA_2$, caused the pressure and pulse rate to rise to the pre-injection levels, whereas cutting the vagi while the pressure was elevated prior to injections of $PGA_2$ did not alter the arterial pressure to the same extent. These findings supported an indirect action of $PGA_2$ dependent on the intact vagi in this hypertensive state.

The earlier observations of Carlson and Oro (1966), plus the more recent results described by Kannegiesser and Lee (1971), and Leach *et al.*

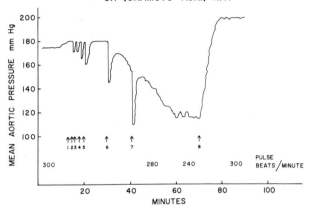

PROSTAGLANDIN A₂ I.V. IN ANESTHETIZED
SH (OKAMOTO—AOKI) RAT

Fig. 15. The response of the arterial pressure of the anesthetized SH rat of Okamoto and Aoki to intravenous injections of PGA₂ is shown as reproduced from a direct tracing. The conditions were: male SH rat, age 235 days, weight 380 gm, anaesthetic pentobarbitone intraperitoneally in two doses, 10 mg each (one, before aortic intubation, one before dissection of jugular vein), at 1 vehicle 0.08 ml of saline, at 2 0.16 µg/kg of PGA₂ at 3 0.32 µg/kg of PGA₂, at 4 0.625 µg/kg of PGA₂, at 5, 6 and 7 1.25 µg/kg of PGA₂, at 8 vagi cut. A dose effect was observed for the second, third and fourth doses. The same dose at 5, 6 and 7 gave rise to progressively greater depressor responses. After the dose at 6 and 7 the arterial pressure gradually declined to a low of about 120 mm Hg (original pressure 180 mm Hg). At the same time the pulse rate dropped from 300 to 240. When the vagi were cut at 8 the arterial pressure rose to 200 mm Hg and the pulse returned to 300 beats per minute. The paired control animal received pentobarbitone only. The conditions for the control were: male SH rat, age 237 days, weight 360 gm, pentobarbital 20 mg in two doses, the mean arterial pressure began at 160 mm Hg, became 170 by 40 minutes, 175 by 80 minutes, then 180 mm Hg until 90 minutes when the vagi were cut, thereafter it was 180 mm Hg. The pulse was steady at 300 to 320 beats per minute. Reproduced from Leach *et al.* (1971) with permission of the publisher.

(1971) indicate the need to pursue further the relationship of PGE₂ and PGA₂ to the control of the arterial pressure, especially in terms of possible mechanisms more complex than vasodepression due to direct vascular smooth muscle action.

*Effect of renomedullary prostaglandins on various vascular beds*

The vascular effect of PGE₁ thus far studied are very similar to those of PGE₂ and information on vascular beds, using these two prostaglandins, may be interchanged. At the present time, the same may be said of PGA₁ and PGA₂.

The intravenous infusion of the E prostaglandins in normal subjects causes a marked decrease in total peripheral vascular resistance (PVR) associated with an elevation in heart rate, stroke volume, cardiac output and venous return (Nakano and McCurdy, 1967) (Figure 16). The net effect is one of a hyperkinetic circulation while the arterial pressure is lowered. Less consistent but similar results have been noted with the A prostaglandins (Hickler *et al.*, 1964).

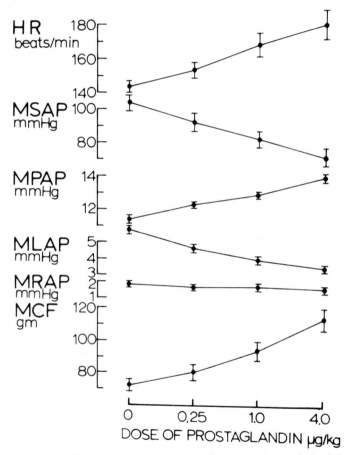

Fig. 16. PGE₁ at the doses indicated was infused into dogs and the following parameters were evaluated: heart rate (HR), mean systemic arterial pressure (MSAP), mean pulmonary arterial pressure (MPAP), mean left atrial pressure (LAP), mean right atrial pressure (MRAP) and myocardial contractile force (MCF). Reproduced from Nakano and McCurdy (1967) by permission of the authors and publisher.

(a) *In vitro* arterial effect:

Strong and Bohr (1968) determined the effects of prostaglandins ($E_1$, $E_2$, $A_1$ and $F_{2\alpha}$) on isolated strips of various arteries at doses of $10^{-11}$ to $10^{-5}$ gm/ml within the bathing fluid.

These compounds caused contraction of the aorta which became more pronounced with increasing dose. Similar results were noted using $PGE_1$, $E_2$ and $A_1$ and coronary artery strips. Strips of resistance arteries (mesenteric, renal and skeletal muscle sources) yielded a biphasic response, lower doses caused relaxation and higher doses caused contraction. Alpha and beta-adrenergic blockage and blockade with atropine, antihistamines and d-lysergic acid diethylamide failed to prevent the relaxation and contraction of the strips from these resistance arteries.

(b) Effect on vascular bed of extremities:

The cumulative experience with prostaglandins of the E and A series indicates the ability of these compounds, when infused directly into major arteries of entry, to cause marked arterial vasodilation in the extremities and a decrease in PVR (Lee, 1967; Nakano, Perry and Denton, 1968; Smith, McMorrow, Covino and Lee, 1968; Holmes, Horton and Main, 1963; Beck *et al.,* 1968; von Euler, 1936). The effect involves vessels of muscles and skin (Daugherty, Schwinghamer, Swindall and Haddy, 1968). The influence of $PGF_{2\alpha}$ has been subject to some variable interpretation as well as species difference. In the cat, $PGF_{2\alpha}$ dilates resistance vessels of the extremity. In the dog, $F_{2\alpha}$ increases PVR and decreased the blood flow but the mechanism of action is in dispute; some contended a venopressor effect (Ducharme *et al.,* 1968), others a direct action on resistance vessels (Nakano and McCurdy, 1968b).

(c) Effect on mesenteric and splenic beds:

A and E prostaglandins, including $PGE_2$ and $PGA_2$, following intra-arterial infusion, causes a profound vasodilatation of the mesenteric arterial system (Nakano *et al.,* 1968). Similar dilatation also occurs in the splenic arterial bed (Davies, Horton and Withrington, 1968). Neither response is opposed by alpha or beta-adrenergic blockage nor blockade of histamine, serotonin and acetylcholine receptors. This pronounced response led to the suggestion that splanchnic vasodilation was the main cause of the hypotensive effect of these prostaglandins (Smith *et al.,* 1968). These recent results support earlier results in the cat reported by von Euler (1939).

$PGF_{2\alpha}$ infused into the superior mesenteric artery of dogs caused an increase in PVR and a decrease in blood flow (Price, Shehadeh, Neumann and Jacobson, 1968). In part, this appeared due to constriction of hepatic veins (Nakano and Cole, 1968). Once more the F compound appeared to oppose the vascular action of the E and A compounds.

(d) Effect on coronary arterial system:

The E and A compounds cause coronary vasodilation and an increase in coronary blood flow (Vergroesen, de Boer and Gottenbos, 1967; Nakano, 1968). The effect of $PGF_{2\alpha}$ is controversial (Maxwell, 1967; Hollenberg, Walker and McCormick, 1968).

(e) Effect on pulmonary vasculature:

The pulmonary vascular bed seems also to afford a contrast between the action of the E and A prostaglandins and $PGF_{2\alpha}$. The E and A compounds increase pulmonary arterial pressure, apparently secondary to an increase in venous return and inflow load into the lungs (Nakano and McCurdy, 1968b; Ducharme *et al.*, 1967; Ducharme *et al.*, 1968). Although earlier observations were consistent with an increase in pulmonary vascular resistance, more recent measurements indicate a lowering of resistance in these vascular beds. $PGF_{2\alpha}$ seems to cause pulmonary vasoconstriction and by this means an increase in pulmonary arterial pressure (Änggård and Bergström, 1963; Hyman, 1968; Said, 1968).

(f) Effect on cerebral vasculature:

Infused into the carotid artery of dogs and rhesus monkeys, $PGF_{2\alpha}$ increased cerebrovascular tone seemingly due to vasoconstriction. This effect was not prevented by serotonin and noradrenaline blockade. $PGE_1$ caused vasodilatation and $PGA_1$ had no effect (White, Denton and Robertson, 1971). Spasm of cerebral vessels is a main complication of trauma to the brain and is especially noted following subarachnoid haemorrhage attendant on rupture of aneurysm of the circle of Willis. The brain is rich in prostaglandin which may be released under various conditions (Horton, 1969). These observations raised the issue of whether $PGF_{2\alpha}$ is the mediator of the local spasm following haemorrhage and trauma to the brain.

Infused into the carotid artery, E and A prostaglandins decrease cerebral vascular resistance and increase blood flow while $F_{2\alpha}$ acts conversely (Nakano and McCurdy, 1967; White *et al.*, 1971). The influence of carotid artery infusion on the systemic arterial pressure appears to be dose dependent (Alpert and Hickler, 1971), at lower doses causing no effect while at higher doses apparently increasing sympathetic tone and raising the systemic arterial pressure.

In summary, the response of various vascular beds to renomedullary prostaglandins appears consistent. Most results indicate a vasodilatory local effect by the E and A compounds apparently due to direct action on arterial and arteriolar vascular smooth muscle. This vascular dilatation is accompanied by a decrease in vascular resistance and an elevation of blood flow. The vascular beds so responding include those of the limbs, abdominal viscera, heart, lungs and brain. $PGF_{2\alpha}$, in general, acts conversely; i.e., it increases PVR and decreases the blood flow through most of these vascular beds. The site of action of $F_{2\alpha}$ remains somewhat controversial; the question is whether it acts mainly by venoconstriction or whether some increase in the tone of resistance vessels occurs.

## 7. EFFECT ON RENAL VASCULATURE AND
## RENAL FUNCTION

Renomedullary extracts containing VDL from the rabbit infused directly into the renal artery of anaesthetized trained dogs elevated the total renal blood flow (Hickler, Birbari, Kamm and Thorn, 1966). By the krypton-85 washout technique of Barger, it was demonstrated that the cortical renal flow increased by one-third while the medullary flow decreased by one-fourth. At the same time, the ureteral urine flow increased. During these observations, the mean aortic pressure dropped. These early studies demonstrated an active renocortical vasodilatation. After $PGA_2$ was identified it was infused into the renal artery under the same circumstances (Lee, 1968). The increase of renocortical flow and decrease of renomedullary flow was again noted and this was confirmed by autoradiography and sialastic injection. Infusion of $PGE_1$ into the renal artery of the dog also causes a pronounced vasodilatation and depression of the PVR (Nakano and McCurdy, 1967). Alpha-adrenergic blockade does not prevent this effect.

Prostaglandin of the E and A series, when injected directly into the renal artery of the dog, caused a significant rise in urinary sodium excretion, urinary volume, osmolar clearance, free water clearance and renal plasma flow. Urinary potassium excretion also increased (Herzog, Johnston and Lauler, 1968; Johnston, Herzog and Lauler, 1971). PAH extraction decreased. These changes occurred while the mean aortic pressure and glomerular filtration rate remained unchanged. The natriuretic effect was interpreted as occurring somewhat distal to the proximal segment (Figure 17). Atropine, vasopressin and $\alpha$- or $\beta$-adrenergic blockade failed to prevent these alterations.

The renal effect of $PGA_1$ during intravenous infusion has been evaluated in man with essential hypertension (Carr, 1970; Lee, McGiff, Kannegiesser, Aykent, Mudd and Frawley, 1971b). Low infusion rates (0.1-2.1 $\mu$/kg/min) did not change the systemic blood pressure but resulted in a pronounced increase in renal plasma flow, glomerular filtration rate, urinary flow and urinary sodium and potassium excretion. These results differed from those of Herzog *et al.* (1968) in that the GFR was elevated. At higher infusion rates the systemic arterial pressure fell and this was associated with a reduction in renal plasma flow and GFR, urinary flow and sodium and potassium excretion, all of which returned to near pre-infusion levels. Thus, renal vasodilation and natriuresis could be detected in the absence of a change in systemic blood pressure emphasizing again. the sensitivity of the renal vasculature to this prostaglandin. When the systemic arterial pressure was lowered by higher doses of $PGA_1$, the renal haemodynamic changes and natriuresis were offset and the antihypertensive effect was maintained while renal blood flow remained normal. Thus, the infusion of $PGA_1$ resulted in the production of normotension associated with normal renal blood flow

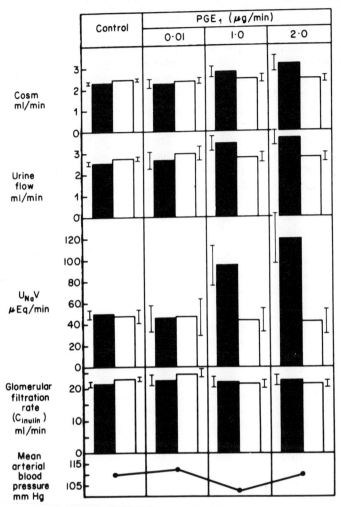

Fig. 17. Demonstrated are effects of the infusion of PGE₁ into the renal artery of dogs (black bars infused left renal artery, clear bars control right kidney). The results represent the mean values and standard error of the mean in 10 experiments. The osmolar clearance, urine flow and sodium excretion changed significantly while the GFR and mean arterial pressure remained unchanged. Reproduced from Johnston *et al.* (1971) by permission of the authors and publisher.

and normal sodium and water excretion but with loss of renal 'autoregulation' (Lee *et al.*, 1971b). This is interesting since other antihypertensive agents tend to compromise renal function as the arterial pressure is lowered. Moreover, prostaglandins are natural products and are synthesized within the kidney. They differ from other vasodilating agents which cause natriuresis (acetylcholine, etc.) in this important respect.

In one study in hypertensive man infused with $PGA_1$ (Carr, 1970), emphasis was placed on enhancement of free water clearance ($CH_2O$) and decrement of solute free water clearance ($T^cH_2O$) as the sodium diuresis proceeded. The sodium diuresis could have resulted from either increased GFR or decreased tubular resorption or both. In view of the increase in the excretion of the percent of filtered sodium, decreased tubular resorption seemed evident. The rise in $CH_2O$ most likely resulted from the increased delivery of sodium to the ascending loop of Henle. The decrement of $T^cH_2O$ was unexplained but could have resulted from a rise in medullary blood flow and reduced papillary tonicity. The latter is somewhat at odds with the krypton-85 washout results.

In summary, several lines of attack indicate that prostaglandins, natural products within the kidney, elevate renal blood flow and, at the same time, effect diuresis, natriuresis and kaliuresis. These effects may occur with doses which do not lower the systemic arterial pressure. Thus prostaglandins are powerful renal vasodilators. They differ from other vasodilators capable of similar action in being readily synthesized by renal tissue.

## 8. RELEASE OF PROSTAGLANDINS INTO THE RENAL VENOUS EFFLUENT

The concept that renomedullary prostaglandins are released into the general circulation is intriguing but inconclusive at the moment. There are some indications that this phenomenon may occur under special and abnormal circumstances. There is, as yet, no indication that the release occurs as part of normal homeostasis. The suggestion that $PGA_2$ released from the kidney into the general circulation may be an effective substance dilating resistance vessels, thus assisting in the prevention of a heightened pressure because it escapes inactivation of its smooth muscle activity by the lung, is offset by the observation of Horton, Thompson, Jones and Poyser (1971) that an isomerization system for the A prostaglandins exists in the plasma of several species. This system causes loss of depressor activity of the A prostaglandins but apparently does not operate against E prostaglandins. The isomerization seems to change the A compound into its inactive B isomer. $PGE_2$, the prevalent renomedullary prostaglandin, loses its depressor activity during traverse through the lungs and is not so attractive as a circulating, directly acting vasodilator.

The meager indications that prostaglandins are released from the kidney result primarily from four observations: (i) Hickler *et al.* (1966) claimed a reduction of VDL in the medulla of kidneys perfused under hypertensive pressure. (ii) McGiff, Crowshaw, Tenagro, Lonigro, Strand,

Williamson, Lee and Ng (1970b), using the Ferrerra–Vane super-fused blood-bathed organ technique (Gaddum, 1953), detected prostaglandin-like substance in the renal venous effluent following renal artery constriction. (iii) Edwards, Strong and Hunt (1969) reported the occurrence of VDL resembling $PGE_2$ in renal venous blood of the effected side in renovascular hypertension of man. The depressor lipid disappeared after surgical correction of the lesion. (iv) McGiff, Crowshaw, Tenagro and Lonigro (1970a) detected prostaglandin-like substance in renal venous effluent following infusion of angiotensin into the renal artery.

These observations are inconclusive since the methods of detection were crude and imprecise. This matter will remain unresolved until the problem of recovery and identification of prostaglandin at nanogram level is solved.

## 9. RENOMEDULLARY PROSTAGLANDINS IN HYPERTENSION

Very few experimental observations are available on the use of renomedullary prostaglandins in the hypertensive state. Although some of these observations suggest a beneficial effect the data available are insufficient for a definitive conclusion. There is need not only for more data from experimental animals but also for data dealing with the hypertensive states of man.

Muirhead, Daniels, Pike and Hinman (1967) reported the prevention of renoprival hypertension and the lowering of renal hypertension of the dog by renomedullary extracts containing VDL (Figure 18). These workers claimed the separation of two lipid moieties from renomedullary extracts; one was acidic and in time was identified as prostaglandin, and the other was neutral (Muirhead, Daniels, Booth, Freyburger and Hinman, 1965). When prostaglandin became available, these agents, including $PGE_2$ and $PGA_2$, prevented canine renoprival hypertension (Muirhead *et al.*, 1967). The lowest dose so active was 5 $\mu$g/kg/day of $PGA_1$ by mouth.

Hickler *et al.* (1966) injected intraperitoneally a rabbit renomedullary extract containing VDL daily into rats having renovascular hypertension. The arterial pressure dropped significantly (200 to about 125 mm Hg) during four courses of treatment in three rats. After cessation of the treatment the pressure returned to prior hypertensive levels over a period of days. These workers also noted a drop in the arterial pressure of similarly hypertensive animals when $PGA_1$ was injected intraperitoneally daily (25-100 $\mu$g) (Alpert and Hickler, 1971). Again, upon cessation of the injection, the pressure returned to the pretreatment level (Figure 19).

In a few observations, Muirhead *et al.* (1967) (Muirhead, Leach, Brooks, Brown, Daniels and Hinman, 1968a) noted a minor drop in

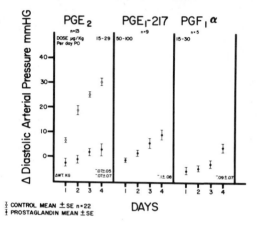

Fig. 18. Prevention of renoprival hypertension of the dog as induced by salt and dietary protein by three prostaglandins is indicated. $PGE_1$-217 is now termed $PGA_1$. Reproduced from Muirhead, Daniels, Pike and Hinman (1967) by permission of the authors and publisher.

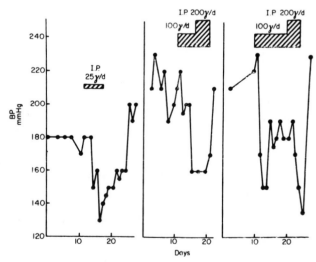

Fig. 19. This figure demonstrates the antihypertensive effect of $PGA_1$ in Goldblatt hypertension of the rat. There are similarities between these responses and those of ANRL. Reproduced from Alpert and Hickler (1971) by permission of the authors and publisher.

arterial pressure when prostaglandins were given daily by mouth to dogs with Goldblatt and Page types of hypertension. These workers observed a more profound effect on the hypertensive state when rats with a single kidney Goldblatt hypertension were injected with $PGE_2$ daily. However, it required a very high dose (over 1 mg/kg/day) for this effect and some animals developed an escape from the effect. A large dose (about 1 mg/kg) intraperitoneally to the hypertensive rabbit caused a drop in arterial pressure, requiring four days or longer to return to pre-injection level (Figure 20).

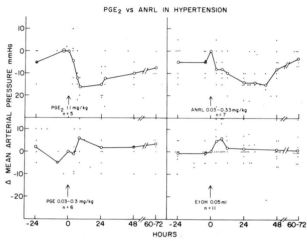

Fig. 20. $PGE_2$ in large dose intraperitoneally (1.1 mg/kg) lowered the arterial pressure of the rabbit having renovascular hypertension in a manner similar to that of ANRL in smaller doses. Reproduced from Muirhead *et al.* (1972b) with permission of the publisher.

More recently, Samova (1969) recorded the ability of both $PGE_2$ and $PGE_1$ to lower the arterial pressure of rats having a modest level of Goldblatt type hypertension. The prostaglandin was given intraperitoneally each day for 30 days (10-15 $\mu$g of $PGE_1$ and 20-30 $\mu$g of $PGE_2$). The average change in pressure for rats on $PGE_1$ was from 172 to 117 mm Hg, and for rats on $PGE_2$ from 155 to 113 mm Hg. The changes were analyzed as significant.

Lee and coworkers infused $PGA_1$ and $PGA_2$ (Lee, 1967; Lee, 1968; Lee *et al.*, 1971b; Westura, Kannegiesser, O'Toole and Lee, 1970) intravenously into patients having essential hypertension. Doses of 5 $\mu$g/kg/min of the pure prostaglandin caused a major drop in arterial pressure associated with tachycardia and increase in cardiac output, interpreted as due to baroceptor mediated reflexes. As soon as the infusion was discontinued, the arterial pressure reverted to prior hypertensive levels. Fichman (1970) noted a pronounced sensitivity in hypertensive anephric patients when low doses of $PGA_1$ were given intravenously (less than 0.5 $\mu$g/kg/min). This arterial pressure sensitivity of renoprival man is in keeping with the sensitivity of renoprival dog (Muirhead *et al.,* 1967).

In summary, the available data on the use of prostaglandins, especially renomedullary prostaglandins, in hypertension, experimental and in man, is much too fragmentary for a definitive interpretation. Thus, the use of these agents for the management of hypertension remains in doubt. Although a definitive answer is not available, there are interesting observations in the literature derived from various laboratories. These suggest a possible beneficial effect on renoprival and renal hypertension. The questions of dose, route and mechanism of action remain unsettled. Obviously, much more work and better standardization are needed in attempts to clarify this matter.

## 10. SPECULATIONS ON THE ACTION OF RENOMEDULLARY PROSTAGLANDINS IN HYPERTENSION

Assuming that renomedullary prostaglandins are concerned with the antihypertensive function of the kidney, several interpretations for their action have been considered.

Lee *et al.* entertained three different possibilities (Lee, Kannegiesser, O'Toole and Westura, 1971a). The first possibility considers that the renal medulla elaborates its depressor prostaglandins ($PGE_2$ and $PGA_2$) into either venous or lymphatic effluent of the kidney and these circulate and cause peripheral arteriolar dilatation. This would suppose a direct arteriolar smooth muscle effect. Splanchnic dilatation was proposed as the main site concerned with lowering the arterial pressure (Lee, 1969). A deficiency of these prostaglandins from this source would conceivably result in the preponderance of a pressor mechanism, increased peripheral vascular resistance and hypertension. As previously mentioned, this proposal will remain speculative until precise methods of measuring minute quantities of prostaglandins are available. The second possibility considers that prostaglandins may be synthesized at or near peripheral arterioles where they would be expected to cause a dilating effect. Following their action they could be degraded, either locally or in the lungs. The third possibility considers that renomedullary prostaglandins regulate the distribution of blood flowing through the kidneys. Since the renal arterial injection of prostaglandin appears to cause a shift of blood flow from the medulla to the cortex, it was reasoned that a local deficiency of prostaglandin might result in an increase in medullary flow and a corresponding decrease in cortical flow. The postulated intrarenal vasoconstriction would then cause the elaboration of pressor agents, such as from the renin-angiotensin system, which then would upset the pressor-depressor balance in favour of hypertension. This concept considers an acquired or genetic deficiency of renal prostaglandins as the basis of the hypertensive state (Figure 21).

Several problems evolve from Lee's speculations. The main renomedullary prostaglandin is $PGE_2$. This prostaglandin is rapidly inactivated as a depressor compound by the lungs (15 hydroxy to 15

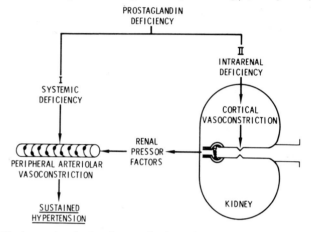

Fig. 21. A postulated role of prostaglandin in the hypertensive state. From Lee *et al.* (1971a) be permission of the author and publisher.

keto conversion). It appears incongruous for $PGE_2$ from the kidney to act on a major vascular bed such as the splanchnic bed and yet be mostly inactivated by the lungs. Besides, $PGE_1$ is more potent as a splanchnic dilator than $PGE_2$, and one would have expected this prostaglandin to be involved in such a mechanism. One can bypass this problem by attempting to assign the antihypertensive action primarily to $PGA_2$ which apparently is not so readily inactivated by the lungs. This contention has its problems also. $PGA_2$ is not readily recovered from the kidney. Mechanisms for inactivating $PGA_2$ may be present in the plasma by converting it to $PGB_2$, a non-depressor metabolite (Horton *et al.*, 1971).

There are problems, also, in the suggestion that renomedullary prostaglandins regulate renocortical blood flow. One can conceive of locally elaborated prostaglandins modulating the state of medullary vessels and by this means the renomedullary blood flow. But, the postulate is based on the ability of prostaglandins injected into the renal artery to cause a pronounced cortical vasodilation. A means of transferring the medullary compound into the cortical area is needed in support of this contention. Such a transfer has not been demonstrated.

The interpretation by Kannegiesser and Lee (1971) of a difference in the depressor action of $PGE_2$ and $PGA_2$ raises the issue of indirect mechanisms for the depressor action of these agents. An indirect action of renomedullary prostaglandins would offset the objection to the above proposed direct mechanisms. An indirect mechanism would explain more clearly the findings of Hickler et al. (1966), Alpert and Hickler (1971), Muirhead et al. (1968a) and Samova (1969) using mainly $PGE_2$ in renovascular hypertension. These workers noted a drop in the pressure of hypertensive rats after daily parenteral injections. It required a period of time for the pressure to be lowered and a period of time for it to return to the pre-injection hypertensive levels. The seeming ability of low doses of $PGA_2$ to lower the pressure of the SH rat over a period of time also speaks for an indirect mechanism. Such a mechanism has not been elucidated.

Additional observations seem to indicate a relationship of renomedullary prostaglandins to the hypertensive state. Although these observations are based on crude techniques of prostaglandin detection, they were derived in different laboratories and complement each other.

Hickler et al. (1966) noted a decrease in extractable VDL, now considered to consist mostly of $PGE_2$, from kidneys perfused under hypertensive pressure. Strong, Boucher, Nowaczynski and Genest (1966) noted an increase in VDL content, considered by them as an E prostaglandin, within an area of ischemia of the kidney related to the hypertensive state. Samova and Dochev (1970) noted an increase in both renin and VDL during the early phase of renal hypertension of the rat. In the late phase, the renin content returned to normal while VDL remained elevated but not as high as earlier. Nekrosova, Nikolaeva and Khukhorev (1968), Nekrasova and Lantsberg (1969), Nekrasova, Serebrovskaya, Lantsberg and Uchitel (1970a) approached the problem differently. These workers studied both the two-kidney and the one-kidney Goldblatt hypertension of the rabbit. With the two-kidney preparation (one kidney clipped, the other intact), the arterial pressure was elevated up to 30 days, at which time the prostaglandin content of the clipped kidney was less than normal while that of the normal kidney was normal. After this time the arterial pressure returned to normal or below normal within 150 to 270 days. At these times, the prostaglandin content of both kidneys was elevated and more so in the clipped kidney. The renin content rose during the first 14 days, then decreased somewhat by the 30th day. In the one-kidney Goldblatt hypertension the prostaglandin content of the ischaemic kidney was depressed despite a marked hypertrophy of this kidney. In a subsequent publication Nekrosova, Puleeva and Khundodze (1970b) demonstrated a reduction of prostaglandin-like substances in kidneys removed from patients with renovascular hypertension while the renin content was elevated when these measurements were compared with those of kidneys from healthy subjects derived immediately after death. Thus, the results in hypertensive man resembled those of rabbits made hypertensive. Nekrosova concluded that the 'inter-reaction of the pressor-depressor function of the kidneys will evidently determine the degree of development of arterial hypertension' and indicated the need for greater understanding in the future of the proposed relationship between the antihypertensive function of the kidney and the pressor function.

The discrepancies of these various studies undoubtedly reflect the crude nature of the assay procedures for VDL and prostaglandins. The work of Strong *et al.* and Samova present us with a paradox, i.e., more VDL in the kidney under conditions of hypertension. The work of Hickler *et al.,* Edwards, Strong and Hunt (1969) and of Nekrosova and his co-workers indicates a flushing out of prostaglandin during the hypertensive state. Improved techniques of detection will no doubt clarify these points.

## 11. ANTIHYPERTENSIVE NEUTRAL RENOMEDULLARY LIPID (ANRL)

*Background:* The prevention of sodium-protein induced renoprival hypertension of the dog by renomedullary transplants (Model No. 2 above) led to a test of crude renomedullary extracts in this same system (Muirhead *et al.,* 1960c). These crude extracts not only prevented this hypertensive state but also evoked an acute depressor effect in animals having this form of hypertension. The prevention of renoprival hypertension of the dog was then used as an assay procedure in attempts to purify and identify the active principle (Muirhead, Hinman and Daniels, 1963; Muirhead, Brooks, Kosinski, Daniels and Hinman, 1966). This proved cumbersome but yielded some worthwhile information albeit not the definitive one.

Extraction of the acidified homogenate (pH 5.5) of dog renal medulla in 55% ethanol in the cold yielded the active principle. The principle was slowly dialyzable. Sephadex chromatography indicated a relatively low molecular weight (<1000). Porcine renal medulla gave similar results. In a few experiments the active principle was derived from human kidneys (Muirhead *et al.,* 1963; Muirhead, *et al.,* 1966).

Next, the aqueous concentrate of the ethanol extract was defatted with Skellysolve B and extracted in ethyl acetate. This extract was run through a counter-current distribution apparatus. The solvent system was prepared by equilibrating benzene, cyclohexane, ethanol and water (5 : 5 : 8 : 2). In a 120-tube arrangement, the active principle was identified between tubes 24 and 45, separating in the lower phase. Using saturated aqueous butanol and single phase paper chromatography, the active principle was derived in an area which did not absorb ultraviolet light above 240 $\mu$. The active principle was not retained by a Dowex-50 resin column. It flocculated out of an aqueous preparation and had oily and wax-like properties. For this reason, it was dissolved in 95% ethanol. It proved active in the renoprival assay when given by mouth (Muirhead et al., 1963).

At this juncture the active principle appeared to be a low molecular weight lipid absorbed by mouth.

In the next steps the principle was further purified by silicic acid column and thin-layer chromatography. The fractions up to this juncture were tested in chronic renal hypertension of the dog (Goldblatt and Page types). Certain fractions proved to lower the arterial pressure of these animals when given either intravenously or by mouth (Muirhead et al., 1966). The response was characteristic. After a lag period of days, the arterial pressure dropped significantly, often to near control levels. As long as the preparation was given, the pressure remained depressed. Upon cessation of treatment, the pressure returned slowly over days to the pre-treatment hypertensive level (Figure 22).

While the antihypertensive renomedullary principle was being tested in hypertensive dogs, Lee et al. (1963) reported on the discovery of the depressor principle from renomedullary extracts which became known as

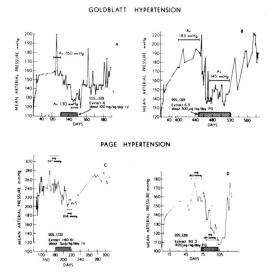

Fig. 22. In these examples pork renomedullary extracts with and without VDL were given to dogs having chronic fixed renal hypertension. The arterial pressure dropped slowly and significantly and remained depressed as long as the extract was given. Upon cessation of the treatment the arterial pressure slowly returned to the pre-treatment hypertensive level. From Muirhead et al. (1966) by permission of the publisher.

the vasodepressor lipid (VDL) and later was identified as consisting mainly of $PGE_2$ (Daniels *et al.*, 1967).

As soon as the VDL activity (Lee *et al.*, 1963) became known to our group, extracts at various levels of refinement were tested in the prepared dog*. The acute vasodepressor effect was encountered in most antihypertensive extracts. The most refined preparation did not elicit this response (Figure 23). One batch of the ethanol and ethyl acetate

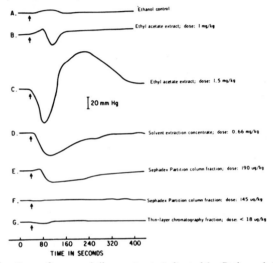

Fig. 23. Fractions of renomedullary extracts indicated by B through E caused an acute vasodepressor effect of the prepared dog while fractions F and G did not. Yet fractions F and G had antihypertensive activity. All fractions were derived from the same batch. These observations among others indicated a separation of two vasoactive and/or antihypertensive lipid moieties from the renal medulla. From Muirhead *et al.* (1965) by permission of the publisher.

extract was purified by further solvent extraction and partition chromatography using a Sephadex column (Muirhead *et al.*, 1965). The column separated the extract into a fraction giving the depressor effect and one devoid of this effect. The fraction devoid of the depressor effect protected against renoprival hypertension. Thus, there appeared to be a separation of the renomedullary lipids into a fraction causing the acute vasodepressor effect and a fraction without this effect but which retained an antihypertensive action. The principle of the latter fraction was termed the antihypertensive neutral renomedullary lipid (ANRL).

*Refinement of ANRL:* Three additional approaches were used to derive ANRL of the rabbit. The first represented a modification of

*According to Dr J. R. Weeks, the dog is more sensitive than the rat for this purpose.

extraction procedures for prostaglandins (Daniels, 1971). Homogenized renal medulla was extracted into acetone, defatted with petroleum ether and extracted into methylene chloride. The acidic lipids were removed with a phosphate buffer (0.2 M, pH 8.0). The neutral lipid was left behind and dried into a waxy substance. This crude preparation prevented canine renoprival hypertension and lowered the pressure of hypertensive rats and dogs (Muirhead, Leach, Daniels and Hinman, 1968b). This method gave variable yields, in part due to variable losses in the petroleum ether. A second method yielded more consistent results (Muirhead, Leach, Byers, Brooks, Daniels and Hinman, 1971). The kidneys were removed from the rabbit carcass shortly after death and placed on ice. Within 15 minutes, the medulla was dissected away from most of the cortex and frozen. The frozen medulla was shipped and processed within one week. The medulla was homogenized in dry ethyl ether and then evaporated to a yellow oil (100 gm tissue yielded about 4 gm of oil). This oil was subjected to silicic acid column chromatography using Hanahan's technique (Morgan, Tinker and Hanahan, 1963). ANRL was derived from the final portion of the 5% ether in hexane fraction containing mainly triglycerides and cholesterol esters. Additional fractions were derived by preparative gas liquid chromatography (GLC) and by means of a modified lipophilic Sephadex LH-20 column. By these means, the active principle was purified from the ether extract level to the lipophilic Sephadex product by 800 times. It still contained a mixture of triglycerides which interfered with ultimate identity (Muirhead et al., 1971).

The third approach was based on the assumption that ANRL was an alkenyl-l-glyceryl ether. This assumption resulted in part from speculative reasons and in part from a study of the fractions derived by preparative GLC. A greater portion of the active preparations consisted of common variety triglycerides. It was determined that the antihypertensive activity appeared to reside in a non-saponifiable fraction of alkali-treated neutral fraction. This finding was compatible with the supposition that the active principle was a glyceryl ether rather than an ordinary triglyceride.

The procedure chosen for the liberation of fatty aldehydes from alkenyl ether was that of Parks, Keeney and Schwartz (1961). Two celite columns were arranged in tandem. The first column contained phosphoric acid which presumably split the aldehydes from the glyceryl ether and the second column contained sodium bisulfite which was capable of forming an addition product, thus trapping the aldehydes present. The effluent, containing the glycerides and alkyl glyceryl ethers, was discarded. Aliquots of the contents of the column were liberated by mild alkali treatment with $Na_2CO_3$ and tested in hypertensive rabbits (see below). This liberated product was unstable and in this respect resembled fatty aldehydes. By this procedure, the yield of the end-product was low and variable (Muirhead *et al.,* 1972c).

The fractions of ANRL beyond the original ether extract were devoid of the acute vasodepressor effect and presumably of prostaglandins. The methods of refinement, especially column chromatography and the derivation of the fatty aldehyde fraction, were such as to exclude prostaglandins in their classical form. What has not been excluded is the possibility that ANRL is related to the prostaglandin moiety. Indeed, under certain conditions, there are similarities in the antihypertensive action of prostaglandins and ANRL (see below).

Antihypertensive action of ANRL: Injected parenterally ANRL derived from rabbit renal medulla dropped the arterial pressure of hypertensive rabbits slowly over a period of 8 to 24 hours (Muirhead *et al.,* 1971). A second dose at 24 hours caused the pressure to remain depressed for an additional variable period of 24 or more hours (Figure 24). The arterial pressure then returned slowly to the pre-injection hypertensive level. This pattern of response was similar to that observed earlier in the hypertensive dog when ANRL containing and not containing VDL (prostaglandin) was used. A similar pattern of

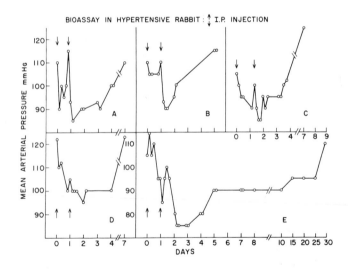

Fig. 24. Effect on the arterial pressure of the hypertensive rabbit by ANRL at various levels of refinement is demonstrated. Two doses were injected intraperitoneally 24 hours apart. In A the ethyl ether extract of renal medulla was used. In B and C the 5% ether in hexane eluate of the silicic acid column was used (first a pool of fractions, then a single fraction). In D the product of the lipophilic Sephadex column and in E the most refined material derived by preparative GLC was injected. The doses changed from 5 mg in A to 7 μg in E. Reproduced from Muirhead *et al.* (1971) by permission of the publisher.

antihypertensive action was observed when the product of the aldehyde-liberating procedures was injected intravenously into hypertensive rabbits (Figure 25). The slowness of the antihypertensive effect was unique and suggested an action through a complex system. The ultimate effect appeared due to a lowering of PVR (Muirhead *et al.*, 1966).

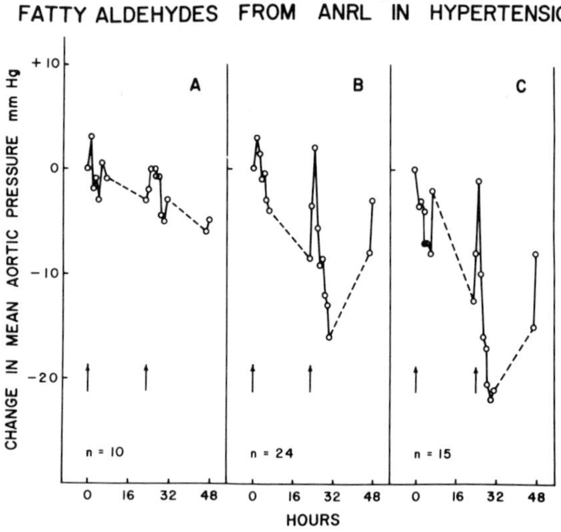

Fig. 25. Fatty aldehydes were derived from ANRL by the Schwartz technique (Parks *et al.*, 1961) and these were immediately injected intravenously into hypertensive rabbits on two occasions 24 hours apart (at arrows of panels B and C). Panel A represents results when the vehicle alone (0.05 ml 95% ethanol) was injected. The mean aortic pressure was measured every hour for five minutes over seven to nine hours by an automated device while the animals remained quietly in specially designed boxes. The control or zero pressure consisted of the average of the pressure for 24 hours before the first injection (mean 105 mm Hg ± 2.2 SE). The broken line represents the overnight stay in the animals' regular cages. In B 24 unselected consecutive results are plotted for comparison with their corresponding controls in A. In C 15 examples of B were arbitrarily selected on the basis that four consecutive blood pressure measurements were more than 10 mm Hg below the control value. Note the gradual lowering of the arterial pressure, especially after a pressor effect noted following the second injection. The differences between B and A at hours 30 and 31 are highly significant (p < .001).

There were similarities between the antihypertensive action of ANRL and that of $PGE_2$ when large doses of the latter were given (Figure 20). The same gradual decline in pressure was observed following the parenteral injection of large doses of $PGE_2$ into the hypertensive rabbit. When $PGE_2$ was antihypertensive in the rat the decline in pressure was also slow. Thus, once more the suggestion of an indirect mechanism appreared attractive, i.e., one other than that causing a direct vasodilating effect on vascular beds.

The antihypertensive renomedullary function and the renomedullary interstitial cell: It was noted above that the lipid vesicles of the renomedullary interstitial cells contained the precursor of renomedullary prostaglandins, arachidonic acid, and, indeed, appeared to contain prostaglandin itself. These vesicles also contained other lipids including cholesterol and neutral lipids.

Muehrcke and associates (1970) studied the state of the renomedullary interstitial cells in DOCA-salt hypertension of the rat and noted a depletion of their lipid droplets during the more advanced phases of the hypertension. It was not possible to conclude whether this depletion was related to the genesis of the hypertension since advanced vascular disease was also present. Tobian *et al.* (1969) and Ishii and Tobian (1969) also detected a depletion of lipid vesicles in salt-loading and Goldblatt types of hypertension of the rat. This depletion occurred while the osmolar gradient of the medulla was lowered. It could not be determined whether the depletion related to the hypertension or the altered osmolar gradient. More recently, Tobian and Azar (1972) evaluated the ability of medullary slices from the kidneys of hypertensive animals to produce prostaglandins and noted the ability of these slices to produce prostaglandin to the same extent as slices of renal medulla from normotensive rats. The studies of Muirhead *et al.* (1972a, b) indicated that the main cell within transplants of fragmented renal medulla which exerted an antihypertensive function had the characteristics of the renomedullary interstitial cells. Moreover, these cells occurred in clusters suggesting local proliferation.

These various observations dealing with the renomedullary interstitial cells and the hypertensive state not only raise the issue of whether these cells are actually involved in the renomedullary antihypertensive function but, if so, whether they mediate this function by secreting either prostaglandins or ANRL, or both, or by some other mechanism.

In summary, the antihypertensive neutral renomedullary lipid (ANRL) is a lipid that can be separated from the renomedullary prostaglandins by extraction and chromatographic procedures. In these procedures ANRL appears to associate with triglycerides. ANRL differs from $PGE_2$ and $PGA_2$ in that it is antihypertensive but does not evoke the acute vasodepressor effect in the prepared animal. The action of ANRL in the hypertensive animal is characteristic, it drops the arterial pressure slowly. Once depressed under the impact of ANRL the arterial pressure usually returns to the pre-treatment hypertensive level slowly. In this respect, the antihypertensive action of ANRL resembles that of transplants of fragmented renal medulla. When evoking an antihypertensive effect in the hypertensive rat and rabbit, $PGE_2$ behaves in a similar manner. However, a possible relationship between ANRL and $PGE_2$ and $PGA_2$ remains speculative.

A procedure which liberates aldehydes from alkenyl ethers yields a principle from ANRL which maintains its antihypertensive activity. Thus, there is a possibility that ANRL is a neutral lipid of the glyceryl alkenyl ether type.

## 12. CONCLUSIONS AND THERAPEUTIC IMPLICATIONS

Two classes of lipids having vasoactive and/or anti-hypertensive activity are extractable from the renal medulla. One lipid appears to consist mainly of $PGE_2$. A small quantity of $PGA_2$ is also extractable but it is uncertain whether this agent is a natural product or a conversion product from $PGE_2$ formed during the extraction procedure. The other renomedullary lipid appears to be a neutral lipid (ANRL) which associates with triglycerides in most extraction procedures. The application of procedures which liberate fatty aldehydes from alkenyl ethers suggested the possibility that the antihypertensive principle of ANRL could be a glyceryl ether. The specific characteristics of ANRL, however, remain unknown and its relationship to the renomedullary prostaglandins is at present unresolved.

With respect to the relationship of $PGE_2$, $PGA_2$ and ANRL to the hypertensive state, the author has used the term 'acute depressor effect' to indicate a depression of the arterial pressure in the normotensive or hypertensive animal which lasts only a few minutes (Lee et al., 1963; Muirhead et al., 1965, 1966). Conversely, the term 'antihypertensive action' was used to indicate a lowering of the arterial pressure of the hypertensive animal over a prolonged period, such as that produced by vasodilators [diazoxide (Finnerty, Kakaviatos, Tackman and Magill, 1963); minoxidil (Gottlieb and Chidsey, 1971)], and drugs which either deplete catecholamine stores or interfere with catecholamine function (Carlson, 1966).

In the doses usually employed the renomedullary prostaglandins $E_2$ and $A_2$ have mainly an acute depressor action on the arterial pressure. This action may be prolonged either by a continuous infusion (Lee et al., 1971a, b) or by the use of very large pharmacological doses (Muirhead et al., 1968a), but at the risk of unwanted effects such as those due to a hyperkinetic circulation and exaggerated intestinal motility. On the other hand, ANRL causes a sustained fall in the arterial pressure lasting from hours to a few days depending on the number of doses employed (Muirhead et al., 1966, 1971). This antihypertensive effect resembles that initiated by the transplantation of fragmented renal medulla (Muirhead et al., 1970a, b). It is important to note that ANRL is not an acute depressor agent even when bolus doses are injected intravenously into the prepared animal (Muirhead *et al.,* 1965, 1968b), neither does ANRL lower the arterial pressure of normal animals in doses which exert an antihypertensive effect in those with a raised blood pressure (Muirhead *et al.,* 1968b). These considerations raise issues concerning the possible physiological, pathological and therapeutic roles of the vasoactive and/or antihypertensive renomedullary lipids.

The demonstration of prostaglandin-like material resembling the E series compounds in the renal venous effluent under certain conditions raises the question whether this outpouring has some regulatory effect on the arterial pressure, renal flow and sodium excretion (Lee *et al.,* 1969, 1971a). In view of the transient nature of this activity within the circulation, due to modifications mediated by lung enzymes (Änggård and Samuelsson, 1964, 1965) and possibly by circulating plasma (Horton *et al.,* 1971), it is possible that this activity is of the short-term compensatory type. The localization of a main synthesizing site of prostaglandins with renomedullary interstitial cells and the apparent ability of these cells to liberate such lipids interstitially as well as into the circulation adds to the attractiveness of this hypothesis. Moreover, a continuous outpouring of the depressor prostaglandins ($E_2$ and possibly $A_2$) into the circulation could have the same effect as that of an intravenous infusion and give rise to a more prolonged effect on the arterial pressure. The outpouring of $PGF_{2\alpha}$ from the kidney could serve to moderate the tone of capacitance vessels (DuCharme and Weeks, 1967, 1968) and serve additionally in the control of the circulation by increasing venous return to the heart and thereby modifying the cardiac output. Such speculations should be subject to definitive tests in the near future when precise measurements of prostaglandins, as by the radioimmune assay, become available. Thus the kidney conceivably could have a unique relationship to circulating prostaglandins and their circulatory effects.

The translation of these considerations to the treatment of hypertension, however, has not so far been possible. This results mainly from the need of either a continuous infusion of depressor prostaglandin or the use of large doses with the possibility of unwanted effects. However, the preliminary indication that $PGA_2$ and $PGE_2$, in proper doses, lower the arterial pressure of the anaesthetized SH rat slowly and over a prolonged period of time is interesting, particularly since the SH rat has been considered as the experimental model most closely resembling essential hypertension of man (Udenfriend and Spector, 1972). ANRL appears as a more attractive regulator of the hypertensive state since it does not appear to alter the arterial pressure of the normotensive animal and, as such, seems subject to intrinsic controls. The problem with ANRL has been the inconsistency of its extraction procedures and purification, and the failure to identify its structure. In view of its seeming potentialities, the search for this principle continues to be of considerable importance.

The kidney appears to exert an antihypertensive function. This function seems to result, in part, from the regulation of sodium and water balance. Sodium and water loads tend to elevate the arterial pressure through haemodynamic changes, i.e., increase in venous return and cardiac output. The latter has been put forward as the sole explanation for renoprival hypertension. The situation appears to be more complex than this since transplanted renal medulla, prostaglandins and ANRL either prevent or significantly blunt this hypertensive state as it occurs in experimental animals. Moreover, transplanted renal medulla prevents or reverts experimental renovascular hypertension. Attention is being focused on the renomedullary interstitial cells as the most likely cells mediating the renomedullary antihypertensive function.

The investigative future of this general area dealing with the antihypertensive functions of the kidney appears bright and promising, partly in view of these considerations but mainly in view of the need to determine with certainty the possible relationships between sodium and water loads and the actions of renomedullary vasoactive and/or antihypertensive lipids. The antihypertensive action of renomedullary cells appears to be unique; that this action is mediated by lipids derived from renomedullary interstitial cells remains to be determined. The most interesting and exciting aspect of these considerations relates to the possibility of deriving agents which may eventually be employed in the control of high blood pressure which are natural products and which exert some degree of feedback control.

## REFERENCES

Alpert, J. S. and Hickler, R. B. (1971). Cardiovascular and renal effects of renomedullary prostaglandins. Kidney Hormones (Ed. J. W. Fisher), pp. 525-561, Academic Press, London.

Änggård, E. (1971). Studies on the analysis and metabolism of the prostaglandins. *Annals of the New York Academy of Sciences,* **180**, 200.

Änggård, E. and Bergström, S. (1963). Biological effects of an unsaturated trihydroxy acid ($PGF_{2\alpha}$) from normal swine lung. *Acta Physiologica Scandinavica,* **58**, 1.

Änggård, E. and Samuelsson, B. (1964). Metabolism of prostaglandin $E_1$ in guinea-pig lung: the structure of two metabolites. *Journal of Biological Chemistry,* **239**, 4097.

Änggård, E. and Samuelsson, B. (1965). Metabolism of prostaglandin $E_3$ in guinea-pig lung. *Biochemistry* (Easton), **4**, 1864.

Bayliss, W. M. (1902). On the local reactions of the arterial wall to changes of internal pressure. *Journal of Physiology, London,* **28**, 220.

Beck, L., Pollard, A. A., Harbo, J. N. and Silver, T. M. (1968). Does prostaglandin mediate sustained dilatation; *Prostaglandin Symposium of the Worcester Foundation* (Eds. P. W. Ramwell and J. E. Shaw), pp. 295-305, Interscience, New York.

Bergström, S. and Sjövall, J. (1957). The isolation of prostaglandin. *Acta Chemica Scandinavica*, 11, 1086.

Bergström, S., Duner, H., von Euler, U. S., Pernow, B. and Sjövall, J. (1959a). Observations on the effects of infusion of prostaglandin E in man. *Acta Physiologica Scandinavica*, 45, 145.

Bergström, S., Eliasson, R., von Euler, U. S. and Sjövall, J. (1959b). Some biological effects of two crystalline prostaglandin factors. *Acta Physiologica Scandinavica*, 45, 133.

Bergström, S. and von Euler, U. S. (1963). The biological activity of prostaglandin $E_1$, $E_2$ and $E_3$. *Acta Physiologica Scandinavica*, 59, 493.

Biron, P. (1968). Vasoactive hormone metabolism by pulmonary circulation. *Circulation Research*, 16, 112.

Blalock, A. and Levy, S. E. (1937). Studies on the etiology of renal hypertension. *Annals of Surgery*, 106, 826.

Bohman, S.-O. and Maunsbach, H. B. (1969). Isolation of the lipid droplets from interstitial cells of the renal medulla. *Journal of Ultrastructure Research*, 29, 569.

Borst, J. G. G. and Borst de Geus, A. (1963). Hypertension explained by Starling's theory of circulatory homeostasis. *Lancet*, 1, 677.

Braun-Menendez, E. and von Euler, U. S. (1947). Hypertension after bilateral nephrectomy in rat. *Nature*, 160, 905.

Braun-Menendez, E., Fasciolo, J. C., Leloir, L. F., Munoz, J. M. and Taquini, A. C. (1946). Renal Hypertension, pp. 209-217, C. C. Thomas, Springfield, Illinois.

Braun-Menendez, E. (1958). The prohypertensive and antihypertensive actions of the kidney. *Annals of Internal Medicine*, 49, 717.

Brooks, B. and Muirhead, E. E. (1971). Rigid clip for standardized hypertension in the rat. *Journal of Applied Physiology*, 31, 307.

Byrom, F. B. and Dodson, L. F. (1949). The mechanism of the vicious circle in chronic hypertension. *Clinical Science*, 8, 1.

Carlson, L. A. and Oro, L. (1966). Effect of prostaglandin $E_1$ on blood pressure and heart rate in the dog. Prostaglandin and related factors 48. *Acta Physiologica Scandinavica*, 67, 89.

Carr, A. A. (1970). Hemodynamic and renal effects of a prostaglandin, $PGA_1$, in subjects with essential hypertension. *American Journal of Medical Science*, 259, 21.

Chanutin, A. and Ferris, E. B. Jr. (1932). Experimental renal insufficiency produced by partial nephrectomy. *Archives of Internal Medicine*, 49, 767.

Crowshaw, K., McGiff, J. C., Strand, J. C., Lonigro, A. J. and Terragno, N. A. (1970). Prostaglandins in dog renal medulla. *Journal of Pharmacy and Pharmacology*, 22, 302.

Daniels, E. G. (1971). Extraction of renomedullary prostaglandins. Kidney Hormones (Ed. J. W. Fisher), pp. 507-524, Academic Press, London.

Daniels, E. G., Hinman, J. W., Leach, B. E. and Muirhead, E. E. (1967). Identification of prostaglandin $E_2$ as the principal vasodepressor lipid of rabbit renal medulla. *Nature (London)*, 215, 1298.

Daugherty, R. M. Jr., Schwinghamer, J. M., Swindall, S. and Haddy, F. J. (1968). The effects of local and systemic infusions of prostaglandin $E_1$ on the skin and muscle vasculature. *Journal of Laboratory and Clinical Medicine*, 72, 869.

Davies, B. N., Horton, E. W. and Withrington, P. G. (1968). The occurrence of prostaglandin $E_2$ in splenic venous blood of the dog following splenic nerve stimulation. *British Journal of Pharmacology and Chemotherapy*, 32, 127.

Dorp, D. van (1971). Recent developments in the biosynthesis and analyses of prostaglandins. *Annals of the New York Academy of Sciences*, 180, 181.

DuCharme, D. W. and Weeks, J. R. (1967). Cardiovascular pharmacology of prostaglandin $F_{2\alpha}$, a unique pressor agent. Proceedings of the 2nd Nobel Symposium, pp. 173-181, Almqvist & Wiksell, Stockholm.

DuCharme, D. W., Weeks, J. R. and Montgomery, R. G. (1968). Studies on the mechanism of the hypertensive effect of prostaglandin $F_{2\alpha}$. *Journal of Pharmacology and Experimental Therapeutics*, 160, 1.

Ducrot, H., Jungers, P., Funck-Brentano, J. L., Perrin, D., Crosnier, J. and Humburger, J. (1960). L'action de la transplantation renale human sur l'hypertension arterielle. L'Hypertension Arterielle (Eds. P. Milliez and Ph. Tcherdakoff), pp. 208-222, L'Expansion Scientifique Francais, Paris.

Ducrot, H., Kleinknecht, D., Jungers, P., Vantelon, J., Auvert, J., Zingraff, I. and Funck-Brentano, J. L. (1970). Blood pressure, hemodynamics, renin and body fluid in renoprival man. Proceedings of the Fourth International Congress of Nephrology, pp. 65-75, Karger, Basel/New York.

Dustan, H. P. and Page, I. H. (1964). Some factors in renal and renoprival hypertension. *Journal of Laboratory and Clinical Medicine*, 64, 948.

Edwards, W. G. Jr., Strong, C. G. and Hunt, J. C. (1969). A vasodepressor lipid resembling prostaglandin $E_2$ ($PGE_2$) in renal venous blood of hypertensive patients. *Journal of Laboratory and Clinical Medicine*, 74, 389.

Euler, U. S. von (1934). Zur Kenntnis der pharmakologishen Wirkungen von Nativsekreten und Extrackten männlicher accessorischer Geschlechtsdrüsen. *Naunun-Schmiedeberes Archives of Experimental Pathology and Pharmacology*, 175, 78.

Euler, U. S. von (1935). Uber die spezifische blutdrucksenkende Substanz des menschlichen Prostata- und Samenblasensekretes. *Klinische Wochenschrift;* 14, 1182.

Euler, U. S. von (1936). On the specific vasodilating and plain muscle stimulating substances from accessory genital glands in man and certain animals (prostaglandin and vesiglandin). *Journal of Physiology (London)*, 88, 213.

Euler, U. S. von (1939). Weitere Untersuchunger über Prostaglandin, die physiologish aktive Substanz gewisser Genitaldrusen. *Skandinavisches Archiv. fur Physiologie*, 81, 65.

Fasciolo, J. D., Houssay, B. A. and Taquini, A. C. (1938). The blood pressure raising secretion of the ischemic kidney. *Journal of Physiology*, 94, 281.

Ferrario, C. M., Page, I. H. and McCubbin, J. W. (1970). Increased cardiac output as a contributory factor in experimental renal hypertension in dogs. *Circulation Research*, 27, 799.

Ferreira, S. H. and Vane, J. R. (1967). Prostaglandins: their disappearance from and release into the circulation. *Nature (London)*, 216, 868.

Fichman, M. P. (1970). Natriuretic and vasodepressor effect of prostaglandin ($PGA_1$) in man. *Clinical Research,* 18, 149.

Finnerty, F. A., Jr., Kakaviatos, N., Tuckman, J., Magill, J. (1963). Clinical evaluation of diazoxide, a new treatment for acute hypertension. *Circulation,* 28, 203.

Floyer, M. A. (1955). Further studies on the mechanism of experimental hypertension in the rat. *Clinical Science,* 14, 163.

Fried, J., Lin, C., Mehra, M., Kao, W. and Dalven, P. (1971). Synthesis and biological activity of prostaglandins and prostaglandin antagonists. *Annals of the New York Academy of Sciences,* 180, 38.

Gaddum, J. H. (1953). Technique of superfusion. *British Journal of Pharmacology,* 8, 321.

Goldblatt, H. (1938). Experimental hypertension induced by renal ischemia. Harvey Lecture. *Bulletin of the New York Academy of Medicine,* 14, 523.

Goldblatt, H., Lynch, J., Hanzal, R. F. and Summerville, W. W. (1934). Studies on experimental hypertension. I. The production of persistent elevation of systolic blood pressure by means of renal ischemia. *Journal of Experimental Medicine,* 59, 347.

Goldblatt, M. W. (1933). A depressor substance in seminal fluid. *Journal of the Society of Chemical Industry,* 52, 1056.

Gomez, A. H., Hoobler, S. W. and Blaquier, P. (1960). Effect of addition and removal of kidney transplant in renal and adrenocortical hypertensive rats. *Circulation Research,* 8, 464.

Gottlieb, T. and Chidsey, C. (1971). Vasodilators in hypertension: A comparative evaluation of minoxidil and hydralazine. *Circulation,* 44: (Suppl. II) 129.

Green, J. A., Lucas, J. and Floyer, M. A. (1970). The effect of the kidney in altering the response of the circulation to fluid loading. *Clinical Science,* 38, 4P.

Grollman, A. (1944). Simplified procedure for inducing chronic renal hypertension in mammal. *Proceedings of the Society of Experimental Biology and Medicine,* 57, 102.

Grollman, A. (1959). A unitary concept of experimental and clinical hypertensive cardiovascular disease. *Perspectives in Biology and Medicine,* 2, 208.

Grollman, A., Muirhead, E. E. and Vanatta, J. (1949). Role of the kidney in pathogenesis of hypertension as determined by a study of the effects of bilateral nephrectomy and other experimental procedures on the blood pressure of the dog. *American Journal of Physiology,* 157, 21.

Guyton, A. C., Coleman, T. G., Bower, J. D. and Harris, J. G. (1970). Circulatory control in hypertension. *Circulation Research,* 27 Suppl. II, 135.

Herzog, J. P., Johnston, H. H. and Lauler, D. P. (1968). Effects of prostaglandins $E_1$, $E_2$ and $A_1$ on renal hemodynamics, sodium and water excretion in the dog. Prostaglandin Symposium of the Worcester Foundation (Eds. P. W. Ramwell and J. E. Shaw), pp. 147-161, Interscience, New York.

Hickler, R. B., Birbari, A. E., Kamm, D. E. and Thorn, G. W. (1966). Studies on a vasodepressor and antihypertensive lipid of rabbit renal medulla. L'Hypertension Arterielle (Eds. P. Milliez and Oh. Tcherdakoff), pp. 188-202, L'Expansion Scientifique Francais, Paris.

Hickler, R. B., Lauler, D. P., Saravis, C. A., Vagnucci, A. I., Steiner, G. and Thorn, G. W. (1964). Vasodepressor lipid from renal medulla. *Canadian Medical Association Journal*, **90**, 280.

Hollenberg, M., Walker, R. S. and McCormick, D. P. (1968). Cardiovascular responses to intra-coronary infusions of prostaglandin $E_1$, $F_{1\alpha}$ and $F_{2\alpha}$. *Archives Internationales de Pharmacodynamie et de Therapie*, **174**, 66.

Holmes, S. W., Horton, E. W. and Main, I. H. (1963). The effect of prostaglandin $E_1$ on responses of smooth muscle to catecholamines, angiotensin and vasopressin. *British Journal of Pharmacology and Chemotherapy*, **21**, 538.

Horton, E. W. (1969). Hypotheses on physiological role of prostaglandins. *Physiological Reviews*, **49**, 122.

Horton, E. W. and Main, I. H. (1963). A comparison of the biological activities of four prostaglandins. *British Journal of Pharmacology and Chemotherapy*, **21**, 182.

Horton, E. W. and Main, I. H. (1965). A comparison of the actions of prostaglandins $F_{2\alpha}$ and $E_1$ on smooth muscle. *British Journal of Pharmacology*, **24**, 470.

Horton, E., Thompson, C., Jones, R. and Poyser, N. (1971). Release of prostaglandins. *Annals of New York Academy of Sciences*, **180**, 351.

Houck, C. R. (1954). Problems in maintenance of chronic bilaterally nephrectomized dog. *American Journal of Physiology*, **176**, 183.

Hyman, A. L. (1968). Active responses in pulmonary veins. *Clinical Research*, **16**, 71.

Ishii, M. and Tobian, L. (1969). Interstitial cell granules in renal papilla and the solute composition of renal tissue in rats with Goldblatt hypertension. *The Journal of Laboratory and Clinical Medicine*, **74**, 1.

Johnston, H. H., Herzog, J. P. and Lauler, D. P. (1971). Local renal tubular action of lipids from kidney. *Kidney Hormones* (Ed. J. W. Fisher), pp. 563-584, Academic Press, London.

Kannegiesser, H. and Lee, J. B. (1971). Difference in haemodynamic response to prostaglandins A and E. *Nature (London)*, **229**, 498.

Katz, L. N., Mendlowitz, M. and Friedman, M. (1938). A study of the factors concerned in renal hypertension. *Proceedings of the Society of Experimental Biology and Medicine*, **37**, 722.

Khairallah, P. A., Page, I. H. and Türker, R. K. (1967). Some properties of prostaglandin $E_1$ action on muscle. *Archives Internationales de Pharmacodynamie et de Therapie*, **169**, 328.

Kolff, W. J. (1958). Reduction of experimental renal hypertension by kidney perfusion. *Circulation*, **17**, 702.

Kolff, W. J. and Fischer, E. R. (1952). Pathologic changes after bilateral nephrectomy in dogs and rats. *Laboratory Investigation*, **1**, 351.

Kolff, W. J. and Page, I. H. (1954). Pathogenesis of renoprival cardiovascular disease in dogs. *American Journal of Physiology*, **178**, 75.

Kolff, W. J., Page, I. H. and Corcoran, A. C. (1954). Pathogenesis of renoprival cardiovascular disease in dogs. *American Journal of Physiology*, **178**, 237.

Leach, B. E., Armstrong, F. B. Jr, Germain, G. S. and Muirhead, E. E. (1971). Antihypertensive action of renomedullary prostaglandins ($PGE_2$ and $PGA_2$) in the spontaneously hypertensive rat (SH rat): Evidence for an indirect blood-pressure lowering effect. *Journal of Laboratory and Clinical Medicine*, **78**, 803.

Ledingham, J. M. (1971). Blood pressure regulation in renal failure. *Journal of the Royal College of Physicians*, **5**, 103.

Ledingham, J. M. and Pelling, D. (1970). Haemodynamic and other studies in the renoprival hypertensive rat. *Journal of Physiology,* 210, 233.

Lee, J. B., Hickler, R. B., Saravis, C. A. and Thorn, G. W. (1963). Sustained depressor effect of renal medullary extract in the normotensive rat. *Circulation Research,* 13, 359.

Lee, J. B., Covino, B. G., Takman, B. H. and Smith, E. R. (1965). Renomedullary vasodepressor substance medullin: Isolation, chemical characterization, and physiological properties. *Circulation Research,* 17, 57.

Lee, J. B., Gougoutas, J. Z., Takman, B. H., Daniels, E. G., Grostic, M. F., Pike, J. E., Hinman, J. W. and Muirhead, E. E. (1966). Vasodepressor and antihypertensive prostaglandins of PGE type with emphasis on the identification of medullin as $PGE_2$-217. *Journal of Clinical Investigation,* 45, 1036.

Lee, J. B. (1967). Chemical and Physiological properties of renal prostaglandins: The antihypertensive effects of medullin in essential human hypertension. Proceedings of the 2nd Nobel Symposium, pp. 197-210, Almqvist & Wiksell, Stockholm.

Lee, J. B., Crowshaw, K., Takman, B. H., Attrep, K. A. and Gougoutas, J. Z. (1967). The identification of prostaglandin $E_2$, $F_{2\alpha}$ and $A_2$ from rabbit kidney medulla. *Biochemical Journal,* 105, 1251.

Lee, J. B. (1968). Cardiovascular implications of the renal prostaglandins. Prostaglandin Symposium of the Worcester Foundation (Eds. P. W. Ramwell and J. E. Shaw), pp. 131-146, Interscience, New York.

Lee, J. B. (1969). Hypertension, natriuresis and the renal prostaglandins. *Annals of Internal Medicine,* 70, 1033.

Lee, J. B., Kannegiesser, H., O'Toole, J. and Westura, E. (1971a). Hypertension and the renomedullary prostaglandins. A human study of the antihypertensive effects of $PGA_1$. *Annals of the New York Academy of Sciences,* 180, 218.

Lee, J. B., McGiff, J. C., Kannegiesser, H., Aykent, Y. Y., Mudd, J. G. and Frawley, T. F. (1971b). Prostaglandin $A_1$: Antihypertensive and renal effects. Studies in patients with essential hypertension. *Annals of Internal Medicine,* 74, 703.

Leonards, J. R. and Heisler, C. R. (1951). Maintenance of life in bilaterally nephrectomized dogs and its relation to malignant hypertension. *American Journal of Physiology,* 167, 553.

McCurdy, R. and Nakano, J. (1966). Cardiovascular effects of prostaglandin $E_1$. *Clinical Research,* 14, 428.

McGiff, J. C., Crowshaw, K., Tenagro, N. A. and Lonigro, A. J. (1970a). Release of a prostaglandin-like substance into renal venous blood in response to angiotensin II. *Circulation Research,* 27, (Supp. I), 121.

McGiff, J. C., Crowshaw, K., Tenagro, N. A., Lonigro, A. J., Strand, J. C., Williamson, M. A., Lee, J. B. and Ng, K. R. (1970b). Prostaglandin-like substances appearing in canine renal venous blood during renal ischemia. *Circulation Research,* 27, 765.

McGiff, J. C., Tenagro, N. A., Strand, J. C., Lee, J. B., Lonigro, A. J. and Ng, K. K. F. (1969). Selective passage of prostaglandins across the lung. *Nature (London),* 223, 742.

Maxwell, G. N. (1967). The effect of prostaglandin $E_1$ upon the general and coronary haemodynamics and metabolism of the intact dog. *British Journal of Pharmacology and Chemotherapy,* 31, 162.

Maxwell, M. H. and Prozan, G. B. (1962). Renovascular hypertension. *Progress in Cardiovascular Disease,* 5, 81.

Merrill, J. P., Giordano, C. and Heetderks, D. K. (1961). The role of the kidney in human hypertension, failure of hypertension to develop in the renoprival subject. *American Journal of Medicine, 31,* 931.

Morgan, T. E., Tinker, D. O. and Hanahan, D. J. (1963). Phospholipid metabolism in kidney. Isolation and identification of lipids of rabbit kidney. *Arch. Biochem. and Biophys., 103,* 54.

Muehrcke, R. C., Mandal, A. K. and Volini, F. I. (1970). A pathophysiological review of the renal medullary interstitial cells and their relationship to hypertension. *Circulation Research, 27* (Supp. I), 109.

Muirhead, E. E., Vanatta, J. and Grollman, H. (1950). Papillary necrosis of the kidney, a clinical and experimental correlation. *Journal of the American Medical Association, 142,* 627.

Muirhead, E. E., Turner, L. B. and Grollman, A. (1951). Hypertensive cardiovascular disease: vascular lesions of dogs maintained for extended periods following bilateral nephrectomy or ureteral ligation. *Archives of Pathology, 51,* 575.

Muirhead, E. E., Jones, F., and Graham, P. (1953). Hypertension following bilateral nephrectomy of the dog: The influence of dietary protein on its pathogenesis with emphasis on its development in the absence of 'extracellular fluid' expansion. *Circulation Research, 1,* 439.

Muirhead, E. E., Stirman, J. A., Lesch, W. and Jones, F. (1956). The reduction of postnephrectomy hypertension by renal homotransplant. *Surgery, Gynecology and Obstetrics, 103,* 673.

Muirhead, E. E., Stirman, J. A. and Jones, F. (1959). Further observations on the potentiation of postnephrectomy hypertension of the dog by dietary protein. *Circulation Research, 7,* 68.

Muirhead, E. E., Jones, F. and Stirman, J. A. (1960a). Hypertensive cardiovascular disease of dog: Relation of sodium and dietary protein to ureterocaval anastomosis and ureteral ligation. *Archives of Pathology, 70,* 108.

Muirhead, E. E., Stirman, J. A. and Jones, F. (1960b). Renal autoexplantation and protection against renoprival hypertensive cardiovascular disease and hemolysis. *Journal of Clinical Investigation, 39,* 266.

Muirhead, E. E., Jones, F. and Stirman, J. A. (1960c). Antihypertensive property in renoprival hypertension of extract from renal medulla. *Journal of Laboratory and Clinical Medicine, 56,* 167.

Muirhead, E. E. (1962). Protection against sodium overload hypertensive disease by renal tissue and medullorenal extract. *Archives of Pathology, 74,* 214.

Muirhead, E. E., Hinman, J. W. and Daniels, E. G. (1963). Canine renoprival hypertension and the antihypertensive function of the kidney. Boorhave Cursus, pp. 88-106, Boorhave Edition, Leiden.

Muirhead, E. E., Daniels, E. G., Booth, E., Freyburger, W. A. and Hinman, J. W. (1965). Renomedullary vasodepression and antihypertensive function. *Archives of Pathology, 80,* 43.

Muirhead, E. E., Brooks, B., Kosinski, M., Daniels, E. G. and Hinman, J. W. (1966). Renomedullary antihypertensive principle in renal hypertension. *The Journal of Laboratory and Clinical Medicine, 67,* 778.

Muirhead, E. E., Daniels, E. G., Pike, J. E. and Hinman, J. W. (1967). Renomedullary antihypertensive lipids and the prostaglandins. Proceedings of the 2nd Nobel Symposium, pp. 183-196. Almqvist and Wiksell, Uppsala.

Muirhead, E. E., Leach, B. E., Brooks, B., Brown, G. B., Daniels, E. G. and Hinman, J. W. (1968a). Antihypertensive action of prostaglandin $E_2$. Prostaglandin Symposium of the Worcester Foundation (Eds. P. W. Ramwell and J. E. Shaw), pp. 183-200, Interscience, New York.

Muirhead, E. E., Leach, B. E., Byers, L. W., Brooks, B. and Pitcock, J. A. (1972c). Antihypertensive function of the renal medulla. 26th Hahnemann International Symposium (in press). Grune & Stratton, New York.

Muirhead, E. E., Leach, B. E., Daniels, E. G. and Hinman, J. W. (1968b). Lapine renomedullary lipid in murine hypertension. *Archives of Pathology,* **85,** 72.

Muirhead, E. E., Brown, G. B., Germain, G. S. and Leach, B. E. (1970a). The renal medulla as an antihypertensive organ. *Proceedings of the Fourth International Congress of Nephrology* (Volume 2), pp. 57-64, Karger, Basel/New York.

Muirhead, E. E., Brown, G. B., Germain, G. S. and Leach, B. E. (1970b). The renal medulla as an antihypertensive organ. *Journal of Laboratory and Clinical Medicine,* **76,** 641.

Muirhead, E. E., Brooks, B., Pitcock, J. A. and Stephenson, P. (1972a). The renomedullary antihypertensive function in accelerated (malignant) hypertension. With observations on renomedullary interstitial cells. *Journal of Clinical Investigation,* **51,** 181.

Muirhead, E. E., Leach, B. E., Byers, L. W., Brooks, B., Daniels, E. G. and Hinman, J. W. (1971). Antihypertensive renomedullary lipids (ANRL). Kidney Hormones (Ed. J. W. Fisher), pp. 485-506, Academic Press, London.

Muirhead, E. E. and Brooks, B. (1971). Antihypertensive action of renal medulla in salt-loading hypertension. *Federation Proceedings,* **30,** 431.

Muirhead, E. E., Brooks, B., Pitcock, J. A., Stephenson, P. and Brosius, W. L. (1972b). Role of the renal medulla in the sodium-sensitive component of renoprival hypertension. Laboratory Investigation (in press).

Muirhead, E. E. and Brooks, B. (1970). Prevention of malignant hypertension of rabbit by renomedullary tissue. *Federation Proceedings,* **29,** 447.

Nakano, J. (1968). Effect of prostaglandin $E_1$, $A_1$ and $F_{2\alpha}$ on cardiovascular dynamics in dogs. Prostaglandin Symposium of the Worcester Foundation (Eds. P. W. Ramwell and J. E. Shaw), pp. 201-213, Interscience, New York.

Nakano, J. and Cole, B. (1968). Cardiovascular effects of prostaglandin $F_{2\alpha}$. *Clinical Research,* **16,** 242.

Nakano, J. and McCurdy, J. R. (1967). Cardiovascular effects of prostaglandin $E_1$. *Journal of Pharmacology and Experimental Therapeutics,* **156,** 538.

Nakano, J. and McCurdy, J. R. (1968a). Hemodynamic effects of prostaglandin $F_{2\alpha}$. *Circulation,* **38** (Suppl. VI), 146.

Nakano, J. and McCurdy, J. R. (1968b). Hemodynamic effects of prostaglandins $E_1$, $A_1$ and $F_{2\alpha}$ in dogs. *Proceedings of the Society for Experimental Biology and Medicine,* **128,** 39.

Nakano, J., Perry, M. and Denton, D. (1968). Effect of prostaglandins $E_1$ ($PGE_1$), $A_1$ ($PGA_1$) and $F_{2\alpha}$ ($PGF_{2\alpha}$) on the peripheral circulation. *Clinical Research,* **16,** 110.

Nekrasova, A. A., Nikolaeva, E. N. and Khukhorev, V. V. (1968). Prostaglandins and the depressor function of the kidneys in the pathogenesis of hypertonia. *Kardiologia,* **8,** 16.

Nekrasova, A. A. and Lantsberg, L. A. (1969). Role of renal prostaglandins in the pathogenesis of hypertension. *Kardiologia,* **9,** 86.

Nekrasova, A. A., Serebrovskaya, Y. A., Lantsberg, L. A. and Uchitel, I. A. (1970). Depressor prostaglandin-like substances and renin in the kidneys during experimental renal hypertonia. *Kardiologia,* **10**, 31.

Nekrasova, A. A., Paleeva, F. M. and Khundadze, S. Sh. (1970). The content of depressor prostaglandin-like substances and the activity of renin in the kidneys in patients suffering from renovascular hypertension. *Kardiologia,* **10**, 88.

Nissen, H. M. (1968). On lipid droplets in renal interstitial cells. II. A histological study on the number of droplets in salt depletion and acute salt repletion. *Zeitschrift fur Zell forschung und Mikrokopische Anatomie,* **85**, 483.

Nissen, H. M. and Bojesen, I. (1969). On lipid droplets in renal interstitial cells. IV. Isolation and identification. *Zeitschrift fur Zell forschung and Mikrokopische Anatomie,* **97**, 274.

Orbison, J. L., Christian, C. L. and Peters, E. (1952). Studies on experimental hypertension in bilaterally nephrectomized dogs. *Archives of Pathology,* **54**, 185.

Osvaldo, L. and Latta, H. (1966). Interstitial cells of the renal medulla. *Journal of Ulstructure Research,* **15**, 589.

Pace-Asciak, C., Morawska, K., Coceani, F. and Wolfe, L. S. (1968). The biosynthesis of prostaglandin $E_2$ and $F_{2\alpha}$ in homogenates of the rat stomach. Prostaglandin Symposium of the Worcester Foundation (Eds. P. W. Ramwell and J. E. Shaw), pp. 371-378, Interscience, New York.

Page, I. H. (1939). Production of persistent arterial hypertension by cellophane perinephritis. *Journal of the American Medical Association,* **113**, 2046.

Page, I. H. and McCubbin, J. W. (1968). Renal Hypertension, pp. 296-305, Yearbook Medical Publishers. Inc., Chicago, Illinois.

Parkes, O. W., Keeney, M. and Schwartz, D. P. (1961). Bound aldehyde in butter oil. *Journal of Dairy Science,* **44**, 1940.

Pickering, G. W. and Prinzmetal, M. (1938). Experimental hypertension of renal origin in the rabbit. *Clinical Science,* **3**, 357.

Price, W. E., Shehadeh, Z., Neumann, D. A. and Jacobson, E. D. (1968). Vasoactive agent in the mesenteric circulation. *Federal Proceedings,* **27**, 282.

Said, S. I. (1968). Some respiratory effects of prostaglandin $E_2$ and $F_{2\alpha}$. Prostaglandin Symposium of the Worcester Foundation (Eds. P. W. Ramwell and J. E. Shaw), pp. 267-277, Interscience, New York.

Samova, L. (1969). Dynamic tracing of the activity of vasodepressor lipid isolated from kidneys of hypertensive animals. *Comptes renders de l'academie bulgare des Sciences,* **22**, 1189.

Samova, L. and Dochev, D. (1970). Changes in the renin activity in rats with experimental hypertension treated with $PGE_1$ and $PGE_2$. *Comptes renders de l'academie bulgare des Sciences,* **23**, 1581.

Selye, H. (1942). Production of nephrosclerosis by overdosage with desoxycorticosterone acetate. *Canadian Medical Association Journal,* **47**, 515.

Skelton, F. R. (1959). Adrenal regeneration and adrenal-regeneration hypertension. *Physiological Reviews,* **39**, 162.

Smith, E. R., McMorrow, J. V., Covino, B. G. and Lee, J. B. (1968). Studies on the vasodilator action of prostaglandin $E_1$. Prostaglandin Symposium of the Worcester Foundation (Eds. P. W. Ramwell and J. E. Shaw), pp. 259-266, Interscience, New York.

Steinberg, D., Vaughan, M., Nestel, P. J. and Bergström, S. (1963). Effects of prostaglandin E opposing those of catecholamines on blood pressure and on triglyceride breakdown in adipose tissue. *Biochemical Pharmacology,* 12, 764.

Strong, C. G., Boucher, R., Nowaczynski, W. and Genest, J. (1966). Renal vasodepressor lipid. *Mayo Clinic Proceedings,* 41, 433.

Strong, C. G. and Bohr, D. F. (1968). Effects of several prostaglandins on isolated vascular smooth muscle. Prostaglandin Symposium of the Worcester Foundation (Eds. P. W. Ramwell and J. E. Shaw), pp. 225-239, Interscience, New York.

Sunahara, F. A. and Kadar, D. (1968). Effects of ouabain on the interaction of autonomic drugs and prostaglandins on isolated vascular tissue. Prostaglandin Symposium of the Worcester Foundation (Eds. P. W. Ramwell and J. E. Shaw), pp. 247-257, Interscience, New York.

Tobian, L., Schonning, S. and Seefeldt, C. (1964). The influence of arterial pressure on the antihypertensive action of a normal kidney. A biological servomechanism. *Annals of Internal Medicine,* 60, 378.

Tobian, L., Ishii, M. and Duke, M. (1969). Relationship of cytoplasmic granules in renal papillary interstitial cells to 'post-salt' hypertension. *Journal of Laboratory and Clinical Medicine,* 73, 309.

Tobian, L. and Azar, S. (1972). Antihypertensive and other functions of the renal papilla. Transactions of the American Association of Physicians, 84, 281.

Udenfriend, S. and Spector, S. (1972). Spontaneously hypertensive rat. *Science (New York),* 176, 1155.

Vergroesen, A. J., de Boer, J. and Gottenbos, J. J. (1967). Effects of prostaglandins on perfused isolated rat hearts. Proceedings of the 2nd Nobel Symposium, pp. 211-218, Almqvist and Wiksell, Stockholm.

Westura, E. E., Kannegiesser, H., O'Toole, J. D. and Lee, J. B. (1970). Antihypertensive effects of prostaglandin $A_1$ in essential hypertension. *Circulation Research,* 27 (Suppl. I), 131.

White, R. P., Denton, I. C. and Robertson, J. F. (1971). Differential effects of prostaglandins $A_1$, $E_1$ and $F_{2\alpha}$ on cerebrovascular tone in dogs and rhesus monkey. *Federation Proceedings,* 30, 625.

Wilson, C. and Byrom, F. B. (1939). Renal changes in malignant hypertension. *Lancet,* 1, 136.

# CHAPTER VII

# Prostaglandins and Respiratory Smooth Muscle

M. F. Cuthbert

Prostaglandin $E_1$ ($PGE_1$) was isolated from the vesicular gland of the sheep and its structure determined by Bergström early in 1962 and shortly after this prostaglandins $E_2$ and $E_3$ ($PGE_2$ and $PGE_3$) were isolated from the same source (Bergström, Ryhage, Samuelsson and Sjövall, 1962a; Bergström, Dressler, Ryhage, Samuelsson and Sjövall, 1962b). It was also noted that the acidic fraction of a lipid extract from the normal lungs of sheep and pigs, stimulated smooth muscle and subsequently the first member of a new series of prostaglandins was isolated, $PGF_{2\alpha}$ (Bergström, Dressler, Krabisch, Ryhage and Sjövall, 1962c). This was found in the lungs of all species examined together with small quantities of $PGF_{3\alpha}$ and $PGE_2$. Bergström also showed that $PGF_{2\alpha}$ isolated from normal lungs was identical to the more active of the two reduction products obtained when $PGE_2$ is treated with sodium borohydride.

In view of the fact that from the earliest stages of identification the lungs were known to be a potent source of prostaglandins, it is somewhat surprising that their effects on respiratory smooth muscle have until recently received little attention.

The object of this chapter is to review the effects of prostaglandins on isolated tracheal and bronchial muscle and their influence on bronchial resistance in experimental animals and healthy and asthmatic volunteers. The possible physiological role of the prostaglandins is considered in relation to their release and metabolism by the lungs and finally some speculations are made on their therapeutic application.

## 1. EFFECTS ON ISOLATED RESPIRATORY SMOOTH MUSCLE

*Animal studies*

The first observations relating to this activity were made by Änggård and Bergström (1963) when they studied the biological effect of $PGF_{2\alpha}$.

These authors found that a number of isolated smooth muscle preparations were contracted by $PGF_{2\alpha}$; including rabbit duodenum, guinea-pig ileum, rat duodenum and colon, hen rectal caecum, guinea-pig uterus and rat uterus. However, the effect of $PGF_{2\alpha}$ in causing contraction of tracheal muscle preparations from cats, rats and guinea-pigs was very weak, even in concentrations of up to 2.5 μg/ml and there was also no effect on the bronchial smooth muscle preparation from the cat.

The first demonstration of the inhibitory effect of the E prostaglandins was made by Main (1964) who studied the effects on isolated tracheal muscle from various species. Tracheal muscle of the cat, monkey and rabbit does not have any intrinsic tone and the relaxant effect was only demonstrable after a contraction had been induced by acetylcholine or other agonists. This is illustrated in Fig. 1. When $PGE_1$ was added to the organ bath before acetylcholine it had no effect but the subsequent contraction to acetylcholine was reduced. However, when $PGE_1$ was added to the bath after the muscle had contracted it produced a relaxation. Doses of $PGE_1$ as small as 1 ng/ml were effective in relaxing the tracheal muscle of the cat. Monkey tracheal muscle was almost as sensitive but that of the rabbit was less sensitive. The absence of intrinsic tone in the cat and rat tracheal muscle and the low potency of $PGF_{2\alpha}$ explains the failure of Änggård and Bergström (1963) to demonstrate effects with this prostaglandin. In contrast the tracheal muscle of the guinea-pig and ferret possesses intrinsic tone and small doses of $PGE_1$ reduced the tone and antagonised acetylcholine. Of the tracheal muscle

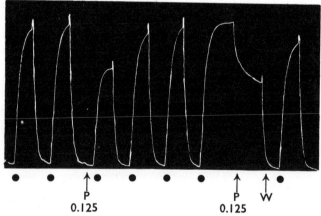

Fig. 1. Responses of a cat isolated trachea preparation, suspended in a 4 ml organ-bath containing Krebs-Henseleit solution. At the dots acetylcholine (0.5 μg/ml) was added. P = prostaglandin $E_1$ (0.125 μg/ml); W = wash. Reproduced from Main (1964) with permission of the author and publisher.

preparations examined, only that of the cat contracted in response to dihydroergotamine. This produced a slow contraction of the muscle which could be inhibited by the addition of $PGE_1$. Contractions of the tracheal muscle of the cat, guinea-pig and ferret induced by barium chloride were similarly inhibited by $PGE_1$.

These results are summarized in Table 1 which shows that small doses of $PGE_1$ relax isolated tracheal smooth muscle from the guinea-pig and

Table 1

Threshold concentrations of prostaglandin $E_1$ causing inhibition in isolated tracheal muscle preparations.

| | *Threshold concentration ($\mu g/ml$) of prostaglandin acting on* | | | | |
|---|---|---|---|---|---|
| | *Contraction due to* | | | | |
| | *Acetyl-choline* | *Dihydro-ergotamine* | *Barium chloride* | *Histamine* | *Inherent tone* |
| *Species* | | | | | |
| Cat | 0.001 | 0.001 | 0.25 | * | * |
| Monkey | 0.02 | * | >2.5 | * | * |
| Rabbit | 0.05 | * | * | * | * |
| Guinea-pig | 0.005 | * | <0.25 | 0.005 | 0.005 |
| Ferret | 0.005 | * | 0.25 | * | 0.005 |
| Sheep | 3.0 | * | 0.05 | * | >1.0 |
| Pig | 0.25 | * | * | * | 2.0 |

Asterisks indicate that no inhibition could be demonstrated since the preparation had no initial tone even in the presence of the stimulant compound added. Values are $\mu g/ml$ of prostaglandin $E_1$ which inhibited tone in the presence of the stimulants indicated. Reproduced from Main (1964) with permission of the author and publisher.

ferret and in other species antagonize contractions produced by a variety of agonists including acetylcholine, histamine, dihydroergotamine and barium chloride. It has also been shown that $PGE_1$ relaxes the isolated tracheal muscle of the dog (Türker and Kharrihalah, 1969). The relative potency of $PGE_1$, $PGE_2$, $PGE_3$, $PGF_{1\alpha}$ and $PGF_{2\alpha}$ in relaxing acetylcholine-induced contractions of isolated cat tracheal muscle is 1.0, 1.0, 0.2, 0.002 and 0.003 respectively (Main, 1964; Horton and Main, 1965).

More recently Horton and Jones (1969) have investigated the action of prostaglandin $A_1$ on the isolated tracheal muscle of the cat. They found that both $PGA_1$ and $PGE_1$ inhibited the contractions caused by acetylcholine and increasing concentrations of both prostaglandins led to a progressive inhibition of the response. Figure 2 shows the shift of the dose-response curves to acetylcholine in the presence of various concentrations of prostaglandins $E_1$ and $A_1$. Although $PGA_1$ was some 30 times less active than $PGE_1$ as an inhibitor of the contractions of the tracheal muscle, its effect was of longer duration (Fig. 3). The time for the inhibition of the contraction to diminish to 50% of its maximum after wash-out of the prostaglandin was $4.2 \pm 0.48$ mins (mean $\pm$ SE, 9 determinations) with $PGE_1$ compared with $13.1 \pm 2.2$ mins (7 determinations) with $PGA_1$.

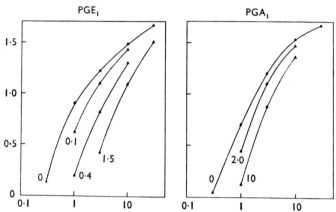

Fig. 2. Culmulative dose-response curves to acetylcholine chloride on the cat tracheal chain preparation in the presence of prostaglandins $E_1$ and $A_1$. Figures adjacent to the curves refer to prostaglandin concentrations in $\mu g/ml$. Ordinate: tension in g. Abscissa: acetylcholine concentration in $\mu g/ml$. Reproduced from Horton and Jones (1969) with permission of the authors and publisher.

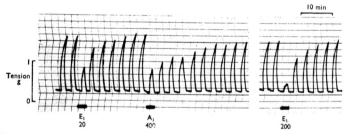

Fig. 3. Inhibition of the response of the cat isolated tracheal chain preparation to acetylcholine chloride by prostaglandins $E_1$ and $A_1$. Acetylcholine chloride 200 ng/ml, was added to the organ-bath for 90 sec every 6 min to produce contractions of the tracheal muscle. Doses of prostaglandins $E_1$ and $A_1$ (ng/ml) were added to the organ-bath 1 min before a dose of acetylcholine. Reproduced from Horton and Jones (1969) with permission of the authors and publisher.

*Human Studies*

Interest in the possible action of the prostaglandins on human respiratory smooth muscle was stimulated by the discovery of $PGE_2$ and $PGF_{2\alpha}$ in the human lung (Änggård, 1965; Karim, Sandler and Williams, 1967). Although most human tissues contain both $PGF_{2\alpha}$ and $PGE_2$ it is interesting that in the lungs $PGF_{2\alpha}$ appears to predominate and concentrations of up to 50 ng/g tissue are found.

The effects of the prostaglandins on isolated human bronchial muscle were first investigated by Sweatman and Collier (1968). Spirally-cut segments of human bronchus possess sufficient intrinsic tone to show relaxant effects without the use of agonists. Both $PGE_1$ and $PGE_2$ relaxed isolated human bronchial muscle although $PGE_1$ appeared to be slightly more potent. In contrast, the application of $PGF_{2\alpha}$ caused a marked contraction after a latent period of up to one minute. During this latent period there was sometimes a slight relaxation of the muscle. This is illustrated in Fig. 4. Thus human bronchial muscle reacts differently from animal bronchial muscle which was weakly relaxed or unaffected by the F prostaglandins (Main, 1964). Sweatman and Collier also found that the addition of $PGE_1$ or $PGE_2$ reduced the contraction caused by $PGF_{2\alpha}$, while the addition of atropine (1 μg/ml) or mepyramine (1 μg/ml) had no effect.

The slow-reacting substance produced in anaphylaxis of the isolated lung (SRS-A) has similar properties to the prostaglandins and since both

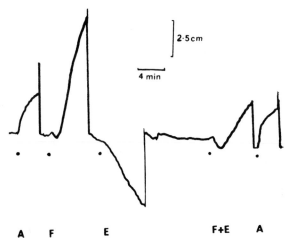

Fig. 4. Human isolated bronchial muscle in a 25 ml bath. Responses to prostaglandins $F_{2\alpha}$ ($PGF_{2\alpha}$) and $E_1$ ($PGE_1$) and to a mixture of the two. A, 10 μg of acetylcholine, F, 20 μg of $PGF_{2\alpha}$; E, 10 μg of $PGE_1$; •, drug added. Recording magnification × 40. Reproduced from Sweatman and Collier (1969) with permission of the authors and publisher.

SRS-A and $PGF_{2\alpha}$ were found to contract isolated human bronchial muscle, Sweatman and Collier (1968) performed experiments to determine whether cross-tachyphylaxis could be induced. It was found that repeated high doses of SRS-A or $PGF_{2\alpha}$ rendered bronchial muscle strips insensitive but that those made insensitive to $PGF_{2\alpha}$ still responded to SRS-A and *vice versa*. $PGE_1$ and $PGE_2$ still relaxed muscle strips which had been rendered insensitive to $PGF_{2\alpha}$ (Fig. 5). These results

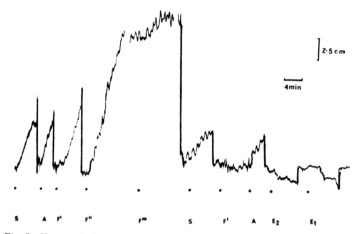

Fig. 5. Human isolated bronchial muscle in a 25 ml bath. Development of tachyphylaxis to $PGF_{2\alpha}$ without loss of response to slow reacting substance in anaphylaxis (SRS-A) or to $PGE_1$ or $PGE_2$. During the first break in the record, exposure to $2 \mu g$ $PGF_{2\alpha}$ continued for 5 min; during the second break in the record, exposure to 20 $\mu g$ $PGF_{2\alpha}$ continued for 15 min. S, 0.25 mg of SRS-A; A, 1 $\mu g$ of acetylcholine; F', 1 $\mu g$; F'', 2 $\mu g$ and F''', 20 $\mu g$ of $PGF_{2\alpha}$; $E_2$, 0.5 $\mu g$ $PGE_2$; $E_1$, 0.5 $\mu g$ of $PGE_1$. Reproduced from Sweatman and Collier (1969) with permission of the authors and publisher.

suggest that SRS-A and $PGF_{2\alpha}$ are different substances. In separate experiments Collier and Sweatman (1968) showed that the contraction of human bronchial muscle caused by $PGF_{2\alpha}$ could be reduced by non-steroidal anti-inflammatory drugs such as fenamates. Vane (1971) has recently presented convincing experimental evidence that non-steroidal anti-inflammatory drugs are potent inhibitors of prostaglandin synthesis but the relationship of these two observations is at present obscure.

Sheard (1968) independently confirmed that $PGE_1$ relaxed isolated human bronchial muscle and also antagonized the contractions caused by histamine. Neither of these effects was abolished by prior treatment of the preparation with propranolol, a beta-adrenoceptor blocking agent, or by phenoxybenzamine, an alpha-adrenoceptor blocking agent. More recently Adolphson and Townley (1970) have shown that while beta-adrenoceptor blockers completely abolish the relaxation of human bronchial muscle produced by isoprenaline, they have no effect either on the relaxation produced by $PGE_1$ or on the contraction produced by $PGF_{2\alpha}$. These observations indicate that at least *in vitro* the action of the prostaglandins is not mediated through stimulation of adrenergic receptors.

## 2. EFFECTS ON BRONCHIAL RESISTANCE

*Animal studies*

In most experiments in intact anaesthetized animals changes in 'bronchial resistance' are assessed from changes of inflation volume using a modification of the method described by Konsett and Rössler (1940). The principle of this method is as follows: Animals are anaesthetized to a sufficient depth to suppress voluntary respiration. The trachea is cannulated and connected to a respiration pump. The lungs are inflated at a constant pressure and the excess air at each stroke of the pump not necessary for inflation of the lungs is deflected to a piston recorder or volumetric pressure transducer. Hence any increase in the resistance to inflation, caused for example by bronchoconstriction, will result in an increase in the volume of air passing to the recorder. Conversely, if resistance to inflation decreases, as in bronchodilatation, more air enters the lungs and less passes to the recorder. Instead of measuring the changes in volume which occur when the lungs are inflated at constant pressure as in the Konsett-Rössler method, an alternative is to measure the changes in intra-tracheal pressure which occur when the lungs are inflated at a constant volume, as originally described by Dixon and Brodie (1903).

It should be emphasized that although changes in the calibre of the bronchioles are the most important factors modifying inflation pressure or volume, effects on the pulmonary vasculature and pulmonary congestion may contribute.

Some interesting observations were made by Änggård and Bergström (1963) following the intravenous injection of $PGF_{2\alpha}$ in anaesthetized cats. Doses of 15-30 $\mu$g/kg increased right ventricular pressure and reduced systemic blood pressure and rate. These changes were regularly accompanied by an increase in bronchial resistance as measured by the Konsett-Rössler method (Fig. 6). The bradycardia was abolished by atropine but this had no effect on the other cardiovascular changes or on the increase in bronchial resistance. These authors were reluctant to attribute this increase in bronchial resistance to a direct constrictor effect on bronchial smooth muscle, perhaps because of their findings

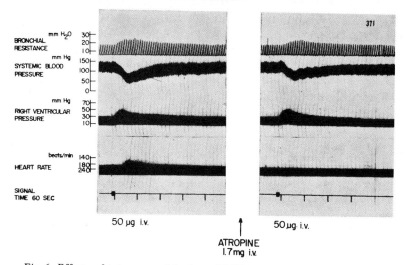

Fig. 6. Effects of intravenous injection of $PGF_{2\alpha}$ before and after atropine. Cat 2.1 kg. Chloralose 100 mg urethane 0.6 g. Note the bradycardia after about 20 sec latency and that it is abolished by atropine. Reproduced from Änggård and Bergström (1963) with permission of the authors and publisher.

that this prostaglandin had little effect on isolated tracheal or bronchial muscle of the cat. They concluded that the increase in bronchial resistance was either a direct effect, or secondary to effects of $PGF_{2\alpha}$ on pulmonary blood vessels leading to pulmonary congestion, or a combination of both.

Despite the fact that E prostaglandins relax the isolated tracheal muscle of the cat, Main (1964) found that the intravenous injection of $PGE_1$ caused an increase in bronchial resistance in the anaesthetized cat even in doses as low as 0.3 μg/kg. Fig. 7 shows that the increase in bronchial resistance was most pronounced after the blood pressure returned to normal. These doses of $PGE_1$ are some 50-100 times lower than those of $PGF_{2\alpha}$ employed by Änggård and Bergström (1963). Experiments in anaesthetized rabbits and guinea-pigs yielded quite opposite results. The intravenous injection of $PGE_1$ in these species antagonized the increase in bronchial resistance induced by histamine or vagal stimulation and sometimes reduced the resting bronchial tone (Fig. 8). In this instance the effect on bronchial smooth muscle *in vitro* and *in vivo* was similar and these observations first suggested that the prostaglandins might have important bronchodilator effects. Rosenthale, Dervinis, Begany, Lapidus and Gluckman (1968) using the Konsett-Rössler technique showed that the intravenous administration of $PGE_2$ in a dose of 4-8 μg/kg completely prevented bronchoconstriction caused

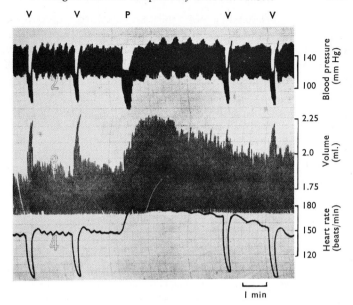

Fig. 7. Cat, 2.8 kg anaesthetized with chloralose and urethane. Upper trace, arterial blood pressure; middle trace, tidal overflow volume; lowest trace, heart rate. V = stimulation of left vagus nerve for 10 sec; P = prostaglandin $E_1$ 10 $\mu$g intravenously. Reproduced from Main (1964) with permission of the author and publisher.

by histamine, 5-hydroxytryptamine, acetylcholine and bradykinin in anaesthetized guinea-pigs. They also demonstrated that the aerosol administration of $PGE_2$ was effective in preventing bronchoconstriction in the unanaesthetized guinea-pig caused by exposure either to a histamine aerosol in normal animals, or to an aerosol of horse serum in passively sensitized animals (Rosenthale *et al.*, 1968, 1970). These observations suggest that as bronchodilators prostaglandins are at least as active given by aerosol as when given intravenously.

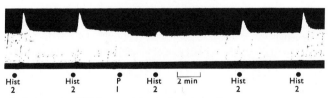

Fig. 8. Guinea-pig, 0.24 kg anaesthetized with urethane. Record of tidal overflow volume. Hist = histamine; P = prostaglandin $E_1$. All doses are in $\mu$g and were injected intravenously. Reproduced from Main (1964) with permission of the author and publisher.

Further understanding of the bronchodilator action of the prostaglandins has come from studies in which a comparison has been made of intravenous and aerosol administration. In preliminary experiments in anaesthetized guinea-pigs using either the Konsett-Rössler or Dixon-Brodie method, Large, Leswell and Maxwell (1969) showed that intravenous injection of $PGE_1$ (0.05-1 $\mu$g) antagonized the bronchoconstriction produced by histamine, 5-hydroxytryptamine, acetylcholine, bradykinin and SRS-A. Subsequent experiments were carried out against histamine-induced bronchoconstriction and a comparison was made between the bronchodilator effects of isoprenaline and $PGE_1$. It was found that the order of potency was similar although $PGE_1$ was slightly less active than isoprenaline and the bronchodilatation was less prolonged (Table 2). By the intravenous route $PGE_1$ was found to have slightly more bronchodilator activity than $PGE_2$ while $PGF_{1\alpha}$ and $PGF_{2\alpha}$ were very weakly bronchodilator in the anaesthetized guinea-pig.

Table 2

Comparison of the bronchodilator effects of $PGE_1$ and isoprenaline by intravenous and aerosol administration in the anaesthetized guinea-pig.

| | Intravenous Administration | | Aerosol Administration (20 inflations) | | |
|---|---|---|---|---|---|
| Dose $\mu$g | Mean inhibition of bronchoconstriction % | | Concentration in generating solution $\mu$g/ml | Mean inhibition of bronchoconstriction % | |
| | Isoprenaline | $PGE_1$ | | Isoprenaline | $PGE_1$ |
| 0.05 | 42 (2) | 20 (1) | 5 | — | 22 (1) |
| 0.1 | 67 (2) | 35 (2) | 10 | — | 53 ± 7.2 (5) |
| 0.2 | 86 (1)* | 58 (1) | 50 | — | 55 ± 11 (4) |
| 0.3 | — | 76 (1) | 100 | 21 ± 4.1 (8) | 67 ± 7.1 (10)§ |
| 1.0 | — | † | 500 | 25 (1) | |
| | | | 1000 | 57 ± 5.9 (11) | |
| | | | 1000 | ‡ | |

* Heart rate + 16 beats/min mean blood pressure + 3 mm (six experiments)

† Heart rate + 14 beats/min blood pressure −8 mm (six experiments)

‡ 360 inflations heart rate + 9 beats/min blood pressure—no change (two experiments)

§ 720 inflations no change in heart rate of blood pressure (two experiments)

Bronchoconstriction was induced by histamine, 5-hydroxytryptamine or bradykinin. Resistance to lung inflation was recorded either by measuring the volume of air entering the lungs at constant inflation pressure, or by recording intra-tracheal pressure with constant volume inflation. Means and standard errors are quoted, where applicable. The number of observations is given in parentheses. Modified from Large, Leswell & Maxwell (1969) with permission of the authors and publisher.

The ratios of activity were 0.6, 0.3, 0.05 and 0.02 respectively (Large and Leswell, personal communication).

A comparison of the bronchodilator effects of $PGE_1$ and isoprenaline (Large *et al.*, 1968) proved more difficult since the actual quantities of drugs reaching the lungs could not be readily determined. A special valve was designed operating through a micro-respiration pump. Aerosols were generated by a Wright's nebulizer. The number of inhalations was standardized and comparison made on the basis of the concentration of prostaglandin or isoprenaline in the aerosol generating solution. As shown in Table 2 and Fig. 9, prostaglandin $E_1$ was 10-100 times more active than isoprenaline when given by aerosol. The duration of the bronchodilator effect was similar with both preparations. By the

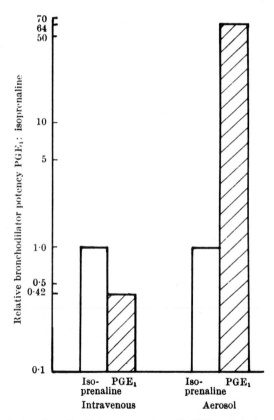

Fig. 9. Relative bronchodilator potencies of $PGE_1$ and isoprenaline in anaesthetized guinea-pigs when administered either intravenously or by aerosol. Reproduced from Large, Leswell and Maxwell (1969) with permission of the authors and publisher.

intravenous route both isoprenaline and $PGE_1$ increased the heart rate and similar effects were obtained with 0.2 $\mu$g isoprenaline and 1 $\mu$g. $PGE_1$. By aerosol administration, however, no tachycardia was detectable when an aerosol containing 100 $\mu$g/ml $PGE_1$ was administered for 10 min; in contrast an aerosol of 1 mg/ml of isoprenaline administered for 5 min produced a marked tachycardia. Results of experiments in which the resistance to inflation was recorded by the Dixon and Brodie method were generally in agreement with those above. Although the bronchodilator responses to aerosols of isoprenaline were inhibited by propranolol there was no inhibition of the bronchodilatation produced by aerosols of $PGE_1$. The anaesthetized monkey was relatively insensitive to both bronchoconstrictor and bronchodilator agents and significant bronchodilator activity could not be demonstrated with either $PGE_1$ or isoprenaline. The bronchodilator activity of $PGE_1$ was confirmed in experiments in the conscious guinea-pig in which aerosol administration was effective in preventing anaphylactic bronchoconstriction (Large et al., 1969). Other workers have also shown that in conscious guinea-pigs, both $PGE_1$ and $PGE_2$ given by aerosol are more potent bronchodilators than isoprenaline (Adolphson and Townley, 1970; Rosenthale et al., 1970) and that the bronchodilatation cannot be abolished by treatment with a $\beta$-adrenoceptor blocker. Adolphson and Townley (1970) have also confirmed the observation that although $PGE_1$ is a more potent bronchodilator than isoprenaline it appears to have less cardiac stimulant effect.

Because of the possibility that the difference in potency between isoprenaline and $PGE_1$ aerosols might be explained on a simple physico-chemical basis, Large and Leswell (personal communication) performed experiments in which changes in surface tension of aerosol solutions had been produced by Triton X, they also generated aerosols from tritiated water and measured the volumes delivered. However, bronchodilator activity was not altered by changes in surface tension and the volumes delivered from isoprenaline and $PGE_1$ aerosols did not differ significantly.

Studies in other animals have shown that there is considerable species variation in the bronchodilator effects of prostaglandin aerosols. Using a sensitive and specific measure of airways resistance, Rosenthale et al. (1970) have investigated the bronchodilator properties of $PGE_2$ and isoprenaline in anaesthetized and artificially ventilated dogs and monkeys. In this method respiratory flow and transpulmonary pressure are measured, the latter being the difference between the pressure in the oesophagus and the pleural cavity. From the relationship of respiratory flow and transpulmonary pressure, pulmonary resistance (the major portion of which is bronchiolar resistance) and compliance (a measure of the rigidity of the lungs) can be calculated. Bronchoconstriction was produced by the inhalation of 1 mg of histamine as an aerosol and all drugs were administered through a nebulizer attached to the inspiratory limb of the respiratory circuit.

The inhalation of histamine produced a marked increase in pulmonary resistance and a fall in compliance. The activity of aerosols of $PGE_2$ and isoprenaline was assessed on their ability to prevent these effects when given immediately before the inhalation of histamine. In dogs isoprenaline was completely effective in preventing the effects of histamine but the activity of $PGE_2$ was weak, more than 50% inhibition being achieved in only 3 of 10 animals with doses up to 2 mg. In contrast both isoprenaline and $PGE_2$ were effective and approximately equipotent bronchodilators in the monkey. In a recent study of the activity of aerosols of $PGE_1$ and $PGE_2$ in the anaesthetized cat (Rosenthale, Dervinis and Kassarich, 1971), using the same technique, have shown both prostaglandins to be highly effective in reversing the increase in pulmonary resistance and fall in compliance induced by histamine, 5-hydroxytryptamine, bradykinin, methacholine or neostigmine. $PGE_1$ was found to be slightly more active than $PGE_2$ and in an aerosol dose of 0.01 $\mu$g both significantly antagonized the effect of histamine. Maximal bronchodilatation usually occurred within 2-3 min and in duration varied between 10-30 min according to the dose. The duration of the bronchodilation appeared to be slightly less prolonged with both $PGE_1$ and $PGE_2$ than with isoprenaline. Cardiovascular effects were insignificant in these experiments. It was concluded that in the cat, both $PGE_1$ and $PGE_2$ are approximately 20 times more potent than isoprenaline as bronchodilators by aerosol administration. This group has recently shown prostaglandin $F_{2\beta}$ to be an effective bronchodilator in experimental animals (Rosenthale, personal communication).

## Human studies

### Aerosol administration of $PGE_1$ and $PGE_2$

When consideration was being given early in 1969 to a study of prostaglandin E aerosols in man, the potent bronchodilator effect of aerosol administration had been described in the guinea-pig but rather inconclusive results were available from other species (Large *et al.*, 1969) and bronchoconstriction was known to occur when $PGE_1$ is given intravenously to the anaesthetized cat (Main, 1964). In view of the possibility of marked species variation it was therefore decided to study the effects of inhalation of an aerosol of $PGE_1$ in healthy non-asthmatic volunteers in order to determine whether this substance produced bronchoconstriction or other adverse effects before proceeding to studies in asthmatic subjects (Cuthbert, 1969; 1971).

Prostaglandin $E_1$ was supplied either as the free acid or triethanolamine salt dissolved in ethyl alchohol and the propellents, dichlorotetraflouroethane and dichlorodiflouromethane, in flasks fitted with aerosol metering valves. The forced expiratory volume in one second ($FEV_1$) was measured with a dry wedge-type spirometer (Vitalograph) as an index of airways resistance and the blood pressure measured by a modified sphygmomanometer. The pulse rate was derived from the electrocardiogram which was monitored continuously. Measurements of $FEV_1$, blood pressure and pulse rate were taken in duplicate at not more than 10 min intervals and the means calculated.

Preliminary studies were performed in six healthy volunteers in which graded doses the free acid of $PGE_1$ (0.275-27.5 µg) were administered by aerosol. No change in heart rate, blood pressure, electrocardiogram or $FEV_1$ was noted but all three subjects who received 27.5 µg found that the inhalation caused coughing and some clearing of the throat. In order to minimise possible subjective effects associated with the inhalation, a comparison was made between $PGE_1$ 55 µg (free acid) and isoprenaline sulphate 550 µg in which the treatments were administered blind in comparison with a placebo aerosol containing ethyl alcohol and propellents only. This study confirmed the irritant effect of the $PGE_1$ aerosol since isoprenaline and placebo aerosols were non-irritant and had no effect on the $FEV_1$ or cardiovascular system. However, inhalation of $PGE_1$ while also not affecting the $FEV_1$ consistently caused coughing and occasional retrosternal soreness and it was considered that this preparation was unsatisfactory for studies in asthmatic subjects.

The absence of any bronchodilator effect with $PGE_1$ or isoprenaline aerosols in healthy subjects was not unexpected since the bronchial smooth muscle of the airways is almost fully relaxed in these subjects and the minimal further bronchodilatation which is possible cannot be detected by measurements of forced expiratory volume or peak expiratory flow.

It was thought possible that the weakly acidic properties of $PGE_1$ might be sufficient to cause irritation of the mucous membrane of the upper respiratory tract. $PGE_1$ was therefore reformulated as the neutral triethanolamine salt and the study repeated in healthy volunteers in comparison with an aerosol of $PGE_1$ (free acid) and a placebo. Inhalation of an aerosol of the triethanolamine salt of $PGE_1$ had no effect on the $FEV_1$ and was better tolerated than the free acid since only two of the five subjects who inhaled 55 µg noted any irritation. The triethanolamine salt was therefore used in studies in asthmatic volunteers.

Preliminary studies showed that small doses of $PGE_1$ (triethanolamine salt) in the range 2.75-27.5 µg caused bronchodilatation in five subjects with reversible airways obstruction. There was a 20-40% increase in the $FEV_1$ and the total duration of the effect was 15-35 min. In two subjects with irreversible airways obstruction the inhalation of $PGE_1$ had no effect. The results of a study in which $PGE_1$ (triethanolamine salt)

55 μg, isoprenaline 550 μg and placebo were administered blind to five asthmatic subjects according to a randomized Latin Square design are shown in Fig. 10 and Table 3. In each subject the inhalation of $PGE_1$ caused an increase in the $FEV_1$ which was similar in both extent and duration to that of isoprenaline. No significant changes occurred in the heart rate, blood pressure or electrocardiogram. There were obvious differences in the time course of the bronchodilatation which occurred

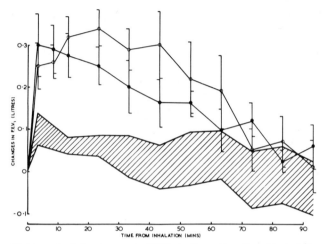

Fig. 10. Record of the changes in $FEV_1$ in five asthmatic subjects following the inhalation of $PGE_1$ (triethanolamine salt) 55 μg (○) and isoprenaline sulphate 550 μg. (●) by metered aerosol. Means ± SE are shown. Shaded area represents mean changes in $FEV_1$ after administration of placebo ± SE. Reproduced from Cuthbert (1969) with permission of the publishers.

after prostaglandin $E_1$ and isoprenaline (Fig. 10). With isoprenaline, maximum values of $FEV_1$ were usually obtained immediately after the inhalation, readings then declining slowly over the subsequent 60-90 min. The effect of $PGE_1$ appeared less rapidly. The time of maximum dilatation was variable but for the five subjects occurred at a mean of approximately 30 min after the inhalation. Although broncho-dilatation appeared to be more persistent after $PGE_1$ than after isoprenaline the overall duration of the effects of the two preparations were very similar. There was a small increase in the $FEV_1$ after the placebo inhalation followed by a slight but progressive fall in $FEV_1$ over the period of the experiment.

Only one of the subjects who took part in the comparative study found the inhalation of $PGE_1$ (triethanolamine salt) to be irritant to the upper respiratory tract but this was not associated with any change in the blood pressure or heart rate. It is interesting to note that although no

Table 3

Comparison of the effect of prostaglandin $E_1$ 55 $\mu$g (triethanolamine salt) and isoprenaline 550 $\mu$g on forced expiratory volume in one second ($FEV_1$) after aerosol administration. The $FEV_1$ before the inhalation is the mean of three paired reading taken at 5 min intervals

| | | Isoprenaline 550 $\mu$g | | | |
| Subject | $FEV_1$ before inhalation | Maximum $FEV_1$ after inhalation | Time of maximum effect (min) | Maximum increase % | Total duration of effect (min) |
|---|---|---|---|---|---|
| 1 | 1.16 | 1.54 | 3rd | 33 | 90 |
| 2 | 2.54 | 3.03 | 3rd | 19 | 70 |
| 3 | 3.53 | 3.8 | 3rd | 7.5 | 80 |
| 4 | 1.29 | 1.65 | 25th | 28 | 130 |
| 5 | 1.09 | 1.28 | 3rd | 17.5 | 55 |

| | | Prostaglandin $E_1$ 55 $\mu$g | | | |
| Subject | $FEV_1$ before inhalation | Maximum $FEV_1$ after inhalation | Time of maximum effect (min) | Maximum increase % | Total duration of effect (min) |
|---|---|---|---|---|---|
| 1 | 1.23 | 1.61 | 13th | 30 | 95 |
| 2 | 2.68 | 3.08 | 13th | 15 | 70 |
| 3 | 3.46 | 3.9 | 38th | 12.5 | 100 |
| 4 | 1.09 | 1.65 | 53rd | 51.5 | 115 |
| 5 | 1.54 | 1.71 | 13th | 11 | 50 |

Reproduced from Cuthbert (1969) with permission of the publisher.

coughing or other irritant effect occurred in most of the asthmatic subjects after the inhalation of $PGE_1$, a feeling of retrosternal 'soreness' or 'roughness', occurring at the same time as the bronchodilator effect was not uncommon. One other asthmatic subject, who had reversible airways obstruction, did cough and experience irritation of the throat for some 10 min following the inhalation of a very small dose of $PGE_1$ (triethanolamine salt). As shown in Fig. 11, there was a slow but progressive fall in the $FEV_1$ and wheezing and bronchospasm was evident when the $FEV_1$ had fallen to 2.3 litres. Inhalation of isoprenaline rapidly reversed the attack. This subject appeared to be particularly sensitive to the irritant effect of inhaled substances since a modest fall in $FEV_1$ occurred after inhalation of the placebo. In this

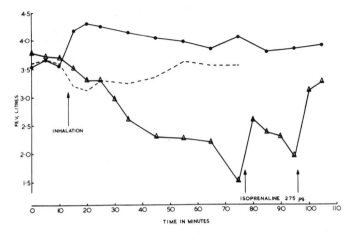

Fig. 11. Record of the $FEV_1$ in one asthmatic subject following the administration of $PGE_1$ (triethanolamine salt) 5.5 $\mu$g ($\triangle$), isoprenaline 550 $\mu$g. ($\circ$) and placebo ( $- - -$ ) by aerosol. At each of the arrows at the right of the figure one inhalation of isoprenaline (275 $\mu$g) was given. Reproduced from Cuthbert (1969) with permission of the publishers.

subject the time course of the progressive fall of $FEV_1$ associated with coughing suggests that the bronchospasm was reflex in origin and secondary to the irritant effect. It seems unlikely that $PGE_1$ has any direct bronchoconstrictor effect in man.

A limited study of the triethanolamine salt of $PGE_2$ has also been carried out (Cuthbert, 1971). In four healthy subjects the effect of aerosol administration of $PGE_2$ was indistinguishable from that of triethanolamine salt of $PGE_1$. The bronchodilator effects of $PGE_2$ by aerosol in two asthmatic subjects were also similar to those described for $PGE_1$. Doses of 5.5-55 $\mu$g produced an 18-40% increase in the $FEV_1$ (Subjects 1 and 2, Table 3) of 40-60 min duration. No irritant effect of the aerosol of $PGE_2$ was noted in either asthmatic subject but from more recent work it seems unlikely that $PGE_2$ offers any advantage over $PGE_1$ in this respect.

The bronchodilator effect of aerosol administration of $PGE_1$ (triethanolamine salt) has been confirmed by Herxheimer and Roetscher (1971). In preliminary studies in healthy volunteers the triethanolamine salt of $PGE_1$ was less irritant on aerosol administration than the free acid. These authors then studied the effect of the inhalation of 100 $\mu$g $PGE_1$ (triethanolamine salt) by metered aerosol in 37 patients with chronic obstructive airways disease, using the non-forced inspiratory vital capacity and the maximum expiratory flow rate (peak flow) as an index of changes in airways resistance. In the majority of patients, the inhalation of $PGE_1$ caused a definite improvement in vital capacity and peak flow which was maximal 30-40 min after the inhalation. These results are in accordance with the study of $PGE_1$ in a small number of asthmatic subjects (Cuthbert, 1969) in which the $FEV_1$ was used to assess changes in airways resistance. Although Herxheimer and Roetscher made no formal comparison between $PGE_1$ and isoprenaline, a number of patients were given isoprenaline or salbutamol (1.15-1.54 mg) from a spirometer circuit immediately before or after the inhalation of $PGE_1$. The results may be summarized as follows: 7 patients had irreversible airways obstruction and were not benefited by $PGE_1$, isoprenaline or salbutamol. Seven other patients given isoprenaline initially showed an improvement in vital capacity and peak flow but the subsequent administration of $PGE_1$ only resulted in further improvement in one patient. In 18 of the remaining 23 patients, the inhalation of $PGE_1$ produced a significant increase in the vital capacity and peak flow. In seven of these patients the response was good (peak flows increased by 13-48%) and in four only moderate (peak flows increased by 6-12%) but no further improvement could be obtained with isoprenaline or salbutamol. In three patients there was a good improvement with $PGE_2$, but isoprenaline resulted in at least an additional 15% increase in peak flow. Four patients showed a good response to $PGE_1$ but isoprenaline or salbutamol were not given. In the remaining five patients there was no significant improvement with $PGE_1$ but a good improvement with isoprenaline.

In this series, 25 of the 37 patients (67%) coughed after the inhalation of $PGE_1$, and this group included all the patients who showed no response to $PGE_1$ but a subsequent improvement on isoprenaline. Perhaps if coughing is troublesome the bronchodilator effect of $PGE_1$ may be prevented in some cases. The prior inhalation of isoprenaline did not prevent the irritant effect of the $PGE_1$ aerosol.

Prostaglandin $E_1$ appears to be an effective bronchodilator in the majority of subjects with reversible airways obstruction but under the conditions used by Herxheimer and Roetscher (1971), isoprenaline or salbutamol can have a more powerful effect.

The bronchodilator effect of both $PGE_1$ and $PGE_2$ have recently been confirmed in studies in which airways resistance was measured by total body plethysmography (Smith and Cuthbert, unpublished observations). In both normal and asthmatic subjects, the inhalation of 55 $\mu$g $PGE_1$ or $PGE_2$ produced falls in airways resistance which were similar to that of the inhalation of 550 $\mu$g isoprenaline. The advantage of this sensitive and more specific method, is that it appears possible to assess the activity of bronchodilator aerosols without recourse to asthmatic subjects.

*Aerosol administration of PGF$_{2\alpha}$*

A preliminary study has been performed in healthy volunteers to investigate the effect of inhaled PGF$_{2\alpha}$ on airways resistance using total body plethysmography (Smith and Cuthbert, 1972a, b).

In all four subjects, the inhalation of PGF$_{2\alpha}$ (40-60 $\mu$g) caused an increase in airways resistance and fall in specific airways conductance; these effects were maximal within 4-6 min and total duration 30-40 min. Wheezing or dyspnoea did not occur. Similar findings have been reported by Hedqvist, Holmgren and Mathé (1971). Both PGE$_2$ (55 $\mu$g) and isoprenaline (550 $\mu$g) given by metered aerosol immediately after the peak effect of PGF$_{2\alpha}$, promptly reversed the bronchoconstriction. Isoprenaline was more effective than PGE$_2$ in this respect. As with the E prostaglandins, inhalation of PGF$_{2\alpha}$ was associated with upper respiratory tract irritation.

The bronchoconstrictor action of PGF$_{2\alpha}$ was not influenced by pre-treatment with several possible antagonists including flufenamic acid by mouth, or by disodium cromoglycate or atropine methonitrate by inhalation (Smith and Cuthbert, unpublished observations).

*Intravenous administration*

Prostaglandins E$_2$ and F$_{2\alpha}$ are becoming increasingly used intravenously for the induction of labour and therapeutic abortion. It would appear important to determine whether the doses of prostaglandins used in these procedures bring about any changes in bronchial smooth muscle tone. On the basis of the animal experiments described, PGF$_{2\alpha}$ would be expected to produce bronchoconstriction when given intravenously, while PGE$_2$ is likely to have bronchodilator activity, though the latter would be difficult to detect in healthy subjects.

Changes in airways resistance have been studied by Smith (1972) in 15 patients who were undergoing termination of pregnancy by intravenous infusion of PGE$_2$ or PGF$_{2\alpha}$. Four of the patients had a family history of asthma, eczema or bronchitis but none suffered from asthma or had any other disease of the heart or lungs at the time of the study. A control group was also included which consisted of 11 women who were undergoing minor gynaecological procedures.

Methods of studying airways resistance such as the FEV$_1$ or peak expiratory flow were abandoned because the patients undergoing termination of pregnancy were often in pain or discomfort and were unable to co-operate sufficiently. For this reason the interruptor method was chosen (Clements, Sharp, Johnson and Elam, 1959) which requires no forced effort on the part of the patient. In principle, the patient breaths in a tidal fashion into a mouthpiece in which the airflow is

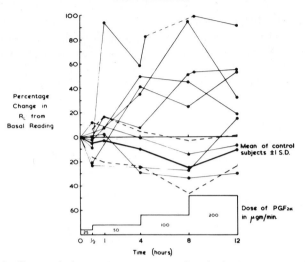

Fig. 12. Changes in lung resistance associated with the intravenous infusion of PGF$_{2\alpha}$ in 8 healthy women undergoing therapeutic abortion. The mean ± one standard deviation (1 SD) for a control group of 11 other women are shown. During the break in the record of one subject receiving PGF$_{2\alpha}$ (at the top of the figure) lung resistance fell to normal when the infusion was discontinued but became elevated again when it was recommenced. Reproduced from Smith (1972) with permission of the author.

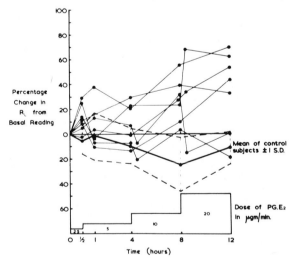

Fig. 13. Changes in lung resistance associated with the intravenous infusion of PGE$_2$ in 7 healthy women undergoing therapeutic abortion. The mean ± one standard (1 SD) for a control group of 11 other women are shown. Reproduced from Smith (1972) with permission of the author.

interrupted 10 times a second by a rotating valve. The mouthpiece pressure is measured at mid-inhalation both before and during interruption of airflow; during interruption the mouthpiece pressure is considered to approximate the alveolar pressure. Pressure at the mouthpiece has previously been calibrated for known rates of flow and, since alveolar pressure and flow can be derived from the measurements, resistance can be calculated. The result obtained by this method is higher than that of airways resistance calculated with the body plethysmograph and approximates to lung resistance. The method seems particularly useful for measuring changes in normal subjects in which airways resistance accounts for approximately 90% of total lung resistance.

Eight patients received intravenous infusion of $PGF_{2\alpha}$ in a step-wise dosage of 25-200 $\mu g/min$ as shown in Fig. 12. In three there was no change in lung resistance compared with the control group. In the other five there was a significant increase in lung resistance although the dose at which the resistance became elevated varied between individual patients. In one patient (see Fig. 12), in whom a marked increase in lung resistance occurred, there was mechanical failure of the infusion apparatus and lung resistance fell to normal but became elevated again within half an hour of recommencing the infusion. No symptoms or signs of bronchospasm could be detected in this or any other patient in this group.

Seven patients received intravenous infusions of $PGE_2$ in doses of 2.5-20 $\mu g/min$. As shown in Fig. 13 there was a small increase in lung resistance due to the infusion of 2.5 $\mu g/min$ and in five patients there was a significant increase in lung resistance which was related to the dose infused. Two patients showed a small increase at 10 $\mu g/min$ which was not maintained on increasing the dose. As in the previous group, no patient complained of breathlessness or cough and there was no evidence of bronchospasm. In all patients the lung resistance returned to normal on discontinuing the infusion.

These results indicate that the intravenous infusion of $PGE_2$ or $PGF_{2\alpha}$ results in an increase in airways resistance in healthy subjects, presumably due to an increase in bronchial smooth muscle tone although a contribution due to some bronchial oedema cannot be excluded. Although none of the subjects had any respiratory difficulty the author suggests that in view of the changes in lung resistance $PGF_{2\alpha}$ or $PGE_2$ should not be infused in patients with pre-existing obstructive airways disease.

An increase in bronchial smooth muscle tone due to intravenous infusion of $PGF_{2\alpha}$ conforms to the known properties of this prostaglandin. The results with the intravenous infusion of $PGE_2$ are unexpected since intravenous and aerosol administration of this prostaglandin is bronchodilator in most species.

## 3. POTENCY IN RELATION TO ROUTE OF ADMINISTRATION

In most studies of the effects on bronchial resistance of prostaglandins administered by aerosol it has been found that $PGE_1$ and $PGE_2$ are more potent bronchodilators than isoprenaline although there is considerable species variation (see Section 2). In human studies small doses of $PGE_1$ and $PGE_2$ given by aerosol are effective bronchodilators. Although no formal comparison has been made the results suggest that both E prostaglandins are more potent than isoprenaline as bronchodilators on a weight basis (Cuthbert, 1969, 1971). In contrast, in the only study of the effects of intravenous prostaglandins on pulmonary function in the human subject (Smith, 1972), both $PGE_2$ and $PGF_{2\alpha}$ caused an increase in airways resistance.

The difference in the bronchodilator activity of the E prostaglandins when administered by intravenous and aerosol routes may be related to their metabolism. Prostaglandins are stable in the blood (Ferreira and Vane, 1967) but their half-life in the circulation is short because they are rapidly inactivated, 90-95% of $PGE_1$ and $PGE_2$ being removed in one circulation through guinea-pig and other animal lungs (Biron, 1968a; Ferreira and Vane, 1967; Piper, Vane and Wyllie, 1970). Similar results have been obtained in the rat, cat and dog and inactivation has also been shown to occur in the hepatic and peripheral vascular beds. In man, radio-active labelled $PGE_1$ disappears rapidly from the circulation after intravenous injection (Granström, 1967) and there is evidence that over 90% is inactivated in pulmonary circulation (Biron, 1968b). The metabolic fate of the prostaglandins is fully discussed in Chapter III.

It seems possible, therefore, that a considerable proportion of infused prostaglandins are inactivated in the pulmonary circulation before it reaches bronchial smooth muscle sites. A more theoretical possibility is that the sites to which prostaglandins must penetrate may be more readily accessible to aerosols than to circulating prostaglandins. If inhaled E prostaglandins are inactivated in the lungs, but slightly later than the initiation of bronchial smooth muscle relaxation, this would account for their unexpected high bronchodilator potency, relatively short duration of action and lack of cardiovascular effects (Large *et al.*, 1969). Variations in the potency of prostaglandins by aerosol in different species might thus reflect differences in their rate of inactivation, the activity of metabolites and accessibility to bronchial smooth muscle.

In the study of the effect of intravenous infusion of large doses of $PGF_{2\alpha}$ and $PGE_2$ on airways resistance in women undergoing therapeutic abortion (Smith, 1972), samples of arterial blood were taken at various times during the infusions, but no $PGF_{2\alpha}$ or $PGE_2$ was detected. To explain the increase in airways resistance with $PGE_2$ in this situation this author considered the possibility that inactivation rapidly takes place in the pulmonary circulation, with the release of active bronchoconstrictor metabolites which are returned to the lungs by the systemic circulation. This suggestion may also be of relevance in the effect of infused prostaglandins on the pregnant uterus. Since none of the infused prostaglandins can be detected in the arterial blood the active substance may similarly be an unidentified metabolite.

## 4. MECHANISM OF ACTION

From the previous discussion it is evident that prostaglandins of the E series in general relax isolated tracheal and bronchial smooth muscle and cause bronchodilatation while prostaglandins of the F series contracted isolated tracheal and bronchial muscle and cause bronchoconstriction. The evidence for the underlying pharmacological mechanism will now be considered.

In isolated tracheal muscle from various animals $PGE_1$ antagonises the contractions produced by acetylcholine, histamine, dihydroergotamine and barium sulphate and also inhibits the intrinsic tone (Main, 1964). $PGE_1$ also inhibits the intrinsic tone of isolated human bronchial muscle (Sweatman & Collier, 1968; Sheard, 1968). Both $PGE_1$ and $PGE_2$ given intravenously or by aerosol similarly antagonize bronchoconstriction caused by a number of agonists including histamine, 5-hydroxytryptamine, acetylcholine, bradykinin and SRS-A in various animal species and bronchoconstriction caused by passive sensitization in the guinea-pig (Main, 1964; Rosenthale *et al.*, 1968, 1970; Large *et al.*, 1969; Adolphson and Townley, 1970). These observations suggest that the E prostaglandins relax bronchial smooth muscle itself rather than act as an antagonist to any particular substance causing contraction.

The bronchodilator effect of $PGE_1$ cannot be abolished by the treatment of isolated bronchial smooth muscle preparations with $\alpha$ or $\beta$-adrenoceptor blockers such as phenoxybenzamine and propranolol (Sheard, 1968; Adolphson and Townley, 1970), neither is the contraction of isolated human bronchial muscle due to $PGF_{2\alpha}$ antagonized by atropine or mepyramine (Sweatman and Collier, 1968). Similar results have been obtained with intact animal preparations in which the bronchodilator effect of $PGE_1$ or $PGE_2$, intravenously or by aerosol, has been unaffected by $\beta$-adrenoceptor blockers, reserpine, atropine and hexamethonium, or by such procedures as vagotomy, pithing or adrenalectomy (Änggård and Bergström, 1963; Rosenthale *et al.*, 1968, 1970; Large *et al.*, 1969; Adolphson and Townley, 1970). The increase in bronchial resistance induced with $PGF_{2\alpha}$ in the anaesthetized cat is not affected by vagotomy or by atropinization (Änggård and Bergström, 1963).

The effects of the E prostaglandins are therefore not mediated by adrenoceptor stimulation or by the release of catecholamines from the adrenal medulla or by central or ganglionic stimulation. The action of the F prostaglandins cannot be due to the stimulation of cholinergic nerves or to the liberation of histamine. All the available evidence therefore suggests that all the prostaglandins have a direct action on bronchial smooth muscle.

There has recently been much interest in the relationship of the cyclic adenosine-3',5'-monophosphate system (cyclic AMP system) and the mechanism of action of the prostaglandins. This is fully discussed in Chapter IV but is briefly considered here since it may have relevance to the action of prostaglandins on bronchial smooth muscle.

Cyclic AMP seems to be closely related to hormonal function. On this hypothesis (Butcher, 1968; Sutherland, Robison and Butcher, 1968) the exciting hormone, called the 'first messenger', activates adenyl cyclase in the cell membrane which catalyzes the transformation of adenosine monophosphate to cyclic adenosine-3',5'-monophosphate (cyclic AMP). As the 'second messenger', cyclic AMP acts intracellularly to bring about the specific response of the cell; this may be a physiological response, e.g. lipolysis or smooth muscle relaxation, or involve the synthesis of other hormones, e.g. thyroxine. Cyclic AMP is in turn broken down to 5'-AMP by phosphodiesterase. Changes in intracellular cyclic AMP can be brought about either by activation or inhibition of adenyl cyclase or by activation or inhibition of phosphodiesterase.

The E prostaglandins stimulate adenyl cyclase and increase intracellular cyclic AMP in many experimental situations. Interest in the possible role of the cyclic AMP system to bronchial smooth muscle function arose when it was found that two substances with bronchodilator activity affect cyclic AMP levels in the rat epidymal fat pad. Adrenaline stimulates adenyl cyclase and increases intracellular cyclic AMP while theophylline and other methyl xanthines have a similar action on cyclic AMP brought about by the inhibition of phosphodiesterase. Moreover, adrenaline and theophylline act synergistically (Vaughan and Steinberg, 1963; Butcher, Ho, Meng and Sutherland, 1963).

Some preliminary observations have been reported with lung tissue. Both an adrenaline-sensitive adenyl cyclase system (Klainer, Chi, Freidberg, Rall and Sutherland, 1962) and phosphodiesterase are present in subcellular fractions of lung tissue (Butcher and Sutherland, 1962). More recently, Sutherland *et al.* (1968) have shown that caffeine, a methyl xanthine, and adrenaline act synergistically in increasing cyclic AMP levels in the rat lung. Unfortunately, the effect of the prostaglandins on cyclic AMP in the lung is not yet known and is complicated by the presence of different tissues in lung slices and the lack of knowledge of changes in cyclic AMP levels in different cell types.

However, it is possible that variations in the tone of bronchial smooth muscle are associated with changes in intracellular cyclic AMP since Adolphson, Kennedy, Reeb and Townley (1971) have shown that dibutyryl-3',5'-cyclic adenosine monophosphate produces relaxation in isolated guinea-pig tracheal muscle and that this effect is potentiated by theophylline. If E prostaglandins cause an increase in cyclic AMP in bronchial smooth muscle cells this may be their mechanism of inducing bronchodilatation.

## 5. PHYSIOLOGICAL AND PATHOLOGICAL INVOLVEMENT

There is no definite evidence that the prostaglandins are involved in normal or abnormal pulmonary function and the title of this section is entirely presumptive. However, it is relevant to consider briefly the distribution, synthesis and release of prostaglandins under experimental conditions and to speculate on their importance.

Prostaglandins are naturally-occurring substances which have been extracted from most tissues examined although there is some doubt whether they exist in tissues as formed substances or are synthesized from precursors during extraction. Early in their discovery prostaglandins were found in the lungs, notably of sheep (Bergström *et al.,* 1962) and later of the guinea-pig (Änggård, 1965). The distribution of prostaglandins in the lungs is interesting since unlike many other tissues, the lungs of most species contain higher concentrations of $PGF_{2\alpha}$ than of $PGE_2$. Karim, Hillier and Devlin (1968) carried out a systematic survey of prostaglandins $E_1$, $E_2$, $F_{1\alpha}$ and $F_{2\alpha}$ in six widely used laboratory animals. No prostaglandins were detected in the lungs of the dog. In rat, guinea-pig and chicken lungs the concentration of $PGF_{2\alpha}$ was high (30-375 ng/g tissue) compared with that of $PGE_2$ (2.5-6.6 ng/g) while in rabbit lung the concentration of both these prostaglandins was low ($PGF_{2\alpha}$ 8 ng/g; $PGE_2$ 5.4 ng/g respectively). In cat lung the proportions were reversed, 1.5 ng/g $PGF_{2\alpha}$ and 15.5 ng/g $PGE_2$ being found respectively. The highest concentration and greatest preponderance of $PGF_{2\alpha}$ was found in the guinea-pig ($PGF_{2\alpha}$ 375 ng/g; $PGE_2$ 2.5 ng/g respectively). Prostaglandins $E_2$ and $F_{2\alpha}$ have also been detected in human pulmonary tissues (Änggård, 1965; Karim *et al.,* 1967) and the distribution in human lung is similar to that in most animals with a preponderance of $PGE_{2\alpha}$. In human bronchial muscle lower concentrations were found with slightly higher amounts of $PGE_2$ (see Table 2, Chapter III). No $PGE_1$ or $PGF_{1\alpha}$ was found in pulmonary tissues of any of the species examined. There is as yet no information available on the distribution of prostaglandins in the lungs or bronchi of asthmatic subjects.

The presence of prostaglandins in human and animal pulmonary tissues does not necessarily imply a physiological function and it is important to demonstrate their release when the tissue is stimulated in some physiological way. A number of diverse stimuli have been shown to release prostaglandins from isolated perfused lungs of the guinea-pig (Piper and Vane, 1971). These include challenge of lungs sensitized to ovalbumen, embolization of the lungs by particles or air, mechanical stimulation, infusion of histamine or 5-hydroxytryptamine and positive pressure ventilation. Prostaglandins can also be released from a chopped-lung preparation or by simple agitation, whether the tissue has been sensitized or not. Piper and Vane (1971) point out that the feature common to all these procedures is probably cellular distortion or damage and that the release of prostaglandins may follow any disturbance of the cell membrane. Many tissues from which the release of prostaglandins has been demonstrated, including the spleen and lungs, release more prostaglandins than can be extracted (Gilmore, Vane and Wyllie, 1968; Ramwell and Shaw, 1970) and it is concluded that the release occurs as a result of stimulation of prostaglandin synthesis.

What physiological interpretation can be advanced to account for the apparently rapid synthesis of prostaglandins by the lung? Because both a potent bronchoconstrictor, $PGF_{2\alpha}$ and a potent bronchodilator, $PGE_2$ , occur or may be readily synthesized, it is tempting to consider that the prostaglandins are somehow responsible for the regulation of normal bronchial smooth muscle tone, either acting as intracellular hormones or being released from cells but having a strictly localized effect. Such a function would necessitate the differential synthesis of E and F prostaglandins in response to variations in bronchial smooth muscle tone. Unfortunately there is as yet no evidence to support this concept of a local regulatory function. However, some indirect observations are worth consideration. Karim et al. (1968) failed to detect any prostaglandins in dog lung; this finding could be related to the weak bronchodilator effect of $PGE_2$ in this species (Rosenthale et al., 1970). Conversely, the lungs of the guinea-pig contain a high proportion of $PGF_{2\alpha}$ related to $PGE_2$ and in this species E prostaglandins are particularly effective bronchodilators (Large et al., 1969). These findings may be fortuitous but suggest that the presence of the prostaglandins is related to their ability to affect bronchial smooth muscle tone. This might conceivably operate through a species variation in the effects of the prostaglandins on cyclic AMP.

Prostaglandins may also be involved in the physiological relationship between the ventilation and perfusion of areas of lung. This suggestion is entirely speculative but it is possible to envisage that such substances, which have powerful effects on bronchial and vascular smooth muscle, may produce proportional changes in ventilation and pulmonary blood flow. In acute experiments, it has been demonstrated that embolization of pulmonary artery branches with particles is accompanied by marked bronchoconstriction (Clarke, Graf & Nadel, 1970) and the release of prostaglandins (Lindsey & Wyllie, 1970). In experimental pulmonary embolism, Thomas, Stein, Tanabe, Rege & Wessler (1964) have shown that 5-hydroxytryptamine is released from platelets in this situation and it seems likely that prostaglandins released as a result of embolisation or from platelets (Smith and Willis, 1971) are also important mediators although their exact role has yet to be determined. Prostaglandins are also released in anaphylactic reactions but it is again difficult to determine their contribution to the bronchoconstriction because other highly active substances, such as histamine and SRS-A, are released at the same time.

The relationship of the prostaglandins to bronchial asthma is similarly obscure. If prostaglandins in the lungs are indeed involved in the normal regulation of bronchial smooth muscle tone, it may be speculated (Horton, 1969) that the overproduction of the bronchoconstrictor $PGF_{2\alpha}$ from arachidonic acid at the expense of the relaxant $PGE_2$ might contribute to the bronchospasm and the increase in sensitivity of respiratory smooth muscle which occurs in bronchial asthma. An alternative suggestion if that E prostaglandins may be converted to F prostaglandins in the lungs, although this is unlikely to occur in normal biosynthesis. Another possibility is that the defect in bronchial asthma is not in the relationship of the prostaglandins but is due to a maladjustment of the cyclic AMP system (Sutherland *et al.*, 1968) since a reduced intracellular concentration of cyclic AMP, a failure of activation of adenylcyclase or increased activity of phosphodiesterase would probably all function to increase bronchial smooth muscle tone. The prostaglandins might well be involved if they are shown to stimulate or inhibit adenylcyclase in this, as in other situations.

For a number of years, Collier and his co-workers have made a study of the antagonism by non-steroidal anti-inflammatory drugs of substances believed to be involved in allergic reactions (see Collier, 1969, 1971). An interaction between these drugs and the prostaglandins was first suggested when it was shown that the fenamates, phenylbutazone and aspirin effectively antagonize the contraction of isolated human bronchial muscle induced by $PGF_{2\alpha}$ (Collier and Sweatman, 1968); this antagonism appeared to be selective since there was no block of the relaxant effect of prostaglandins $E_1$ or $E_2$. A clue to an effect of the non-steroidal anti-inflammatory drugs on prostaglandin synthesis was provided when it was found that aspirin and sodium salicylate antagonize the bronchoconstrictor effect of arachidonic acid, a prostaglandin E precursor, in both isolated human bronchial muscle and in the guinea-pig *in vivo* (Jacques, 1965; Berry, 1966).

Vane (1971) has recently advanced convincing evidence that

indomethacin, aspirin and salicylate, in that order of potency, are effective inhibitors of the synthesis of both $PGE_2$ and $PGF_{2\alpha}$ in cell-free homogenates of guinea-pig lung, perhaps by competing with arachidonic acid for active enzyme sites. Indomethacin and aspirin were effective in low concentrations, 0.27 and 6.3 $\mu$g/ml respectively giving 50% inhibition of synthesis; levels which are well within the range achieved in the plasma in therapeutic doses. Sodium salicylate was 10-30 times less effective. It is interesting that the order of potency of aspirin and sodium salicylate in inhibiting prostaglandin synthesis is similar to their order of potency in antagonizing the bronchoconstrictor effect of bradykinin in the guinea-pig (Collier and Shorley, 1960; Collier, 1969); this raises the possibility that bradykinin, and perhaps other mediators released in anaphylaxis, produce bronchospasm by stimulating the synthesis and release of prostaglandin $F_{2\alpha}$. However, the relationship of aspirin and other anti-inflammatory drugs to the treatment of bronchial asthma is not clear. Amidopyrine and phenazone (Herxheimer and Stresemann, 1961), phenylbutazone (Von Rechenberg, 1962), aspirin (Pearson, 1963) and indomethacin (Jackson, Raymer and Etter, 1968) have all been reported to be of benefit to asthmatic patients although the response is variable and these drugs have never become established in treatment. In view of the recent findings of Vane (1971) it seems possible that the beneficial effects of this group of drugs in asthma may be due to inhibition of the synthesis of $PGF_{2\alpha}$ and perhaps other mediators.

The definition of the non-steroidal anti-inflammatory drugs as powerful inhibitors of prostaglandin synthesis, provides a new approach to the study of these substances in the maintenance of bronchial smooth muscle tone in isolated tissues and in the whole organism. This is complicated however, by the fact that $PGE_2$ and $PGF_{2\alpha}$ have different and mutually antagonistic actions on bronchial smooth muscle and the development of selective inhibitors may well be necessary before their individual contributions can be determined.

A number of compounds which block the effects of the prostaglandins on various smooth muscle preparations have recently been synthesized (see Bennett and Posner, 1971). One of the most interesting of these prostaglandin antagonists is polyphloretin phosphate, which has been shown to block the contraction of isolated human bronchial muscle due to $PGF_{2\alpha}$ while leaving the relaxant effect of $PGE_2$ unaffected (Mathé, Strandberg and Åström, 1971).

## 6. THERAPEUTIC POSSIBILITIES

In our present state of knowledge it does not appear that the prostaglandins have any immediate therapeutic application in respiratory disease but it is appropriate to consider the advantages and defects of the preparations already tested in man and to outline possible future developments.

Prostaglandins $E_1$ and $E_2$ have been shown to be effective bronchodilators when given by aerosol to asthmatic subjects and this activity is detectable with delivered doses as small as 2-5 $\mu$g; Animal and limited human data supports the view that both $PGE_1$ and $PGE_2$ are considerably more active than isoprenaline on a weight basis by the aerosol route. The E prostaglandins are rapidly metabolized in the lungs in experimental animals and if this also occurs in man it may be the reason why doses which cause substantial bronchodilatation do not appear to have any effect on the cardiovascular system. Inactivation in the lungs may also account for the relatively short bronchodilator action which is comparable to that of isoprenaline.

Despite their several advantages it seems unlikely that any natural prostaglandin will prove to be a bronchodilator of therapeutic value. The main reason for this statement is that all the aerosol preparations of E prostaglandins so far studied in man are irritant to the upper respiratory tract (Cuthbert, 1969, 1971; Herxheimer and Roetscher, 1971). Although the coughing and clearing of the throat which occurs after inhalation is not usually troublesome and does not prevent bronchodilatation from taking place, in one asthmatic subject a particularly marked irritant effect was followed by a progressive reduction of $FEV_1$ and bronchospasm. Prostaglandins are weak acids and an aerosol of the neutral triethanolamine salt was better tolerated but was not entirely free from irritant effects. It is not yet clear whether this local effect on the upper respiratory tract is a characteristic feature of the prostaglandin molecule or is limited to the naturally-occurring E and F prostaglandins. Another problem is that the E prostaglandins are not particularly stable in alcoholic solution as pressurized aerosols and slowly lose their activity over a period of several months.

The first objective would appear to be the development of a preparation which has acceptable properties as a bronchodilator. An approach to this problem is suggested by the properties of the A prostaglandins (Horton and Jones, 1969) which although of low potency as bronchodilators pass through the pulmonary circulation of experimental animals without significant loss of activity. If a prostaglandin analogue can be prepared which is stable, does not cause irritation on inhalation and is not rapidly inactivated in the lungs it might well prove to be an extremely effective bronchodilator. Another approach is by modification of the formulation. All the prostaglandin aerosols so far tested have been in the form of an alcoholic solution with propellents; since very small doses have been found effective it is likely that nanogram quantities are actually reaching the bronchiolar smooth muscle and producing relaxation. Formulation of prostaglandins in a micronized form is a possible method of improving their deposition in the airways which has been successfully employed in the formulation of isoprenaline and salbutamol aerosols.

Although the relationship of the E and F prostaglandins to the regulation of bronchial smooth muscle is obscure, it is conceivable that a hypothetical deficiency of E prostaglandins in bronchial asthma might be corrected by their prophylactic use.

Another objective of potential therapeutic importance is the development of compounds which block the effects or prevent the synthesis of specific prostaglandins, in particular those of the F series. The compounds at present available are either relatively non-specific and are unsuitable for administration to man. However, this area will undoubtedly be one of intense investigation over the next few years and may lead to an understanding of the role of the prostaglandins in the maintenance of bronchial smooth muscle tone and to the synthesis of compounds of value in the treatment of bronchospasm.

# REFERENCES

Adolphson, R. L., Kennedy, T. J., Reeb, R. and Townley, R. G. (1969). Effect of beta-adrenergic blockade and prostaglandin $F_{2\alpha}$ on isoproterenol and theophylline bronchodilatation. *Journal of Allergy,* **43**, 176.

Adolphson, R. L. and Townley, R. G. (1970). A comparison of the bronchodilator activities of isoproterenol and prostaglandin $E_1$ aerosols. *Journal of Allergy,* **45**, 119.

Änggård, E. (1965). The isolation and determination of prostaglandins in lungs of sheep, guinea pig, monkey and man. *Biochemical Pharmacology,* **14**, 1507.

Änggård, E. and Bergström, S. (1963). Biological effects of an unsaturated trihydroxy acid ($PGF_{2\alpha}$) from normal swine lung. *Acta Physiologica Scandinavica,* **58**, 1.

Bennett, A. and Posner, J. (1971). Studies on prostaglandin antagonists. *British Journal of Pharmacology,* **42**, 584.

Bergström, S., Dressler, F., Krabisch, L., Ryhage, R. and Sjövall, J. (1962c). The isolation and structure of a smooth muscle stimulating factor in normal sheep and pig lungs. *Arkiv för Kemi,* **20**, 63.

Bergström, S., Dressler, F., Ryhage, R., Samuelsson, B. and Sjövall, J. (1962a). The isolation of two further prostaglandins from sheep prostate glands. *Arkiv för Kemi,* **19**, 563.

Bergström, S., Ryhage, R., Samuelsson, B. and Sjövall, J. (1962b). The structure of prostaglandin E, $F_1$ and $F_2$. *Acta Chemica Scandinavica,* **16**, 501.

Berry, P. A. (1966). Ph.D. thesis. *Council for National Academic Awards, London,* 91.

Biron, P. (1968a). Vasoactive hormone metabolism by the pulmonary circulation. *Clinical Research,* **16**, 112.

Biron, P. (1968b). *La Presse,* Montreal, 21st December.

Butcher, R. W. (1968). Role of cyclic AMP in hormone actions. *New England Journal of Medicine,* **279**, 1378.

Butcher, R. W., Ho, R. J., Meng, H. C. and Sutherland, E. W. (1965). Adenosine 3',5'-monophosphate in biological materials. II. Measurement of adenosine 3',5'-monophosphate in tissues and role of cyclic nucleotide in lipolytic response of fat to epinephrine. *Journal of Biological Chemistry,* **240**, 4515.

Butcher, R. W. and Sutherland, E. W. (1962). Adenosine 3',5'-phosphate in biological materials. I. Purification and properties of cyclic 3',5'-nucleotide phospho-diesterase and use of this enzyme to characterize adenosine 3',5'-phosphate in human urine. *Journal of Biological Chemistry,* **237**, 1244.

Clarke, S. W., Graf, P. D. and Nadel, J. A. (1970). *In vivo* visualisation of small-airway constriction after pulmonary microembolism in cats and dogs. *Journal of Applied Physiology,* **29**, 646.

Clements, J. A., Sharp, J. T., Johnson, R. P. and Elam (1959). Estimation of pulmonary resistance by repetitive interruption of airflow. *Journal of Clinical Investigation,* **38**, 1262.

Collier, H. O. J. (1969). A pharmacological analysis of aspirin. *Advances in Pharmacology and Chemotherapy,* **7**, 333. Academic Press.

Collier, H. O. J. (1971). Prostaglandin and aspirin. *Nature (London),* **232**, 17.

Collier, H. O. J. and Shorley, P. G. (1960). Analgesic antipyretic drugs as antagonists to bradykinin. *British Journal of Pharmacology and Chemotherapy,* **15**, 601.

Collier, H. O. J. and Sweatman, W. J. F. (1968). Antagonism by fenamates of prostaglandin $F_{2\alpha}$ and of slow reacting substance on human bronchial muscle. *Nature (London),* **219**, 864.

Cuthbert, M. F. (1969). Effect on airways resistance of prostaglandin $E_1$ given by aerosol to healthy and asthmatic volunteers. *British Medical Journal,* **4**, 723.

Cuthbert, M. F. (1971). Bronchodilator activity of aerosols of prostaglandins $E_1$ and $E_2$ in asthmatic subjects. *Proceedings of the Royal Society of Medicine* **64**, 15.

Dixon, W. E. and Brodie, T. G. (1903). Contributions to the physiology of the lungs. Part 1. The bronchial muscles, their innervation and the action of drugs upon them. *Journal of Physiology,* **190**, 41P.

Ferreira, S. H. and Vane, J. R. (1967). Prostaglandins: their disappearance from and release into the circulation. *Nature (London),* **216**, 868.

Gilmore, N. J. R., Vane, J. R. and Wyllie, J. H. (1968). Prostaglandins released by the spleen. *Nature (London),* **218**, 1135.

Granström, E. (1967). On the metabolism of prostaglandin $E_1$ in man. *Progress in Biochemical Pharmacology,* **3**, 89.

Hedqvist, P., Holmgren, A and Mathé, A. A. (1971). Effect of prostaglandin $F_{2\alpha}$ on airway resistance in man. *Acta Physiologica Scandinavica,* **82**, 29A.

Herxheimer, H. and Roetscher, I. (1971). Effects of prostaglandin $E_1$ on lung function in bronchial asthma. *European Journal of Clinical Pharmacology,* **3**, 123.

Herxheimer, H. and Streseman (1961). Anti-asthmatic effect of phenazone and amidopyrine. *Nature (London),* **192**, 1089.

Horton, E. W. (1969). Hypotheses on physiological roles of prostaglandins. *Physiological Reviews,* **49**, 122.

Horton, E. W. and Jones, R. L. (1969). Prostaglandins $A_1$, $A_2$ and 19-hydroxy $A_1$; their actions on smooth muscle and their inactivation on passage through the pulmonary and hepatic portal vascular beds. *British Journal of Pharmacology,* **37**, 705.

Horton, E. W. and Main, I. H. M. (1965). A comparison of the actions of prostaglandins $F_{2\alpha}$ and $E_1$ on smooth muscle. *British Journal of Pharmacology*, **24**, 470.

Jackson, R. H., Raymer, W. J. and Etter, R. L. (1968). New therapy in bronchial asthma. An evaluation of Ponstel (mefenamic acid) in chronic bronchial asthma and pulmonary emphysema. *Journal of the Kanszs Medical Society*, **4**, 474.

Jacques, R. (1965). Arachidonic acid, an unsaturated fatty acid which produces slow contractions of smooth muscle and causes pain. Pharmacological and biochemical characterisation of its mode of action. *Helv. Physiol. Pharmacol. Acta*, **23**, 156.

Karim, S. M. M., Hillier, K. and Devlin, J. (1968). Distribution of prostaglandins $E_1$, $E_2$, $F_{1\alpha}$ and $F_{2\alpha}$ in some animal tissues. *Journal of Pharmacy and Pharmacology*, **20**, 749.

Karim, S. M. M., Sandler, M. and Williams, E. D. (1967). Distribution of prostaglandins in human tissues. *British Journal of Pharmacology and Chemotherapy*, **31**, 340.

Klainer, L. M., Chi, Y. M., Freidberg, S. L., Rall, T. W. and Sutherland, E. W. (1962). Adenyl cyclase: IV. Effects of neurohormones on the formation of adenosine $3',5'$-phosphate by preparations from brain and other tissues. *Journal of Biological Chemistry*, **237**, 1239.

Konsett, H. and Rössler, R. (1940). Versuchsanordnung zu Untersuchungen an der Bronchialmuskulatur. *Naunyn-Schmiedeberg's Archiv für experimentelle Pathologie und Pharmakologie*, **195**, 71.

Large, B. J., Leswell, P. F. and Maxwell, D. R. (1969). Bronchodilator activity of an aerosol of prostaglandin $E_1$ in experimental animals. *Nature (London)*, **224**, 78.

Lindsey, H. E. and Wyllie, J. H. (1970). Release of prostaglandins from embolized lungs. *British Journal of Surgery*, **57**, 738.

Main, I. H. M. (1964). The inhibitory actions of prostaglandins on respiratory smooth muscle. *British Journal of Pharmacology*, **22**, 511.

Mathé, A. A., Strandberg, K. and Åström, A. (1971). Blockade by polyphloretin phosphate of the prostaglandin $F_{2\alpha}$ action on isolated human bronchi. *Nature New Biology*, **230**, 215.

Pearson, R. S. B. (1963). In: *Salicylates* (Eds. A. St.J. Dixon, B. K. Martin, M. J. H. Smith and P. H. N. Wood), p. 170. Churchill, London.

Piper, P. J. and Vane, J. R. (1971). The release of prostaglandins from lung and other tissues. *Annals of the New York Academy of Sciences*, **180**, 363.

Piper, P. J., Vane, J. R. and Wyllie, J. H. (1970). Inactivation of prostaglandins by the lung. *Nature (London)*, **225**, 600.

Ramwell, P. W. and Shaw, J. E. (1970). Biological significance of prostaglandins. In: *Recent Progress in Hormone Research*, **26**, 139. Academic Press, New York and London.

Rosenthale, M. E., Dervinis, A., Begany, A. J., Lapidus, M. and Gluckman, M. I. (1968). Bronchodilator activity of prostaglandin $PGE_2$. *Pharmacologist*, **10**, 175.

Rosenthale, M. E., Dervinis, A., Begany, A. J., Lapidus, M. and Gluckman, M. I. (1970). Bronchodilator activity of prostaglandin $E_2$ when administered by aerosol to three species. *Experientia*, **26**, 1119.

Rosenthale, M. E., Dervinis, A. and Kassarich, J. (1971). Bronchodilator activity of the prostaglandins $E_1$ and $E_2$. *Journal of Pharmacology and Experimental Therapeutics*, **178**, 541.

Sheard, P. (1968). The effect of prostaglandin $E_1$ on isolated bronchial muscle from man. *Journal of Pharmacy and Pharmacology*, **20**, 232.

Smith, A. P. (1972). Effect of intravenous infusion of graded doses of prostaglandins $E_2$ and $F_{2\alpha}$ on lung resistance in patients undergoing termination. *Clinical Science.* In press.

Smith, A. P. and Cuthbert, M. F. (1972a). Prostaglandins and resistance to $\beta$-adrenoceptor stimulants. *British Medical Journal*, **2**, 166.

Smith, A. P. and Cuthbert, M. F. (1972b). The antagonistic action of prostaglandin $F_{2\alpha}$ and $E_2$ aerosols on bronchial muscle tone in man, *British Medical Journal*, **3**, 212.

Smith, J. B. and Willis, A. L. (1971). Aspirin selectively inhibits prostaglandin production in human platelets. *Nature New Biology*, **231**, 235.

Sutherland, E. W., Robison, G. A. and Butcher, R. W. (1968). Some aspects of biological role of adenosine $3',5'$-monophosphate (cyclic AMP). *Circulation*, **37**, 279.

Sweatman, W. J. F. and Collier, H. O. J. (1968). Effects of prostaglandins on human bronchial muscle. *Nature*, **217**, 69.

Thomas, D., Stein, M., Tanabe, G., Rege, V. and Wessler, S. (1964). Mechanism of bronchoconstriction produced by thromboemboli in dogs. *American Journal of Physiology*, **206**, 1207.

Türker, R. and Khairallah, P. A. (1969). Prostaglandin $E_1$, action on canine isolated tracheal muscle. *Journal of Pharmacy and Pharmacology*, **21**, 498.

Vane, J. R. (1971). Inhibition of prostaglandin synthesis as a mechanism of action for aspirin-like drugs. *Nature New Biology*, **231**, 232.

Vaughan, M. and Steinberg, D. J. (1963). Effect of hormones on lipolysis and esterification of free fatty acids during incubation of adipose tissue *in vitro*. *Journal of Lipid Research*, **4**, 193.

Von Rechenberg, H. K. (1962). In: *Phenylbutazone*, p. 147. Arnold, London.

*CHAPTER VIII*

# Prostaglandins and the Gastro-intestinal Tract

I. H. M. Main

Since their discovery by Goldblatt (1933) and von Euler (1934), prostaglandins have been known to contract isolated smooth muscle from the gastro-intestinal tract. The use of such smooth muscle for biological assay has played an important role not only in the development of techniques leading to the isolation and chemical characterization of prostaglandins but also in the identification and estimation of low concentrations in biological tissues and fluids. The latter studies have provided evidence that prostaglandins are widely distributed and are of potential physiological importance in most animal tissues, including those of the human gastro-intestinal tract.

The effects of prostaglandins on the gastro-intestinal tract are by no means confined to contraction of isolated smooth muscle. Recent studies have revealed interesting qualitative differences between the effects of different prostaglandins on longitudinal and circular muscle and have shown that certain members have potent effects on gastric, pancreatic and intestinal secretion. Moreover, diarrhoea and vomiting are amongst the most prominent side effects associated with the clinical use of the prostaglandins.

The object of this chapter is to review the actions and modes of action of prostaglandins on gastro-intestinal motility and secretion, to consider the possibility that such pharmacological actions may reflect physiological or pathological roles and to assess the potential therapeutic value of prostaglandins or their antagonists in the treatment of gastro-intestinal disease.

## 1. EFFECTS OF PROSTAGLANDINS ON GASTRO-INTESTINAL MOTILITY *IN VITRO*

### The use of gastro-intestinal smooth muscle for biological assay

Rabbit jejunum and guinea-pig ileum were among the first isolated tissues to be employed for the detection and assay of prostaglandins in extracts of semen and reproductive tract. In some early studies, prostaglandin content was expressed as units of biological activity though such animal units are too variable for precise quantitative studies. Following the preparation of a barium salt of a prostaglandin extracted from sheep seminal vesicles it became possible to carry out quantitative assays in terms of this stable laboratory standard. Nevertheless, where standard or unknown consist of a mixture of different prostaglandins the results of biological assay vary according to the proportion of the different prostaglandins present and their relative potencies on the particular assay preparation used. Differences in the relative and absolute potencies of prostaglandins were first demonstrated by Bergström, Eliasson, von Euler and Sjövall (1959b) who found that E prostaglandins were much more potent than F prostaglandins on the guinea-pig ileum whereas on the rabbit jejunum, F prostaglandins were more potent.

The characteristic features of the structure-activity relationships of different prostaglandins on gastro-intestinal smooth muscle are similar to those in most other biological preparations. In general, prostaglandins within each series are qualitatively similar though there are a few exceptions which will be noted later. The relative potency of prostaglandins within each series is usually as follows:

$$E_1 = E_2 > E_3 ; \quad F_{1\alpha} < F_{2\alpha} > F_{3\alpha}$$

Prostaglandins of different series (E, F, A) may show marked quantitative and qualitative differences, for example, the E prostaglandins may relax while F prostaglandins contract circular intestinal muscle. Prostaglandins of the A series are much less potent than the E or F prostaglandins on gastro-intestinal smooth muscle though they have potent effects on gastric secretion. Other naturally occurring prostaglandins including those of the A and B series, the 19-hydroxy derivatives, the precursors and most metabolites of prostaglandins are usually much less active than $PGE_1$ on gastro-intestinal smooth muscle.

In the search for sensitive assay preparations, smooth muscle from different regions of the gastro-intestinal tract in many species ranging from the goldfish to the fruit bat has been studied. A critical assessment of the suitability of four such preparations commonly used for quantitative biological assay was made by Weeks, Schultz and Brown (1968) who considered not only the absolute sensitivity to prostaglandins but the ease of performance and the precision of the assay. The jird colon was considered to be more satisfactory for precise quantitative biological assay than the rat fundus strip, rabbit jejunum and guinea-pig colon. It was at least as sensitive as the others and had the additional advantage of being insensitive to fatty acid hydroperoxides which contract several other preparations, especially the guinea-pig ileum.

Although chemical and physico-chemical methods, capable of detecting nanogram quantities (including those prostaglandins which do not affect smooth muscle) are now available, biological assay continues to be of value for studying structure-activity relationships of prostaglandins and potential antagonists. The technique of parallel quantitative assay employing two or more tissues which differ widely in their response to different prostaglandins may be used, in conjunction with chromatographic evidence, to assist in the identification of small amounts of prostaglandins in biological tissues or fluids (Horton and Main, 1967). The blood-bathed organ technique using serially superfused preparations such as rat stomach strip, rat colon and chick rectum (Vane, 1969) has proved of immense value in studying the release and fate of circulating prostaglandins.

### Effects on longitudinal and circular smooth muscle *in vitro*

Prostaglandins E and F contract isolated whole segments of gastro-intestinal smooth muscle from most species tested. The few exceptions include the rat duodenum which may contract (Horton, 1963) or relax (Khairallah, Page and Türker, 1967) to $PGE_1$, the toad intestine (duodenum, jejunum and ileum) which relaxes to $PGE_1$ (Ng, Sit and Wong, 1970) and the guinea-pig colon (Bennett and Fleshler, 1969) and rat jejunum (Bergström *et al.*, 1959b) in which contraction may be preceded by relaxation. Qualitative differences in the contractile responses to E compounds and F compounds have also been observed. In the isolated rabbit jejunum, the response to $PGF_{2\alpha}$ is slower in onset and reaches its peak more slowly than the response to $PGE_1$ (Horton and Main, 1965).

Closer investigation, using longitudinal or circular muscle preparations, has shown that prostaglandins may cause either contraction or relaxation depending on the type of smooth muscle used. Strips from the body of the human stomach cut parallel to the longitudinal fibres were contracted by $PGE_1$ and $PGE_2$ in concentrations as low as 2 ng/ml (Bennett, Murray and Wyllie, 1968a). Strips from the antrum were much less sensitive.

In marked contrast to their effects on longitudinal muscle, $PGE_1$ and $PGE_2$ inhibited spontaneous activity of human circular muscle strips in concentrations as low as 4-10 ng/ml. On a molar basis, $PGE_1$ and $PGE_2$ were several times more potent than adrenaline. Higher concentrations of E prostaglandins also inhibited the response of circular muscle to acetylcholine.

Circular muscle from ileum and colon of several species including guinea-pig, rat and man are also inhibited by E series prostaglandins (Bennett, Eley and Scholes, 1968b; Bennett and Fleshler, 1970). The effect of $PGE_1$ on circular muscle of the guinea-pig and rat ileum was demonstrated as inhibition of the contractions produced by potassium since these preparations are very insensitive to acetylcholine. The effect of $PGE_1$ and $PGE_2$ (0.15-0.6 $\mu g/ml$) on circular muscle strips from human jejunum and ileum varied. In three experiments only relaxation or inhibition of acetylcholine-induced contraction was observed, while in four experiments, a small initial contraction was followed by a long lasting relaxation during which responses to acetylcholine were depressed. The effect of $PGE_1$ and $PGE_2$ on circular muscle of the colon in guinea-pig, rat and human (Bennett and Fleshler, 1970) and dog (Vanasin, Greenhough and Schuster, 1970) is similar to that on the ileum, i.e. relaxation or inhibition of contraction, though occasionally circular muscle of the human colon responds with a contraction (Bennett and Fleshler, 1970).

Prostaglandins of the F series ($PGF_{1\alpha}$ and $PGF_{2\alpha}$) cause contraction of both longitudinal and circular muscle of ileum and colon in guinea-pig, rat and man (Bennett and Fleshler, 1970) and of the dog colon (Vasasin *et al.*, 1970).

Thus in several species muscle from different regions of the gut has a similar pattern of responses to E and F prostaglandins. Longitudinal muscle is contracted by both, whereas circular muscle is contracted by F prostaglandins but is usually relaxed by E prostaglandins.

## Effects on peristalsis *in vitro*

Qualitative differences in the effects of E and F prostaglandins on circular muscle have also been demonstrated in whole segments of guinea-pig ileum in which peristalsis was induced by raising the intraluminal pressure (Bennett, Eley and Scholes, 1968c).

In the Trendelenburg preparation or the intraluminally perfused ileum, serosally administered $PGE_1$ inhibited the pressure changes caused by circular muscle peristaltic contractions and reduced the propulsion of fluid along the gut. $PGE_1$ also inhibited the contractile response of the circular muscle but not that of the longitudinal muscle to co-axial stimulation (Kottegoda, 1969). Intraluminal administration of $PGE_1$ was without effect on longitudinal muscle but in some experiments reduced peristaltic responses of circular muscle and propulsion of fluid through the gut (Bennett *et al.*, 1968c).

The effects of the F prostaglandins differ from those of E series in that they increase peristaltic contractions of the circular muscle (Bennett and Fleshler, 1970). This is consistent with the results obtained using isolated intestinal strips.

## Mechanism of action of prostaglandins on smooth muscle *in vitro*

Pharmacological analysis indicates that prostaglandins usually act directly on smooth muscle, though in some gastro-intestinal preparations part of their effects may be mediated by nervous mechanisms or by the release of pharmacologically active substances.

The inhibitory effects of E compounds on circular muscle and the stimulatory effect of F compounds on circular and longitudinal muscle of all preparations studied (including human stomach, intestine and colon) appears to be due entirely to a direct action on the muscle, since these effects are not affected by a variety of pharmacological agents including tetrodotoxin, hyoscine, adrenoceptor blocking drugs and 5-hydroxytryptamine antagonists.

The mechanism by which E prostaglandins contract longitudinal muscle varies according to the species and the region of gut. Although only a direct action has been demonstrated in longitudinal muscle from human stomach and colon, the contractile response to E compounds in certain other tissues, including human and guinea-pig ileum and dog colon, may be mediated in part by a nervous mechanism. Contractions of the guinea-pig ileum are always reduced but not abolished by atropine (Horton, 1965), hyoscine or tetrodotoxin (Bennett *et al.*, 1968b) or procaine (Harry, 1968). Contractions of the human ileum are reduced by hyoscine in some preparations but not in others. The nervous component, when present, is not blocked by hexamethoneum suggesting an action on postganglionic cholinergic nerves.

It has been suggested that in some situations the effects of $PGE_1$ may be partly mediated by release of amines. The tendency for the rat isolated intestine to relax in response to $PGE_1$ appears to be greater in the duodenum than in the ileum. Khairallah *et al.* (1967) found that a combination of $\alpha$- and $\beta$-adrenoceptor blocking drugs converted the inhibitory response of the duodenum to $PGE_1$ into a contraction which could then be blocked by the 5-hydroxytryptamine (5-HT) antagonist, bromolysergic acid diethylamide (BOL). Although local release of catecholamines might account for the duodenal inhibition by $PGE_1$, the evidence that $PGE_1$ causes duodenal contraction by release of 5-HT is less convincing. Contractions induced by $PGE_2$, $PGF_{2\alpha}$ and $PGA_1$ in preparations which relax to $PGE_1$, were not abolished by BOL in concentrations just sufficient to block contractions induced by 5-HT (Main, unpublished). Moreover, $PGE_1$ and $PGE_2$ (10-900 $\mu$g/kg/sc) did not alter the levels of 5-HT in rat gastro-intestinal tract (Thompson and Angulo, 1968). Circular muscle of the toad isolated intestine resembles the rat duodenum in that it is relaxed by $PGE_1$ but contracted by $PGE_2$ (Ng et al., 1970). However, the inhibitory response to $PGE_1$ is not abolished by adrenoceptor blocking agents suggesting that, as in all other circular muscle studied, the relaxation is caused by a direct action on smooth muscle.

Contractions of the rat fundus are potentiated by a miscellaneous group of drugs including procaine, bretylium, dichloroisoprenaline, ascorbic acid and by raised $Ca^{++}$ concentrations (Coceani and Wolfe, 1966). Responses are inhibited by lowered $Ca^{++}$ concentrations and by cyanide, azide, carbon monoxide and low $pO_2$, indicating the importance of oxygen for prostaglandin-induced contractions of this preparation.

Anoxia does not however block responses of the guinea-pig colon to prostaglandins (Bennett and Fleshler, 1970) showing that not all smooth muscle is equally sensitive to lack of oxygen.

The precise mechanism by which prostaglandins contract or relax smooth muscle is unknown. They do not appear to act directly on the contractile mechanism since glycerinated smooth muscle from the rabbit intestine which contracted in response to $Ca^{++}$ or ATP did not respond to $PGE_1$ (Miyazaki, Ishizawa, Sunano, Syuto and Sakagami, 1967). Other studies suggest that prostaglandins may act by altering the ion permeability of the plasma membrane. In smooth muscle (Coceani, Dreifuss, Puglisi and Wolfe, 1969) and epithelial tissues such as frog skin (Ramwell and Shaw, 1970), prostaglandins displace membrane $Ca^{++}$ which may result in an influx of $Na^+$. Whether the response of smooth muscle is a direct consequence of $Na^+$ influx, or is secondary to an effect of $Na^+$ influx on adenyl cyclase and intracellular cyclic AMP levels, remains to be established.

Any hypothesis which attempts to explain the effects of prostaglandins on smooth muscle must account not only for the contractile effects which are associated with increased electrical activity (increased frequency and amplitude of slow waves and spiking) but also for the inhibitory effects on circular muscle where such electrical activity may be absent (Vanasin et al., 1970).


## 2. EFFECTS ON GASTRO-INTESTINAL MOTILITY IN VIVO

### Studies in animals

Intravenous injection of an impure mixture of prostaglandins resulted in increased intestinal motility, as judged by direct observation through an abdominal window in an anaesthetized rabbit and by the production of semi-fluid faeces in mice (von Euler, 1966). Pure prostaglandins can also affect motility and cause diarrhoea in several species including man.

Prostaglandin $E_1$, which has a net vasodilator effect on total gastric vasculature under resting conditions (Nakano and Prancan, 1972), inhibited vagally-stimulated motor activity (induced by 2-deoxyglucose) in the innervated antral pouch of the unanaesthetized dog (Chawla and Eisenberg, 1969). In the anaesthetized rat, $PGE_1$ or $E_2$ (1-2 $\mu$g/kg) injected intravenously or intra-arterially contracted longitudinal intestinal muscle and increased intraluminal pressure (Bennett *et al.*, 1968c). These responses were unlikely to be due to the associated fall in blood pressure, since equidepressor doses of histamine did not affect motility. Since *in vitro,* longitudinal muscle is contracted and circular muscle is relaxed by $PGE_1$, the increase in intraluminal pressure *in vivo* suggests that the stimulant effect on longitudinal muscle is greater than the inhibitory effect on circular muscle. It is also possible, however, that circular muscle responds differently *in vivo,* or that blood-borne $PGE_1$ or a metabolite, causes contraction of circular muscle, whereas serosally-applied $PGE_1$ causes inhibition. In the anaesthetized guinea-pig the effects of E prostaglandins were very variable (Bennett *et al.*, 1968c). Longitudinal muscle was either contracted, relaxed or unaffected and intraluminal pressure was either increased, decreased or unchanged. The relaxation of longitudinal muscle was unaffected by blocking the $\alpha$- and $\beta$-adrenoceptors. Relatively high doses of F compounds (approx. 10 $\mu$g/kg), injected intra-arterially, increased intraluminal pressure (Bennett and Fleshler, 1970).

In the anaesthetized dog, $PGF_{2\alpha}$ (0.1-1 $\mu$g/kg/min) injected into the superior mesenteric artery, consistently increased jejunal motility and tone as measured by pressure changes in intraluminal balloons (Shehadeh, Price and Jacobson, 1970). $PGF_{2\alpha}$ usually caused an initial fall in superior mesenteric arterial blood flow, though this response was very variable. In contrast, $PGE_1$ (0.01-1 $\mu$g/kg/min) consistently inhibited jejunal motility and increased blood flow. The inhibitory effect of $PGE_1$ cannot readily be attributed to its potent vasodilator properties, since intestinal motility was increased by acetylcholine (dilator) and angiotensin (constrictor) but was decreased by noradrenaline (constrictor).

In the unanaesthetized dog, $PGE_1$ (1 $\mu$g/kg/min i.v.) inhibited vagally-stimulated motor activity (induced by 2-deoxyglucose) in an innervated antral pouch (Chawla and Eisenberg, 1969), while in the anaesthetized rat, intravenous infusion of $PGE_1$ inhibited the intense phasic motility of the stomach during vagal stimulation with either 2-deoxyglucose or insulin (Main, unpublished).

These results suggest that gastro-intestinal motility and intraluminal pressure are usually increased by $PGF_{2\alpha}$ but may be either increased or decreased by E compounds. However, the effects vary with the species and possibly with the particular experimental conditions.

## Studies in humans

The first indication that prostaglandins might have an effect on the gastro-intestinal tract in man was the observation that E prostaglandins caused abdominal cramps during intravenous infusion in some subjects (Bergström, Duner, von Euler, Pernow and Sjövall, 1959a). Although this observation has been confirmed on several occasions (Carlson, Ekelund and Orö, 1968), the nature of these cramps has not been investigated. More recently diarrhoea and vomiting have been reported to occur during administration of prostaglandins for induction of labour and especially during induction of abortion where higher doses are required.

Direct evidence that prostaglandins affect motor function in humans was first obtained from experiments designed primarily to study the effect of orally administered $PGE_1$ on gastric secretion induced by pentagastrin (Horton, Main, Thompson and Wright, 1968). $PGE_1$ was administered orally in total doses of 0.8-3.2 mg. Two-fifths of the total dose was given 15 min prior to pentagastrin injection and further doses of one-fifth of the total dose were given 0, 15 and 30 min after the injection. Although $PGE_1$ did not inhibit acid secretion, effects on gastro-intestinal motility including bile reflux and passage of loose faeces were observed in all subjects.

*Bile Reflux.* In three subjects who received oral $PGE_1$ in doses of 20, 25 and 40 $\mu g/kg$, large amounts of bile were present in the aspirated samples of gastric juice, particularly those collected 30 and 45 min after pentagastrin (Horton *et al.,* 1968). In two of these subjects, bile was detected in the sample collected 15 min after administration of prostaglandin, that is, before the pentagastrin had been injected (Table 1). In none of the subjects was any bile observed in the gastric

Table 1

Effect of oral $PGE_1$ on the presence of bile in pentagastrin–induced gastric secretion and on intestinal motility in man. Reproduced from Horton *et al.* (1968) with permission of the publisher.

| Subject Number | Dose of PGE (µg/Kg) | Presence of Bile in Gastric Juice | | Increase in Intestinal Motility | |
|---|---|---|---|---|---|
| | | Control (Pentagastrin only) | $PGE_1$ | Control (Pentagastrin only) | $PGE_1$ |
| 1 | 10 | 0 | 0 | nil | + |
| 1 | 40 | 0 | +++ | nil | +++ |
| 2 | 20 | 0 | +++ | nil | + |
| 3 | 25 | 0 | ++ | nil | ++ |

juice secreted in response to pentagastrin when prostaglandin had not been administered.

More recently, Classen, Koch, Bickhardt, Toff and Demling (1971) reported that intravenous infusion of $PGE_1$ (0.17-0.23 $\mu$g/kg/min) for 30 min during the gastric secretory response to pentagastrin resulted in the presence of bile in one subject during the first 15 min and in another subject during the second 15 min period. In all eight subjects bile was present in samples collected after the $PGE_1$ infusion had stopped. Bile was also present in gastric juice from gastric fistula dogs during parenteral administration of $PGE_1$ 1 $\mu$g/kg/min (Robert, personal communication) though in the experiments of Jacobson (1970) in which the same dose of $PGE_1$ was used, the presence of bile was not reported.

*Intestinal motility and transit.* In five experiments on fasted subjects in which $PGE_1$ was administered orally, the passing of loose faeces was observed between two and four hours later (Horton *et al.,* 1968). Following the dose of 40 $\mu$g/kg the faeces were completely liquid. From one hour after the prostaglandin administration until defaecation occurred, sensations of increased intestinal motility were noted and there were sometimes mild colicky pains.

These subjective observations were followed up by Misiewicz, Waller, Kiley and Horton (1969) who studied the effects of oral $PGE_1$ on intestinal transit and motility in four healthy volunteers using objective techniques.

Intraluminal pressures were measured simultaneously in the small intestine, or proximal colon, by radiotelemetering capsules and in the distal colon via air-filled balloons connected to pressure transducers. Transit through the small or large intestine was measured by two methods. Firstly, a radiochemical source was incorporated into the radiotelemetering capsules and a collimated scintillation counter coupled to a ratemeter was used to locate the position of the capsule in relation to bony landmarks. The second method involved the ingestion of radio-opaque polythene pellets and the subsequent fluoroscopic determination of the number of pellets in each stool.

In three volunteers the capsule and pellets were swallowed at 8 p.m. on the night before the tests and two hours after a standard breakfast, recordings were started. The fourth volunteer ingested the capsule on the morning of the study and the test was performed in the fasting state, in order to measure small intestinal as well as distal colonic activity. Following a 30 min control period, $PGE_1$ or a placebo were administered orally and recording continued for 2½ hours. Stool specimens were collected until radio-opaque pellet count was complete.

Symptoms of increased gastro-intestinal motility were experienced by all four volunteers following oral ingestion of 2 mg $PGE_1$. The

symptoms, which included mild to severe colic and desire to defaecate
were most marked in the first three volunteers and were never observed
in control experiments. They occurred after a delay of ½-2 hours and
continued for 1-6 hours after the end of the recording period. All
subjects had loose stools, and a characteristic feature in the first three
volunteers was the passage of fragments of normal faeces accompanied
by a quantity of clear fluid. The fourth volunteer, who took $PGE_1$ while
fasting, had very mild symptoms though his subsequent bowel
movements were looser than usual.

A marked increase in propulsive activity of small and large intestines,
as indicated by movements of the radiocapsules, followed the ingestion
of $PGE_1$ in three of the four volunteers. For example, in the second
volunteer the capsule was in the terminal ileum during the control
period, but 60 min after ingestion of $E_1$ it had passed into the colon and
after a short period in the proximal bowel, the capsule was propelled
rapidly through the ascending and transverse colon to the descending
colon. Throughout the placebo experiments, the capsule remained in the
right colon.

Transit rates, as measured by elimination of radio-opaque pellets, were
markedly increased in all four experiments with $E_1$ compared with the
placebo controls. The results are shown in Fig. 1.

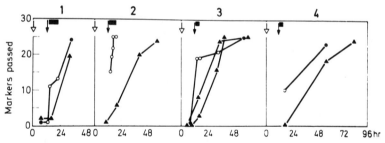

▲  Control experiments
●  $PGE_1$ experiments, formed stools
○  $PGE_1$ experiments, loose stools
▽  Time of ingestion of pellets
▼  Time of ingestion of test material
▣  Approximate duration of subjective symptoms.

Fig. 1. Effect of oral $PGE_1$ (2 mg) on cumulative elimination-rate of radio-opaque
pellets in the stools of four human subjects. Reproduced from Misiewicz *et al.* (1969)
with permission of the authors and publisher.

An analysis of the intraluminal pressure records showed that $E_1$
caused an increased number of progressive pressure waves in the left
colon, but had no consistent effect on other variables of intestinal
motility.

## Mechanism of action of $PGE_1$ on human gastro-intestinal motility

The presence of large quantities of bile in gastric contents of man and dog within a few minutes of administration of $PGE_1$ suggests a reflux of duodenal contents rather than stimulation of bile secretion, though studies on bile secretion have not yet been reported. Bile reflux may be due to relaxation of the pyloric sphincter since $PGE_1$ relaxes the circular muscle of the human stomach *in vitro* (Bennett *et al.,* 1968a) and, in doses similar to those which cause bile reflux, inhibits antral motility in dogs (Chawla and Eisenberg, 1969). The possibility that $PGE_1$ has a simultaneous action on duodenal and gall bladder motility cannot be excluded though in the cat, $PGE_2$ perfused through the lumen of the proximal jejunum did not release cholecystokinin into the circulation (Berry and Flower, 1971).

The mechanism by which oral $PGE_1$ produced a marked increase in propulsive activity and transit rates cannot be readily deduced from the experiments in humans. One possibility is that $PGE_1$ is acting directly on smooth muscle of intestine and colon either from within the lumen of the gut after penetrating the mucosa, or via the blood stream following absorption. Such effects would not necessarily be predicted from *in vitro* experiments on human or animal tissues. $PGE_1$ either has no effect, or inhibits propulsive activity when applied to the serosal or mucosal surface of the intraluminally perfused guinea-pig ileum and inhibits intestinal motility when injected intra-arterially in the dog. Moreover, in the experiments of Misiewicz *et al.* (1969) the rapid propulsion of the radiotelemetered capsule through the human colon after $PGE_1$ administration was unaccompanied by marked changes in colonic pressure activity. This result is in marked contrast to other experiments using various stimuli in which, despite much more marked increase in colonic activity, the capsule remained stationary (see Misiewicz *et al.,* 1969).

An alternative possibility which is suggested by the presence of clear fluid in faecal putput following oral $PGE_1$ is that the increase in intestinal transit rate is secondary to an increased volume of fluid in the gut. This is supported by the observation that, in the dog, $PGE_1$ has potent effects on the transport of water and electrolytes across the intestinal mucosa (Pierce, Carpenter, Elliot and Greenhough, 1971).

## 3. EFFECTS OF PROSTAGLANDINS ON INTESTINAL WATER AND ELECTROLYTE TRANSPORT

In dogs with chronic Thiry-Vella jejunal loops, $PGE_1$ infused into the lumen of the loop in doses of 2-24 $\mu$g/min (1-12 $\mu$g/ml) produced a dose-dependent inhibition of net water and electrolyte absorption (Pierce *et al.,* 1971). Net absorption was reduced to zero during infusion of 24 and 100 $\mu$g/min but returned to control values (net absorption of approximately 400 $\mu$l/cm$^2$/h) within 30-60 min of ending the infusion.

Infusion of PGE$_1$ into the superior mesenteric artery produced a much greater effect than similar doses administered into the jejunal lumen (Fig. 2). Net isotonic fluid secretion into the loop occurred with a dose of 2 $\mu$g/min and maximum secretory responses to PGE$_1$ were obtained with a dose of 24 $\mu$g/min (net secretion approximately 300 $\mu$l/cm$^2$/h).

PGA$_1$ and PGF$_{2\alpha}$ injected intra-arterially produced effects qualitatively similar to those of PGE$_1$. PGF$_{2\alpha}$ was even more potent than PGE$_1$ or PGA$_1$ and in some dogs produced effects in doses as low as 0.2 $\mu$g/min. The effects of PGA$_1$ and PGF$_{2\alpha}$ infused into the jejunal lumen were not investigated.

Of particular interest was the finding that the electrolyte composition of jejunal fluid secreted in response to prostaglandins was very similar to that induced by cholera enterotoxin (C.E.), though the rapid time-course of action contrasted with the delayed onset and prolonged duration of action of C.E. Both stimuli increased intestinal mucus secretion, though PGF$_{2\alpha}$, unlike C.E., increased the plasma protein concentration of jejunal secretion. The maximum rate of net fluid secretion induced by intra-arterial prostaglandins was always less than the maximum response to mucosally applied C. E. but there was a significant correlation between the magnitude of the response to prostaglandins and C.E. in the same dog.

These effects are unlikely to be secondary to their haemodynamic activity since PGE$_1$ and PGF$_{2\alpha}$ have very similar effects on fluid and

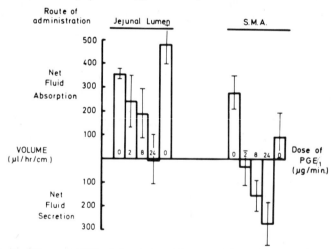

Fig. 2. Effect of PGE$_1$ infused into the jejunal lumen or into the superior mesenteric artery on net jejunal fluid transport in dog Thiry-Vella jejunal loops. Modified from Pierce *et al.* (1971) with permission of the authors.

electrolyte transport in doses which have qualitatively different effects on splanchnic blood flow (Nakano and Cole, 1969; Shehadeh *et al.,* 1970). A primary effect on the mucosa is suggested by experiments on the isolated rabbit ileal mucosa in which serosally applied $PGE_1$ and $PGA_2$ stimulated active chloride secretion and inhibited sodium absorption (Greenhough, Pierce, Al Awqati and Carpenter, 1969; Al Awqati, Field, Pierce and Greenough, 1970b).

The effects of prostaglandins on ion transport and short-circuit current in rabbit and human isolated ileal mucosa are similar to those produced by C.E., theophylline and dibutyryl cyclic AMP (Al Awqati, Cameron, Field and Greenberg, 1970a). The observation that prostaglandins and C.E. markedly increase gut mucosal adenyl cyclase activity (Kimberg, Field, Johnson, Henderson and Gershon, 1971; Sharp and Hynie, 1971) suggests that both act by increasing the intracellular concentration of cyclic AMP which in turn stimulates an increase in fluid and electrolyte secretion from the intestinal mucosa. In man, studies using a multi-lumen tube technique have shown that $PGE_1$, administered intraluminally, decreases net fluid and electrolyte absorption from perfused jejunal segments (Matuchansky and Bernier, 1971).

These results support the hypothesis that the increased intestinal transit rate and diarrhoea following oral or parenteral administration of prostaglandins in man are secondary to a net secretion of intestinal fluid resulting in a greatly increased volume of gut contents. The extent to which direct actions on intestinal or colonic smooth muscle contribute to these effects is difficult to assess and may depend partly on the route of administration. In dogs, defaecation which may occur shortly after starting an intravenous infusion of $PGE_1$ is unlikely to be mediated by increased mucosal secretion.

Orally administered $PGE_1$ may act directly on the mucosal surface to stimulate secretion, though in the dog, mucosal application is less effective than intra-arterial injection. Small amounts of prostaglandins may be absorbed and reach the mucosa or muscle via the bloodstream, though in the experiments of Horton *et al.* (1968) and Misiewicz *et al.* (1969) in humans, no changes of systemic arterial blood pressure or pulse rate were reported.

Prostaglandins administered into the rat jejunum are fairly rapidly metabolized by the mucosa prior to partial absorption (Parkinson and Schneider, 1969). Moreover, in man a significant proportion (20%) of metabolites formed from parenterally administered prostaglandins are excreted in bile and are present in faeces. (Granström, 1967). Although the known metabolites are usually much less active than $PGE_1$ on most biological systems tested (Änggård, 1966) the possibility that metabolites acting either via the bloodstream or from within the lumen of the tract may contribute to the observed effects on intestinal motility and electrolyte transport warrants further investigation.

## 4. EFFECTS OF PROSTAGLANDINS ON GASTRIC SECRETION

### Studies in animals

The inhibitory effects of prostaglandins on gastric secretion in the dog were first reported by Robert and his colleagues (Robert, Nezamis and Phillips, 1967; Robert, Phillip and Nezamis, 1968b; Robert, 1968). Prostaglandin $E_1$ injected intravenously or subcutaneously inhibited the secretory response to histamine, food and pentagastrin in Heidenhain and Pavlov pouch dogs. $PGE_1$ also inhibited the responses to 2-deoxyglucose, carbachol and reserpine in dogs with gastric fistulae. All secretory parameters (volume, acid and pepsin output) were inhibited.

The effect of $PGE_1$ on steady submaximal secretory responses to histamine, pentagastrin or food (Fig. 3) was dose-dependent, Nezamis, Robert and Stowe (1971). For any dose of $PGE_1$, the maximum inhibition occurred after 30-45 mins and was maintained throughout the period of infusion. Secretion returned to normal within 1-2 hours of ending the $PGE_1$ infusion. The effective dose varied somewhat depending on the dog and the intensity of stimulus used. A dose of 1 $\mu$g/kg/min almost completely inhibited secretion induced by food or a submaximal dose of histamine (1 mg/kg/hr). The $ED_{50}$ (the dose inhibiting acid output by 50%) was approximately 0.5 $\mu$g/kg/min regardless of the stimulus used. In some experiments where the higher doses of $PGE_1$ (1 $\mu$g/kg/min) were used, defaecation, urination and vomiting occurred. Similar effects were noted by Rudick, Gonda, Dreiling and Janowitz (1971).

$PGE_2$ also inhibited secretion induced by food or histamine and its effects were qualitatively and quantitatively similar to those of $PGE_1$. In contrast, $PGF_{2\alpha}$ (1 $\mu$g/kg/min), tested only against histamine-induced secretion, was completely without effect. $PGA_1$ (1 $\mu$g/kg/min) did not affect histamine-induced secretion, but was more potent than $PGE_1$ in inhibiting secretion induced by food ($ED_{50}$ 0.1 $\mu$g/kg/min) suggesting that in the dog, $PGA_1$, unlike $PGE_1$, has some degree of selectivity of action against differing secretory stimuli. The characteristics of onset and inhibition of $PGA_1$ were similar to those of $PGE_1$ (Fig. 4).

In the rat, prostaglandins administered either parenterally or from within the lumen of the stomach can inhibit gastric secretion. $PGE_1$ (0.1 ml/min; 5-10 $\mu$g/ml), perfused through the lumen of the stomach in the anaesthetized rat inhibited spontaneous acid secretion and the secretory response to pentagastrin, histamine or direct vagal stimulation (Ramwell and Shaw, 1968). Perfusion of 9-10, dihydroxystearic acid had no effect either on spontaneous or on pentagastrin-stimulated secretion, showing that inhibition is not a non-specific effect of hydroxy-

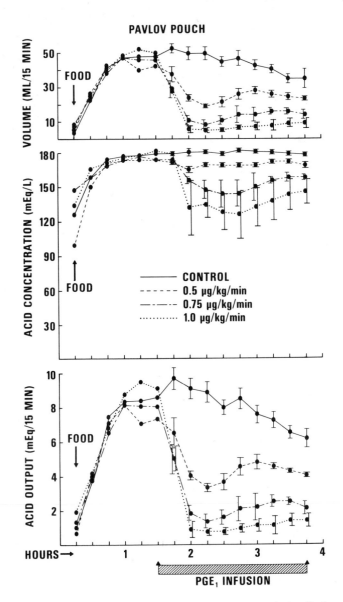

Fig. 3. Effect of various doses of $PGE_1$, infused intravenously in a Pavlov pouch dog, on gastric secretion stimulated with food. Control curve: mean of five studies. Each of the $PGE_1$ curves: mean of three studies. Vertical bars ± S.E. of mean. Reproduced from Nezamis *et al.* (1971) with permission of the authors and publisher.

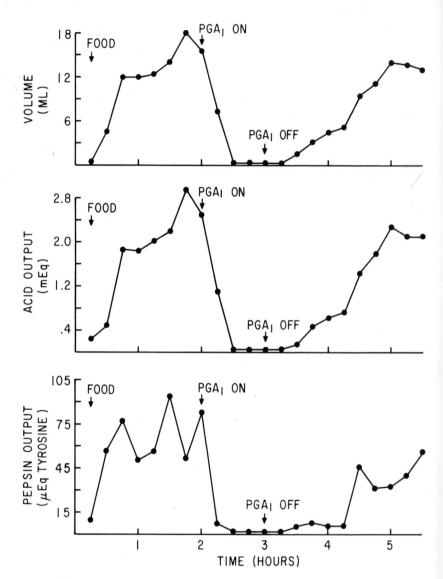

Fig. 4. Effect of PGA$_1$ (0.3 µg/kg/min i.v.) in a Pavlov pouch dog, on gastric secretion stimulated with food. Reproduced from Robert (1968) with permission of the author and publisher.

unsaturated fatty acids. $PGE_1$, $PGA_1$ and $PGA_2$ are also effective inhibitors of pentagastrin-induced secretion when administered intra-luminally (Main and Whittle, unpublished observations). Intravenous infusion of $PGE_1$ and $PGE_2$ caused a dose-dependent inhibition of the secretory responses to histamine, pentagastrin, 2-deoxyglucose and insulin (Main, 1969 and unpublished). Doses of 2-4 $\mu$g/kg/min completely inhibited the near maximal secretory response to penta-gastrin within 30-40 minutes of starting the infusion. On ending the infusion, secretion usually returned to the former level within 60 mins.

$PGA_1$ and $PGA_2$ (4-8 $\mu$g/kg/min), though less potent than $PGE_1$ and $PGE_2$, inhibited pentagastrin-induced secretion in the rat and in contrast to the dog, were effective inhibitors of histamine-induced secretion (Fig. 5). $PGF_{1\alpha}$ and $PGF_{2\alpha}$, in similar doses did not inhibit secretion.

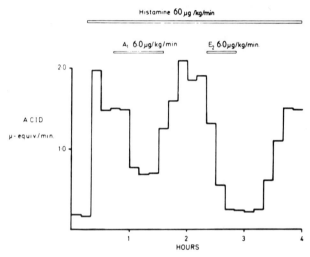

Fig. 5. Effect of $PGA_1$ (6.0 $\mu$g/kg/min i.v.) and $PGE_2$ (6.0 $\mu$g/kg/min i.v.) on gastric acid secretion stimulated by histamine (60 $\mu$g/kg/min i.v.) in the urethane-anaesthetized rat. (Main, unpublished observations.)

Intravenous injection of inhibitory doses of E and A prostaglandins into the rat was always accompanied by a fall in arterial blood pressure, but during prolonged infusions, while acid secretion was still inhibited, blood pressure tended to recover slowly towards the previous level. On stopping the infusion, blood pressure sometimes rose to a higher level than before. This post-infusion 'rebound' phenomenom was most marked following inhibition of histamine-induced secretion induced by the infusion of $PGA_1$ and may be compared with the rebound following intravenous infusion of $PGA_1$ in man (Christlieb, Dobrzinsky, Lyons and Hickler, 1969).

In the pylorus-ligated rat, subcutaneous injection of $PGE_1$ inhibited gastric secretion (volume, acid and pepsin output) collected during the four hours following ligation (Robert, Nezamis and Phillips, 1968a). The effect was dose-dependent, the $ED_{50}$ being approximately 250 $\mu g/kg$ when injected at 0 and 2 hours following ligation, and 0.5-1.0 $\mu g/kg/min$ when administered by subcutaneous infusion for 6 hours starting 2 hours before ligation. Larger doses of $PGE_1$ (2.5 mg/kg), which almost totally inhibit gastric secretion when injected subcutaneously, were ineffective when administered directly into the upper jejunum (Robert, personal communication) (Table 2). $PGE_1$ and a number of prostaglandin

Table 2

Effects of $PGE_1$ administered subcutaneously or intrajejunally on gastric secretion in the rat. The $PGE_1$ was injected immediately following pyloric ligation and the gastric contents were examined three hours later. (Robert, unpublished observations).

|  | Subcutaneous | | Intrajejunal | |
|---|---|---|---|---|
|  | Saline | $PGE_1$ 2.5 mg/kg | Saline | $PGE_1$ 2.5 mg/kg |
| No. of Animals | 6 | 5 | 5 | 6 |
| Gastric Juice | | | | |
| Volume (ml/3 h) | 4.9 | 0.9* | 3.3 | 3.7 |
| Acid | | | | |
| Concentration (mEq/L) | 118 | 7* | 103 | 94 |
| Output (mEq/3 h) | 0.59 | 0.01* | 0.36 | 0.39 |

*'p' < 0.01

analogues inhibited both basal and pentagastrin-induced acid secretion in rats with ligation of both pylorus and oesophagus (Lippmann, 1970). As yet no synthetic analogue has been reported to be more active than the naturally occurring prostaglandins.

### Effect on ulcer formation in rats

The effect of $PGE_1$ on gastric ulcers produced by pyloric ligation (Shay ulcers) or by administration of prednisolone (steroid-induced ulcers) was studied by Robert *et al.* (1968a). The percentage mortality 21 hours after pyloric ligation was reduced from 65% in controls to 14% and 0% in rats receiving subcutaneous infusion of $PGE_1$ 1 and 2 $\mu g/kg/min$ respectively.

The incidence of Shay ulcers was reduced from 100% to 78% and 65% with a more marked reduction in severity of ulcers, while the incidence of gastro-oesophageal perforation was reduced from 90% to 29% and 21% respectively.

The same doses of $PGE_1$ infused throughout the four day period of prednisolone treatment, strongly inhibited the incidence and severity of steroid-induced ulcers.

The incidence and severity of duodenal ulcers produced by constant subcutaneous infusion for 24 h of a combination of two of the following gastric secretagogues, histamine, carbachol and pentagastrin, was reduced or abolished by simultaneous subcutaneous infusion of $PGE_2$, 3-6 µg/kg/min (Robert, Stowe and Nezamis, 1971).

Although the mechanism of anti-ulcer effect is unknown, it seems likely that there may be a causal relationship between inhibition of gastric acid secretion and inhibition of ulcer formation.

## 5. EFFECTS OF PGs ON GASTRIC SECRETION IN HUMANS

### Oral administration

The effect of oral $PGE_1$ on gastric secretion was studied by Horton *et al.* (1968). Gastric contents were collected at 15 min intervals during a control period and for 1 hr following the injection of pentagastrin (6 µg/kg s.c.). In four experiments on three subjects, $PGE_1$ (in total doses of 10, 20, 25 and 40 µg/kg) was administered orally in divided doses and was present in the stomach continuously for 1 hour, from 15 min before to 45 min after the pentagastrin injection. In none of the experiments was there any reduction in volume or acid output when compared with the control experiments in the same subjects (Table 3). The mean concentration of acid was similar despite evidence of bile reflux following oral $PGE_1$.

When $PGE_1$ from the same batch was perfused through the lumen of the rat stomach in a concentration of 6 µg/ml, the response to pentagastrin (9 µg/kg/hr i.v.) was inhibited by up to 45%. During the four experiments on humans the concentration of $PGE_1$ in the stomach at the beginning of each 15 min collection period was at least 13, 22, 24 and 50 µg/ml respectively and on this basis, $PGE_1$ would have been expected to produce inhibition in humans. However, the conditions of the two investigations were different and a direct comparison cannot be made.

Only 30-80% of administered $PGE_1$ was recovered in the aspirated gastric samples (as judged by assay on smooth muscle). Although some prostaglandin may have been absorbed into the bloodstream, there was no change in pulse rate or blood pressure during these experiments, nor was there any potentiation of the slight to marked flushing seen after the pentagastrin injections. The possibility that some of the loss was due to

Table 3

Effect of oral prostaglandin $E_1$ on pentagastrin-induced gastric secretion in man. Volume and acid refer to the total samples aspirated during the first hour after pentagastrin injection. Reproduced from Horton *et al.* (1968) with permission of the publisher.

| Subject Number | Dose of PGE$_1$ (ug/Kg) | | Gastric secretion | |
|:---:|:---:|:---:|:---:|:---:|
| | Administered | Recovered | Vol (ml) | Acid (m-equiv.) |
| 1 | - | - | 184 | 8.8 |
| 1 | - | - | 175 | 14.5 |
| 2 | - | - | 140 | 11.4 |
| 3 | - | - | 148 | 14.9 |
| 1 | 10 | 3 | 170 | 10.0 |
| 1 | 40 | 11 | 241 | 15.4 |
| 2 | 20 | 7 | 314 | 24.8 |
| 3 | 25 | 13 | 241 | 18.0 |

metabolism in the gastric mucosa, or conversion into $PGA_1$ in the acid environment of the stomach, was not excluded.

These results showed that oral $PGE_1$ did not inhibit gastric secretion in doses which had marked effects on gastro-intestinal motility. They did not exclude the possibility that secretion might have been affected if higher doses had been used or if the prostaglandin had been given parenterally.

## Parenteral administration

The effect of $PGE_1$ on basal acid secretion was studied in six subjects by Classen, Koch, Deyhle, Weidenhiller and Demling (1970). Although there was considerable variation between individuals, $PGE_1$ in a dose of 300 μg (0.14-0.17 μg/kg/min) infused intravenously over 30 mins, caused a significant inhibition in basal acid output compared with the previous control period. Side effects were observed in all subjects. These included nausea, vomiting, headache and, in one case, marked hypotension.

Intravenously administered $PGE_1$ also inhibits secretion induced by pentagastrin (Classen, Koch, Bickhardt, Topf and Demling, 1971). In eight subjects, pentagastrin (2 μg/kg/h) was infused intravenously for 2 hr. $PGE_1$ (0.17-0.23 μg/kg/min, 460 μg total) administered during the third half hour of the experiment caused a significant reduction in volume and acid output (Fig. 6). There was no change in acid concentration. Maximum inhibition of secretion occurred in the period from 15 to 45 min after starting the infusion. In three subjects the lowest output was reached in the 15 min following the end of the $PGE_1$ infusion, whereas in the other five subjects, maximum inhibition was reached during the second 15 min period of $PGE_1$ infusion and secretion partially recovered during the next collection period.

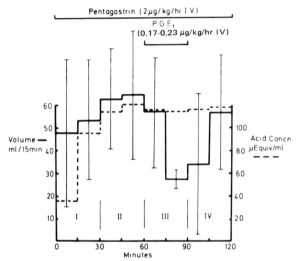

Fig. 6. Effect of $PGE_1$ (0.17-0.23 $\mu g/kg/min$ i.v.) on gastric secretion stimulated by pentagastrin (2 $\mu g/kg/h$ i.v.) in eight human subjects. Modified from Classen *et al.* (1971) with permission of the authors.

During the infusion of $PGE_1$ there was a rise in pulse rate but no consistent change in systemic arterial blood pressure. In addition to the presence of bile in gastric juice from all eight subjects, five subjects experienced a strong desire to evacuate the bowels. Other side effects included muscular pain in the upper arm proximal to the site of injection (8), headache (6), dizziness (8), facial flushing (5), epigastric pain (1) and nausea (1).

The effects of intravenous $PGA_1$ on histamine-stimulated secretion were studied by Wilson, Phillips and Levene (1971). After a steady submaximal secretory response to histamine (15 $\mu g/kg/hr$) had been established, $PGA_1$ (0.5-0.6 and 1.0-1.25 $\mu g/kg/min$ respectively in two groups of nine subjects) was infused intravenously for 30 mins. This resulted in a 23% and 30% reduction in volume output and a 21% and 25% reduction in acid output of gastric secretion collected during the first and second 15 min infusion periods respectively (Fig. 7). During the first half hour following the ending of $PGA_1$ infusion, volume and acid outputs had already returned to control values. In three other subjects

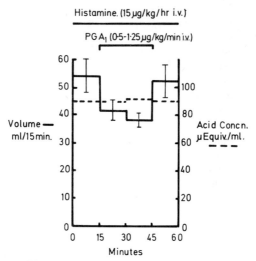

Fig. 7. Effect of PGA₁ (0.5-1.25 μg/kg/min i.v.) on gastric secretion stimulated by histamine (15 μg/kg/h i.v.) in 17 human subjects. Modified from Wilson *et al.* (1971) with permission of the authors.

PGA₁ either had no effect or caused slight or marked inhibition of basal acid secretion.

The interesting observation that subjects receiving the lower dose of PGA₁ had a greater reduction in gastric secretion than those receiving the higher dose may well be related to the fact that, by chance, the latter group had a significantly higher secretory output than the former. Another possibility is that at the higher dose levels, a second mechanism which opposes inhibition comes into play.

PGA₁ was well tolerated in all subjects. Side-effects included transient flushing superimposed on that caused by histamine, and, in one subject at the higher dose level, nausea. There was a significant rise in pulse rate and plasma free fatty acids but no consistent changes in the plasma concentration of glucose, cortisol, immuno-reactive insulin, or growth hormone or in systemic arterial blood pressure. The heart-burn present during histamine infusion was abolished by PGA₁ in 11 out of 18 experiments. The possibility that this reflects an action on gastro-oesophageal motility has not yet been investigated.

## Mechanism of action on gastric secretion

Although PGE₁ and PGA₁ sometimes induce vomiting in dogs (Robert *et al.*, 1967, 1968b; Rudick *et al.*, 1971) their inhibitory effects on gastric secretion cannot be secondary to production of nausea since $PGA_1$ inhibited food-induced secretion in non-retching doses but did not reduce histamine-induced secretion even in doses which caused retching. Moreover, pretreatment with the antiemetic drugs atropine or chlorpromazine prevented vomiting but had no effect on the inhibition of histamine-induced secretion by $PGE_1$ (Robert *et al.*, 1968b; Wilson and Levene, 1969).

Unlike some inhibitors of secretion such as secretin or atropine, $PGE_1$ inhibits gastric secretion induced by a wide variety of stimuli including gastrin, histamine, vagal stimulation, carbachol and reserpine. $PGA_1$ is a potent inhibitor of pentagastrin but, like secretin, was reported to be ineffective against histamine (Robert *et al.*, 1967). However, the latter report has not been confirmed by subsequent studies in the dog (Robert, personal communication) nor does the interesting analogy with secretin apply to rat (Main, unpublished observations) or man (Wilson *et al.*, 1971) since in both these species, $PGA_1$ inhibits histamine-induced secretion. These results imply that prostaglandins act on some mechanism which is common to all these secretory stimuli.

The hypothesis that the inhibitory effect of prostaglandins is brought about indirectly by a reduction in gastric mucosal blood flow received some support from experiments on Heidenhain pouch dogs, treated with chlorpromazine to prevent vomiting, in which inhibition of secretion by $PGE_1$ (1-2 $\mu$g/kg/min) was accompanied by a marked reduction ,in mucosal blood flow as measured by the aminopyrine clearance technique (Wilson and Levene, 1969). Jacobson (1970) using the same technique in gastric fistula dogs confirmed these results but also demonstrated that, with $PGE_1$, the ratio of mucosal blood flow (clearance of aminopyrine) to secretion was unchanged during inhibition of pentagastrin-induced secretion and rose slightly during inhibition of histamine-induced secretion. In contrast, inhibition of secretion by noradrenaline was associated with a marked fall in the ratio of clearance to secretion. These results suggest that, with noradrenaline, the reduction in mucosal blood flow is the limiting factor for gastric secretion whereas with $PGE_1$ reduction in blood flow cannot be the cause but is rather the consequence of reduced secretion resulting from a direct inhibitory effect on some aspect of the secretory process.

In the anaesthetized rat, studies using a $^{14}$C-aniline clearance technique indicated that complete inhibition of high rates of pentagastrin or histamine-induced acid secretion by $PGE_1$ or $PGE_2$ is accompanied by a reduction in mucosal blood flow (Main and Whittle, 1972 and unpublished observations). However, in all experiments, during inhibition of secretion, the ratio of mucosal blood flow to acid rose markedly. When inhibitory doses of prostaglandins were injected intravenously or were perfused through the gastric lumen, during basal

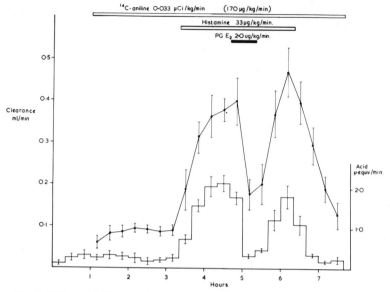

Fig. 8. Effect of PGE$_2$ (2 $\mu$g/kg/min i.v.) on $^{14}$C aniline clearance and gastric acid secretion during intravenous infusion of histamine (33 $\mu$g/kg/min) in the urethane-anaesthetized rat. Mean of four experiments (± S.E.). Reproduced from Main and Whittle (1972) unpublished observations.

secretion or low-rates of pentagastrin-induced secretion, only a rise in mucosal blood flow was observed. The results show that the E prostaglandins have a direct vasodilator action on the mucosa and support the conclusion that their inhibitory effects on acid secretion are not mediated by a reduction in gastric mucosal blood flow.

Conclusive evidence that prostaglandins can act directly was provided by Way and Durbin (1969) who observed that PGE$_1$ inhibited pentagastrin- or histamine-induced secretion in the bullfrog isolated gastric mucosa, where blood flow cannot be a factor.

The hypothesis that the effects of prostaglandins may be mediated by an action on the adenyl cyclase-cyclic AMP system is suggested by the observations that, in a variety of tissues, prostaglandins increase or decrease intracellular concentrations of cyclic AMP (Butcher and Baird, 1968) which may be a mediator of the gastric secretory response to gastrin and histamine (Harris, Nigon and Alonso, 1969). Of particular interest was the observation that in the bullfrog isolated gastric mucosa, PGE$_1$ inhibited secretion induced by gastrin and histamine but not that induced by added cyclic AMP (Way and Durbin, 1969). This supports the hypothesis that PGE$_1$ acts by inhibiting adenyl cyclase and preventing the increase in intracellular cyclic AMP concentration.

In contrast, $PGE_1$, perfused through the lumen of the rat stomach *in vivo*, inhibited the response to cyclic AMP administered by the same route (Ramwell and Shaw, 1968), raising the possibility that $PGE_1$ may inhibit secretion by two different mechanisms. The apparent difference between the *in vitro* and *in vivo* results is unlikely to be due to changes in gastric circulation since $PGE_1$, administered intraluminally, in doses which did not affect systemic arterial blood pressure, inhibited pentagastrin-induced secretion and increased mucosal blood flow (Main and Whittle, unpublished observations).

Intravenous injection of cyclic AMP in the dog did not stimulate basal secretion but, like $PGE_1$, inhibited histamine-induced secretion (Wilson and Levine, 1969). Whether inhibition produced by cyclic AMP was secondary to the observed fall in blood flow or resulted from a direct effect on mucosal metabolism was not established. In the rat, cyclic AMP (i.v.) potentiated pentagastrin-induced secretion and increased mucosal blood flow (Main and Whittle, unpublished observations). Thus, the relationship between the effects of prostaglandins and the possible role of cyclic AMP in gastric secretion is still obscure. A report that that adenyl cyclase activity in guinea-pig gastric mucosa is stimulated by $PGE_1$ and histamine but not by gastrin (Perrier and Laster, 1969) does little to clarify the position.

$PGE_1$ itself stimulated acid secretion from the frog isolated gastric mucosa but partially inhibited the response to pentagastrin (Shaw and Ramwell, 1969). These effects were observed whether $PGE_1$ was added to the mucosal or serosal surfaces. An analogous situation is found in the toad bladder and rabbit kidney tubules where $PGE_1$ itself increased water permeability but inhibited the response to vasopressin (Orloff, Handler and Bergström, 1965; Orloff and Grantham, 1967).

Stimulation of acid secretion in the frog mucosa *in vitro* was correlated with increased oxygen consumption, suggesting an interdependence of $PGE_1$ action on oxidative metabolism (Shaw and Ramwell, 1969). Since $PGE_1$ increased sodium transport from the mucosal surface into the cells and oxygen consumption was dependent on the presence of sodium in the incubation medium, its effects on oxidative metabolism are related to its effect on sodium transport and short circuit currents in the gastric mucosal membrane (Ramwell and Shaw, 1970).

## 6. EFFECTS ON PANCREATIC SECRETION

Recent studies in dogs with chronic duodenal fistulae have shown that $PGE_1$ (0.5-5.0 $\mu g/kg/min$ i.v.) reduced the volume and bicarbonate concentration of pancreatic juice secreted either in the resting state or in response to secretin or secretin and pancreozymin (PZ) (Rudick *et al.*, 1971). The $ED_{50}$ for inhibition of bicarbonate output (1.8 µg/kg/min) was higher than for inhibition of gastric secretion (0.5 µg/kg/min) though the time course of these effects was similar.

In marked contrast to its effect on bicarbonate output, and in spite of reducing the total volume of secretion, $PGE_1$ increased both the concentration and output of enzymes as measured by protein content. However, even large doses of $PGE_1$ were unable to match the maximal secretory response to pancreozymin.

*Mechanism of action*

The typical hyperbolic relationship between bicarbonate concentration and flow rate was maintained during inhibition by $PGE_1$ suggesting that the reduction in bicarbonate concentration is not a selective effect but depends on the rate of secretion. Although the doses of $PGE_1$ which inhibit volume and bicarbonate are sufficient to cause a fall in systemic arterial blood pressure, there is no evidence that a reduction in pancreatic blood flow is the limiting factor for secretion, nor would this account for the observed increase in enzyme output.

Whether or not these effects of $PGE_1$ are mediated by an action on adenyl cyclase cannot be decided on existing evidence. Although both $PGE_1$ and PZ stimulate adenyl cyclase in whole pancreas (Rudick *et al.*, 1971), the reported effects of exogenously administered cyclic AMP on pancreatic secretion are contradictory. It is of interest, however, that theophylline, which may act by inhibiting phosphodiesterase thus allowing the intracellular concentration of cyclic AMP to increase, inhibits basal and secretin-stimulated volume output, decreases bicarbonate and increases chloride concentration, and greatly increases enzyme output, effects which are very similar to those of $PGE_1$ (Guelrud, Rudick and Janowitz, 1971).


## 7. PHYSIOLOGICAL ROLE OF PROSTAGLANDINS IN THE GASTRO-INTESTINAL TRACT

Although prostaglandins have a variety of potent effects on the gastro-intestinal tract, such pharmacological actions do not necessarily reflect physiological roles. Prostaglandins are unlikely to act as circulating hormones because of their rapid removal from the circulation, but they may act locally in the tissues where they are formed.

Prostaglandins are present in all regions of the human gastro-intestinal tract so far investigated. The distribution of prostaglandins between different layers or cell types has not been determined in most regions, though in the human stomach there is a higher concentration of prostaglandins (mainly $PGE_2$) in the mucosa than in the smooth muscle (Bennett *et al.*, 1968a). The amount of prostaglandin which can be extracted from a tissue is, however, a less meaningful indicator of physiological function than the rate of turnover. Prostaglandins are released from frog isolated intestine perfused through the vascular system and the output is increased by acetylcholine and DMPP which stimulate increased motility; by arachidonic acid, the precursor of $PGE_2$ and $F_{2\alpha}$, and by phospholipase A, which splits precursors from membrane phospholipids (Bartels, Kunze, Vogt and Wille, 1970).

The release of prostaglandins from the serosal and mucosal surfaces of the rat isolated stomach is greatly increased by vagal or transmural nerve stimulation which cause muscle contraction (Bennett, Freidman and Vane, 1967; Coceani, Pace-Asciak and Wolfe, 1967). Moreover, the amount released can greatly exceed the total amount extractable from the tissues. Whether this is derived from nerves, contracting muscle or deformed cells is not known, though some prostaglandin is still released after denervation by cold storage.

A role for the prostaglandins in the control of gut motility is suggested by their release during increased muscle activity and by their potent effects on smooth muscle *in vitro* and *in vivo*, though in view of their opposing actions on circular muscle it is difficult to predict the effect of a locally released mixture of E and F compounds. Prostaglandins are released by mechanical deformation of cells and could play a part either in the active increase in tension when smooth muscle is stretched or in the process by which storage organs like stomach and gall bladder accommodate to stretch so that tension in the smooth muscle does not increase in proportion to filling (Piper and Vane, 1971). Low concentrations of indomethacin reduce or abolish both the tone of the isolated rabbit jejunum and the output of prostaglandins, suggesting that smooth muscle tone is maintained by continuous generation of prostaglandins (Ferreira, Herman and Vane, 1972). Whether such prostaglandin release is of physiological importance or is due to the trauma of isolating the tissue remains to be established.

Other possibilities are that prostaglandins act as chemical transmitters of the nerve-mediated, atropine-resistant contractions which have been demonstrated in the guinea-pig ileum (Ambache and Freeman, 1968) and colon (Bennett and Fleshler, 1969) or that an E prostaglandin mediates the inhibitory response of circular muscle in the peristaltic reflex (Kottegoda, 1969).

Evidence available at present is insufficient to substantiate the hypothesis that prostaglandins modulate the effects of hormones and transmitters on smooth mucle by a negative feedback mechanism involving the adenyl cyclase system similar to that proposed for other types of tissue by Bergström (1967). Although inhibition of intestinal muscle by adrenaline is accompanied by increased concentrations of cyclic AMP (Beuding, Butcher and Hawkins, 1966) the effects of different prostaglandins on longitudinal or circular smooth muscle adenylcyclase have not been reported. Prostaglandins might also modulate the effects of sympathetic and parasympathetic nervous activity by a negative feedback mechanism involving reduced transmitter release (Wennmalm and Hedquist, 1971).

A possible role as negative feedback inhibitors of gastric secretion is suggested by the potent inhibitory effects of E and A prostaglandins and by the increased release of prostaglandins, mainly E compounds, into the perfused lumen of the rat stomach during vagal stimulation or pentagastrin administration (Shaw and Ramwell, 1968), though the amounts released into the perfusate are very small (1-3 ng $PGE_1$ equiv./ min) compared with the amount required to inhibit secretion (1 $\mu$g $PGE_2$/min; 10 $\mu$g/ml). In humans, very low or undetectable amounts were present in secretion stimulated by pentagastrin, though the possibility that any E prostaglandin released might have been converted to an A prostaglandin in the acid environment was not excluded (Horton *et al.*, 1968). These results cannot, however, be taken as conclusive evidence against the hypothesis that prostaglandins are negative feedback inhibitors since prostaglandins may be rapidly metabolized in the mucosa and their concentration at the site of action is not known.

The potent, though sometimes qualitatively different effects of the E and F prostaglandins on vascular smooth muscle suggests a possible role in the local regulation of blood flow in the gastro-intestinal tract. For example, the E prostaglandins may contribute to functional vaso-dilatation in the gastric mucosa.

It is of interest that during stimulation of secretion by theophylline and cyclic AMP in the rat there is more F than E prostaglandin released (Shaw and Ramwell, 1968), since F compounds have little of no inhibitory effect on gastric secretion. This result emphasizes that, in situations where there are marked quantitative or even qualitative differences between the effects of E and F prostaglandins, factors affecting the relative as well as the total amount of prostaglandins released, may be of particular importance both in normal conditions and in pathological conditions which might be associated with abnormal prostaglandin metabolism.

## 8. PATHOLOGICAL ROLES OF PROSTAGLANDINS

Prostaglandins have been implicated in the pathogenesis of diarrhoea in several clinical conditions. Williams, Karim and Sandler (1968) provided evidence that diarrhoea in patients with medullary carcinoma of the thyroid may be mediated by prostaglandins released into the circulation. Relatively high concentrations of $PGE_2$ (18-674 ng/g) and $PGF_{2\alpha}$ (17-844 ng/g) were present in tumour tissue from 4 out of 7 cases though the patient with the highest tissue levels had no diarrhoea.

Of greater significance was the finding that prostaglandins were present in blood from two patients with diarrhoea whereas none were detected in blood from healthy control subjects or from patients with diarrhoea of known cause. Moreover, in one patient, with persistent diarrhoea of unknown origin, there was a much higher concentration in blood draining during the tumour (41.5 ng/ml $PGE_2$ and 120 ng/ml $PGF_{2\alpha}$) than in central venous blood (3.3 ng/ml $PGE_2$ and 7.1 ng/ml $PGF_{2\alpha}$) and peripheral venous blood (0.8-2.4 ng/ml $PGE_2$ and 0.4-5.9 ng/ml $PGF_{2\alpha}$). This is consistent with the rapid inactivation of prostaglandins by the lungs.

Raised levels of prostaglandins were also found in neural crest tumours and in tumours derived from fore- and mid-gut (Sandler, Karim and Williams, 1968). The three highest concentrations of $PGF_{2\alpha}$ which were present in a ganglioneuroma (480 ng/g), a bronchial carcinoid (420 ng/g) and an $\alpha$ cell islet tumour (524 ng/g), were all associated with diarrhoea, but high concentrations of $PGF_{2\alpha}$ (e.g. 194, 256, 282 and 412 ng/g) in phaeochromocytoma were never associated with diarrhoea. The latter results cannot necessarily be taken as evidence against the hypothesis since raised tissue levels do ,not always imply increased release of prostaglandins into the circulation and in the only two cases of phaeochromocytoma in which venous blood draining the area of the tumour was examined, no prostaglandins could be detected.

Intravenous administration of prostaglandins in humans can cause increased gastro-intestinal motility and diarrhoea (Karim and Filshie, 1970). Moreover, the passage of clear fluid and faeces following oral prostaglandins in man (Misiewicz *et al.*, 1969) suggests that the diarrhoea may result from increased intestinal fluid secretion. It is therefore of interest that the highest concentration of $PGF_{2\alpha}$ (6 ng/ml) found in peripheral venous blood in patients with medullary carcinoma of the thyroid (Williams *et al.*, 1968) is of the same order as the arterial blood concentration required to stimulate net intestinal fluid secretion in the dog (10 ng/ml i.e. 2 $\mu$g/min injected into the superior mesenteric arterial blood flow of 200 ml/min) (Pierce *et al.*, 1971). These results suggest that circulating prostaglandins acting on the intestinal mucosa may be partly or wholly responsible for the diarrhoea associated with certain tumours. However, in contrast to the results of Williams *et al.* (1968), van Dorp (1971) found no increase in blood prostaglandin levels in patients with medullary carcinoma of the thyroid. This result emphasizes that a causal relationship between circulating prostaglandins released from tumours and diarrhoea, is far from established.

There is, as yet, little evidence to implicate circulating prostaglandins in other gastro-intestinal disorders, though it has been suggested that the increased intestinal activity observed in women during menstruation might be due to release of prostaglandins from the endometrium (Pickles, 1967). The unlikely possibility that the achlorhydria which is sometimes associated with the carcinoid syndrome might be due to circulating prostaglandins, has not been investigated.

Abnormal formation or metabolism of prostaglandins within the tissues of the gastro-intestinal tract might result in a variety of functional disorders, especially if prostaglandins have a local regulatory role in motor and secretory processes. For example, in the gastric mucosa, a reduction in the amount of prostaglandin formed or an alteration in the proportion of E to F compounds formed might contribute to the development of peptic ulcer. Gastro-intestinal irritation associated with the use of aspirin and indomethacin may possibly result from a local inhibition of prostaglandin synthesis. Another important possibility is that the profuse watery diarrhoea of cholera may be mediated by greatly increased formation of prostaglandins in the intestinal mucosa (Bennett, 1971).

## THERAPEUTIC APPLICATION

The inhibitory effect of prostaglandins on the formation of gastric and duodenal ulcers in the rat and on gastric secretion in rat, dog and man, suggests that they may be of potential value in the treatment of peptic ulcer in man. However, the realization of this potential is likely to depend on the discovery of an orally-effective synthetic prostaglandin with greater selectivity and duration of action than any of the known naturally-occurring substances. Although $PGE_1$ and $PGA_1$ injected intravenously can inhibit gastric secretion in man, orally-administered $PGE_1$ does not inhibit secretion in doses which cause bile reflux and increased intestinal motility. The effects of orally administered $PGA_1$ have not yet been reported, though a prostaglandin with some of the characteristics of a $PGA_1$ having less effect on gastro-intestinal smooth muscle and a longer half-life in the circulation than $PGE_1$ seems more likely to fulfill these requirements. A fuller understanding of the mode of action of the antisecretory, antiulcer prostaglandins in rat and dog would assist the rational development of an orally-effective, synthetic analogue for the treatment of peptic ulcer in man.

There is at present no obvious therapeutic application for the potent effects of prostaglandins on gut motility and on intestinal fluid and electrolyte transport, though it is of interest that the reduction in plasma volume during intravenous infusion of $PGA_1$ to hypertensive patients

(Lee, 1971) may have been due in part to decreased intestinal absorption, resulting in a shift of fluid from plasma to intestinal lumen. A synthetic prostaglandin which possessed only the inhibitory effects of the E compounds on circular smooth muscle might conceivably be used to delay gastric emptying or to inhibit intestinal peristalsis.

If prostaglandins have physiological or pathological roles in the gastro-intestinal tract, it may prove desirable, under certain conditions to increase or decrease the activity of the prostaglandin system. In theory this could be achieved in a variety of ways, for example by increasing or decreasing the availability of precursors, or by altering the activity of the synthesizing or metabolizing enzymes. Aspirin and indomethacin are potent inhibitors of prostaglandin synthesis *in vitro* (Vane, 1971) and *in vivo* (Ferreira, Moncado and Vane, 1971) and might be of value in the treatment of diarrhoea associated with increased prostaglandin formation. The recent discovery that aspirin-like drugs reduce or abolish the intestinal fluid loss caused by cholera enterotoxin in the rat (Jacoby and Marshall, 1972), is therefore of considerable interest. Although these results do not prove that prostaglandins mediate the intestinal secretory response to cholera enterotoxin, they emphasize the importance of testing new aspirin-like drugs and other inhibitors of prostaglandin synthesis on fluid loss in human cholera.

The activity of the prostaglandin system could also be altered by specific antagonists which block the effect of released prostaglandins. Of the many compounds examined, a few, including a debenzoxazepine hydrazide derivative, SC 19220 (Sanner, 1969), certain 7-oxaprosta-glandins (Fried, Santhanakrishnan, Himizu, Lin, Ford, Rubin and Grigas, 1969) and polyphloretin phosphate (PPP), have been shown to antagonize some of the effects of prostaglandins on some gastro-intestinal smooth muscle preparations. Although both SC 19220 (Sanner, 1971) and PPP (Eakins, 1971) inhibit $PGE_2$-induced diarrhoea in mice, their potency and specificity as antagonists is limited and they are not suitable for administration to humans.

It is to be hoped that substances which selectively block the effects of either one or other type of prostaglandins both *in vitro* and *in vivo* will soon become available. Such drugs are likely to prove of value, not only in the treatment of prostaglandin-mediated diarrhoea but also as pharmacological tools for testing the many hypotheses on the physiological and pathological roles of the prostaglandins.

## REFERENCES

Ambache, N. and Freeman, M. A. (1968). Atropine-resistant longitudinal muscle spasms due to excitation of non-cholinergic neurones in Auerbach's plexus. *Journal of Physiology (London)*, **199**, 705.

Änggård, E. (1966). The biological activities of three metabolites of prostaglandins $E_1$. *Acta Physiologica Scandinavica*, **66**, 509.

Al Awqati, Q., Cameron, J. L., Field, M. and Greenough, W. B. (1970a). Responses of human ileal mucosa to choleragen and theophylline. *Journal of Clinical Investigation*, **49**, 2a.

Al Awqati, Q., Field, M., Pierce, N. F. and Greenough, W. B. (1970b). Effect of prostaglandin $E_1$ ($PGE_1$) on electrolyte transport in rabbit ileal mucosa. *Journal of Clinical Investigation*, **49**, 2a.

Bartels, J., Kunze, H., Vogt, W. and Wille, G. (1970). Prostaglandin: Liberation from and formation in perfused frog intestine. *Naunyn-Schmiedebergs Archiv für experimentalle Pathologie und Pharmakologie*, **266**, 199.

Bartels, J., Vogt, W. and Wille, G. (1968). Prostaglandin release from and formation in perfused frog intestine. *Naunyn-Schmiedebergs Archiv für experimentalle Pathologie und Pharmakologie*, **259**, 153.

Bennett, A. (1971). Cholera and Prostaglandins. *Nature (London)*, **231**, 536.

Bennett, A., Friedman, C. A. and Vane, J. R. (1967). Release of prostaglandin $E_1$ from the rat stomach. *Nature (London)*, **216**, 873.

Bennett, A., Murray, J. G. and Wyllie, J. H. (1968a). Occurrence of prostaglandin $E_2$ in the human stomach, and a study of its effects on human isolated gastric muscle. *British Journal of Pharmacology and Chemotherapy*, **32**, 339.

Bennett, A., Eley, K. G. and Scholes, G. B. (1968b). Effects of prostaglandins $E_1$ and $E_2$ on human, guinea-pig and rat isolated small intestine. *British Journal of Pharmacology*, **34**, 630.

Bennett, A., Eley, K. G. and Scholes, G. B. (1968c). Effect of prostaglandins $E_1$ and $E_2$ on intestinal motility in the guinea-pig and rat. *British Journal of Pharmacology*, **34**, 639.

Bennett, A. and Fleshler, B. (1969). Action of prostaglandin $E_1$ on the longitudinal muscle of the guinea-pig isolated colon. *British Journal of Pharmacology*, **35**, 351P.

Bennett, A. and Fleshler, B. (1970). Prostaglandins and the gastro-intestinal tract. *Gastroenterology*, **59**, 790.

Bergström, S. (1967). Prostaglandins: Members of a new hormonal system. *Science (New York)*, **157**, 382.

Bergström, S., Carlson, L. A. and Weeks, J. R. (1968). The prostaglandins: a family of biologically active lipids. *Pharmacological Reviews*, **20**, 1.

Bergström, S., Duner, H., Euler, U. S. von, Pernow, B. and Sjövall, J. (1959a). Observations on the effects of infusion of prostaglandins E in man. *Acta Physiologica Scandinavica*, **45**, 145.

Bergström, S., Eliasson, R., Euler, U. S. von and Sjövall, J. (1959b). Some biological effects of two crystalline prostaglandin factors. *Acta Physiologica Scandinavica*, **45**, 133.

Berry, H. and Flower, R. J. (1971). The assay of endogenous cholecystokinin and factors influencing its release in the dog and cat. *Gastroenterology*, **60**, 409.

Bueding, E., Butcher, R. W., Hawkins, J., Timms, A. R. and Sutherland, E. W. (1966). Effect of epinephrine on cyclic adenosine $3',5'$-phosphate and hexose phosphates in intestinal smooth muscle. *Biochimica Biophysica Acta.*, **115**, 173.

Butcher, R. W. and Baird, C. E. (1968). Effects of prostaglandins on adenosine $3',5'$-monophosphate levels in fat and other tissues. *Journal of Biological Chemistry*, **243**, 1713.

Carlson, L. A., Ekelund, L. G. and Oro, L. (1968). Clinical and metabolic effects of different doses of prostaglandin E₁ in man. *Acta Medica Scandinavica*, **183**, 423.

Chawla, R. C. and Eisenberg, M. M. (1969). Prostaglandin inhibition of innervated antral motility in dogs. *Proceedings of the Society for Experimental Biology and Medicine*, **132**, 1081.

Christlieb, A. R., Dobrzinsky, S. J., Lyons, C. J. and Hickler, R. B. (1969). Short term PGA₁ infusion in patients with essential hypertension. *Clinical Research*, **17**, 234.

Classen, M., Koch, H., Deyhle, P., Weidenhiller, S. and Demling, L. (1970). Wirkung von Prostaglandin E₁ auf die basale Megensekretion des Menschen. *Klinische Wochenschrift*, **48**, 876.

Classen, M., Koch, H., Bickhardt, J., Topf, G. and Demling, L (1971). The effect of prostaglandin E₁ on pentagastrin-stimulated gastric secretion in man. *Digestion*, **4**, 333.

Coceani, F., Pace-Asciak, C., Volta, F. and Wolfe, L. S. (1967). Effect of nerve stimulation on prostaglandin formation and release from the rat stomach. *American Journal of Physiology*, **213**, 1056.

Coceani, F., Dreifuss, J. J., Puglisi, L. and Wolfe, L. S. (1969). Prostaglandins and membrane function. In: Prostaglandins, Peptides and Amines (Eds P. Mantegazza and E. W. Horton), p. 73, Academic Press, London.

Coceani, F. and Wolfe, L. S. (1966). On the action of prostaglandin E₁ and prostaglandins from brain on the isolated rat stomach. *Canadian Journal of Physiology and Pharmacology*, **44**, 933.

Dorp, D. A. van (1971). Recent developments in the biosynthesis and the analyses of prostaglandins, *Annals of the New York Academy of Sciences*, **180**, 181.

Eakins, K. (1971). Prostaglandin antagonism by polymeric phosphates of phloretin and related compounds. *Annals of the New York Academy of Sciences*, **180**, 386.

Euler, U. S. von (1934). Zur Kenntnis der pharmakologischen Wirkungen von Nativsekreten and Extrackten mannlicher accessorischer Geschlechtsdrüsen. *Naunyn-Schmiedebergs Archiv fur experimentalle Pathologie und Pharmakologie*, **175**, 78.

Euler, U. S. von (1966). Introductory survey: Prostaglandin. *Memoirs of the Society for Endocrinology*, **14**, 3.

Ferreira, S. H., Herman, A. and Vane, J. R. (1972). Prostaglandin generation maintains the smooth muscle tone of the rabbit isolated jejunum. *British Journal of Pharmacology*, **44**, 328P.

Ferreira, S. H., Moncada, S. and Vane, J. R. (1971). Indomethacin and aspirin abolish prostaglandin release from the spleen. *Nature New Biology*, **231**, 237.

Fried, J., Santhanakrishnan, T. S., Himizu, J., Lin, C. H., Ford, S. H., Rubin, B. and Grigas, E. O. (1969). Prostaglandin antagonists: Synthesis and smooth muscle activity. *Nature (London)*, **223**, 208.

Goldblatt, M. W. (1933). A depressor substance in seminal fluid. *Journal of the Society of Chemical Industry*, **52**, 1056.

Granström, E. (1967). On the metabolism of prostaglandin E₁ in man. *Progress in Biochemical Pharmacology*, **3**, 89.

Greenough, W. B., Pierce, N. F., Al Awqati, Q. and Carpenter, C. C. J. (1969). Stimulation of gut electrolyte secretion by prostaglandins, theophylline and cholera exotoxin. *Journal of Clinical Investigation*, **48**, 32a.

Guelrud, M., Rudick, J. and Janowitz, H. D. (1971). Endogenous cyclic AMP and pancreatic enzyme secretion. *Gastroenterology*, **60**, 671.

Harris, J. B., Nigon, K. and Alonso, D. (1969). Adenosine 3′,5′-monophosphate: intracellular mediator for methyl xanthine stimulation of gastric secretion. *Gastroenterology*, **57**, 377-384.

Harry, J. D. (1968). The action of prostaglandin $E_1$ on the guinea-pig isolated intestine. *British Journal of Pharmacology and Chemotherapy*, **33**, 213P.

Horton, E. W. (1963). Action of prostaglandin $E_1$ on tissues which respond to bradykinin. *Nature (London)*, **200**, 892.

Horton, E. W. (1965). Biological activities of pure prostaglandins. *Experientia*, **21**, 113.

Horton, E. W. (1969). Hypotheses on physiological roles of prostaglandins. *Physiological Reviews*, **49**, 122.

Horton, E. W. and Main, I. H. M. (1965). A comparison of the actions of prostaglandins $F_{2\alpha}$ and $E_1$ on smooth muscle. *British Journal of Pharmacology and Chemotherapy*, **24**, 470.

Horton, E. W. and Main, I. H. M. (1967). Identification of prostaglandins in central nervous tissues of the cat and chicken. *British Journal of Pharmacology and Chemotherapy*, **30**, 582.

Horton, E. W., Main, I. H. M., Thompson, C. J. and Wright, P. M. (1968). Effect of orally administered prostaglandin $E_1$ on gastric secretion and gastro-intestinal motility in man. *Gut*, **9**, 655.

Jacobson, E. D. (1970). Comparison of prostaglandin $E_1$ and norepinephrine on the gastric mucosal circulation. *Proceedings of the Society for Experimental Biology and Medicine*, **133**, 516.

Jacoby, H. I. and Marshall, C. H. (1972). Antagonism of cholera enterotoxin by anti-inflammatory agents in the rat. *Nature (London)*, **235**, 163.

Karim, S. M. M. and Filshie, G. M. (1970). Therapeutic abortion using prostaglandin $F_{2\alpha}$, *Lancet*, **1**, 157.

Khairallah, P. P., Page, I. H. and Türker, R. K. (1967). Some properties of prostaglandin $E_1$ action on muscle. *Archives internationales de pharmacodynamie et de thérapie*, **169**, 328.

Kimberg, D. V., Field, M., Johnson, J., Henderson, A. and Gershon, E. (1971). Stimulation of intestinal mucosal adenyl cyclase by cholera enterotoxin and prostaglandins. *Journal of Clinical Investigation*, **50**, 1218.

Kottegoda, S. R. (1969). An analysis of possible nervous mechanisms involved in the peristaltic reflex. *Journal of Physiology (London)*, **200**, 687.

Lee, J. B. (1971). *Annals of the New York Academy of Sciences*, **180**, 238.

Levine, R. A. (1970). The role of cyclic AMP in hepatic and gastro-intestinal function. *Gastroenterology*, **59**, 280.

Lippmann, W. (1970). Inhibition of gastric acid secretion by a potent synthetic prostaglandin. *Journal of Pharmacy and Pharmacology*, **22**, 65.

Main, I. H. M. (1969). Effects of prostaglandin $E_2$ ($PGE_2$) on the output of histamine and acid in rat gastric secretion induced by pentagastrin or histamine. *British Journal of Pharmacology*, **36**, 214P.

Main, I. H. M. and Whittle (1972). The effect of prostaglandin $E_2$ on rat mucosal blood flow as determined by $C^{14}$ aniline clearance. *British Journal of Pharmacology*, **44**, 331P.

Matuchansky, C. and Bernier, J. J. (1971). Effects of prostaglandin $E_1$ on net and unidirectional movements of water and electrolytes across the jejunal mucosa in man. *Gut*, 12, 854.

Misiewicz, J. J., Waller, S. L., Kiley, N. and Horton, E. W. (1969). Effect of oral prostaglandin $E_1$ on intestinal transit in man. *Lancet*, 1, 648.

Miyazaki, E., Ishizawa, M., Sunano, S., Syuto, B. and Sakagami, T. (1967). Stimulating action of prostaglandin on the rabbit duodenal muscle. In: Proceedings of the 2nd Nobel Symposium (Eds S. Bergström and B. Samuelsson), p. 277, Almqvist and Wiksell, Stockholm.

Nakano, J. and Cole, B. (1969). Effects of prostaglandins $E_1$ and $F_{2\alpha}$ on systemic, pulmonary and splanchnic circulation in dogs. *American Journal of Physiology*, 217, 222.

Nakano, J. and Prancan, A. V. (1972). Effect of prostaglandin $E_1$ and $A_1$ on the gastric circulation in dogs. *Proceedings of the Society for Experimental Biology and Medicine*, 131, 1151.

Nezamis, J. E., Robert, A. and Stowe, D. F. (1971). Inhibition by prostaglandin $E_1$ ($PGE_2$) of gastric secretion in the dog. *Journal of Physiology (London)*, 218, 369.

Ng, K. K. F., Sit, K. H. and Wong, W. C. (1970). Relaxant effect of prostaglandin on the isolated intestine of the toad (Bufo melanostictus). *Agents & Actions*, 1, 227.

Nugteren, D. H. (1970). Inhibition of prostaglandin biosynthesis by 8*cis*, 12*trans*, 14*cis*-eicosatrienoic acid and 5*cis*, 8*cis*, 12*trans*, 14*cis*-eicosatetraenoic acid. *Biochimica biophysica Acta*, 210, 171.

Orloff, J. and Grantham, J. (1967). The effect of prostaglandin ($PGE_1$) on the permeability of response of rabbit collecting tubules to vasopressin. In: Proceedings of the 2nd Nobel Symposium (Eds S. Bergström and B. Samuelsson), p. 143, Almqvist and Wiksell, Stockholm.

Orloff, J. Handler, J. S. and Bergström, S. (1965). Effect of prostaglandin ($PGE_1$) on the permeability response of toad bladder to vasopressin, theophylline and adenosine 3',5'-monophosphate. *Nature (London)*, 205, 397.

Parkinson, T. M. and Schneider, J. C. (1969). Absorption and metabolism of prostaglandin $E_1$ by perfused rat jejunum *in vitro*. *Biochimica Biophysica Acta*, 176, 78.

Perrier, C. W. and Laster, L. (1969). Adenyl cyclase activity of guinea-pig gastric mucosa. *Clinical Research*, 17, 596.

Pickles, V. R. (1967). The prostaglandins. *Biological Reviews*, 42, 614.

Pierce, N. F., Carpenter, C. C. J., Elliot, H. L. and Greenough, W. B. (1971). Effects of prostaglandins, theophylline and cholera exotoxin upon transmucosal water and electrolyte movement in the canine jejunum. *Gastroenterology*, 60, 22.

Piper, P. and Vane, J. R. (1971). The release of prostaglandins from lungs and other tissues. *Annals of the New York Academy of Sciences*, 180, 363.

Ramwell, P. W. and Shaw, J. E. (1968). Prostaglandin inhibition of gastric secretion. *Journal of Physiology (London)*, 195, 34P.

Ramwell, P. W. and Shaw, J. E. (1970). Biological significance of the prostaglandins. *Recent Progress in Hormone Research*, 26, 139.

Robert, A. (1968). Antisecretory property of prostaglandins. Prostaglandin Symposium of the Worcester Foundation (Eds P. W. Ramwell and J. E. Shaw), p. 47, Interscience, New York.

Robert, A., Nezamis, J. E. and Phillips, J. P. (1967). Inhibition of gastric secretion by prostaglandins. *American Journal of Digestive Diseases*, 12, 1073.

Robert, A., Nezamis, J. E. and Phillips, J. P. (1968a). Effect of prostaglandin $E_1$ on gastric secretion and ulcer formation in the rat. *Gastroenterology*, 55, 481.

Robert, A., Phillips, J. P. and Nezamis, J. E. (1968b). Inhibition by prostaglandin $E_1$ of gastric secretion in the dog. *Gastroenterology*, 54, 1263.

Robert, A., Stowe, D. F. and Nezamis, J. E. (1971). Prevention of duodenal ulcers by administration of prostaglandin $E_2$ ($PGE_2$). *Scandinavian Journal of Gastroenterology*, 6, 303.

Rudick, J., Gonda, M., Dreiling, D. A. and Janowitz, H. D. (1971). Effects of prostaglandin $E_1$ on pancreatic exocrine function. *Gastroenterology*, 60, 272.

Sandler, M., Karim, S. M. M. and Williams, E. D. (1968). Prostaglandins in amine-peptide-secreting tumours. *Lancet, II*, 1053.

Sanner, J. H. (1969). Antagonism of prostaglandin $E_2$ by 1-acetyl-2-(8)chloro-10,11-dihydro-dibenz (b,f)(1,4) oxazepine-10-carbonyl) hydrazine (SC-19220). *Archives internationales de pharmacodynamie et de thérapie*, 180, 46.

Sanner, J. H. (1971). Prostaglandin inhibition with a dibenzoxazepine hydrazide derivative and morphine. *Annals of the New York Academy of Sciences*, 180, 407.

Sharp, G. W. G. and Hynie, S. (1971). Stimulation of intestinal adenyl cyclase by cholera toxin. *Nature (London)*, 229, 266.

Shaw, J. E. and Ramwell, P. W. (1968). Inhibition of gastric secretion in rats by prostaglandin $E_1$. *Prostaglandin Symposium of the Worcester Foundation* (Eds P. W. Ramwell and J. E. Shaw), p. 55, Interscience, New York.

Shaw, J. E. and Ramwell, P. W. (1969). Direct effect of prostaglandin $E_1$ on the frog gastric mucosa. *Abstracts of the 4th International Congress of Pharmacology*, 109, Karger, Basel and New York.

Shehadeh, Z., Price, W. E. and Jacobson, E. D. (1970). Effects of vasoactive agents on intestinal blood flow and motility in the dog. *American Journal of Physiology*, 216, 386.

Thompson, J. H. and Angulo, M. (1968). The effect of prostaglandins on gastro-intestinal serotonin in the rat. *European Journal of Pharmacology*, 4, 224.

Vanasin, B., Greenhough, W. and Schuster, M. M. (1970). Effect of prostaglandin on electrical and motor activity of isolated colonic muscle. *Gastroenterology*, 58, 1004.

Vane, J. R. (1969). The release and fate of vasoactive hormones in the circulation. *British Journal of Pharmacology*, 35, 209.

Vane, J. R. (1971). The inhibition of prostaglandin synthesis as a mechanism of action for aspirin-like drugs. *Nature (New Biology)*, 231, 232.

Way, L. and Durbin, R. P. (1969). Inhibition of gastric acid secretion *in vitro* by prostaglandin $E_1$. *Nature (London)*, 221, 874.

Weeks, J. R., Schultz, J. R. and Brown, W. E. (1968). Evaluation of smooth muscle bioassays for prostaglandins $E_1$ and $F_{1\alpha}$ *Journal of Applied Physiology*, 25, 783.

Wennmalm, A. and Hedqvist, P. (1971). Inhibition by prostaglandin $E_1$ of parasympathetic neurotransmission in the rabbit heart. *Life Sciences*, 10, 465.

Williams, E. D., Karim, S. M. M. and Sandler, M. (1968). Prostaglandin secretion by medullary carcinoma of the thyroid. *Lancet*, 1, 22.

Wilson, D. E. and Levine, R. A. (1969). Decreased canine gastric mucosal blood flow induced by prostaglandin $E_1$. A mechanism for its inhibitory effect on gastric secretion. *Gastroenterology*, **56**, 1268.

Wilson, D. E., Phillips, C. and Levine, R. A. (1971). Inhibition of gastric secretion in man by prostaglandin $A_1$. *Gastroenterology*, **61**, 201.

# Index

## A

Abortifacients, 167, 172, 173
Abortion, ix, 174, 176, 177, 182, 183, 185, 294
  missed, 191, 192-95
  therapeutic, ix, 270, 271, 274
Absorption, 181
Acetylcholine, 289, 290, 313
ACTH, 87, 88, 153, 157
Adenyl cyclase, 29, 76, 77, 82, 88, 90, 94, 95, 152-55, 160, 161, 276, 279, 299, 310, 312, 313
  and PDase relationship, 155
Adipose tissue, 78, 83, 84, 86
ADP, 92, 93
Adrenal cortex, 153, 157
Adrenal gland, 88
Adrenaline, 84
Airways resistance, 266, 271, 273, 274
Alkyl side chain variations, 28
Alpha-adrenoceptor blocking agents, 258
Anoxia, 292
Antifertility action, 40
Antihypertensive action, 78, 201
  of ANRL, 237
Antihypertensive function, of kidney, 201, 202-3, 242
  of renal medulla, 203-10
Antihypertensive neutral renomedullary lipid (ANRL), 233-42
  antihypertensive action, 237
  fatty aldehydes from, 238
  refinement of, 235
  therapeutic implications, 240-42
Antihypertensive renomedullary function, 239

## B

Antilipolytic action, 28, 82-84
Antilipolytic potency, 78, 81
Arterial hypertension, 233
Aspirin, 162, 317
Asthma, 279-82
Asymmetric centres, 3
ATP, 93, 153, 156
Atropine, 259, 309
Autoxidation, 13

Beta-adrenoceptor blocking agents, 258-59
Bile reflux, 294, 297
Bile secretion, 297
Biological action, 29
Biological assay, gastro-intestinal smooth muscle for, 287-89
Biosynthesis, 5-8, 133
Blood flow, local regulation in, 314
Blood pressure, 15, 16, 25, 218, 242
Brain, 67
Breakdown, 135-37
Bromolysergic acid diethylamide, 291
Bronchial asthma, 279-82
Bronchial resistance, 259-73
  aerosol administration, 261, 264, 265-71
  animal studies, 259-65
  human studies, 265-73
  intravenous administration, 262, 271
  potency in relation to route of administration, 274
Bronchial smooth muscle, 257, 258, 260, 266, 272, 273, 274, 277, 278, 279, 282

Bronchoconstriction, 259-62, 264, 270, 274
Bronchodilatation, 142, 260-66, 268-75, 278, 279, 281
Bronchospasm, 268-69, 279, 281, 282

C

Cahn-Ingold-Prelog Convention, 3
Carbohydrate metabolism, 84-86
Carboxyl side chain variations, 25
Carboxylic acids, 1, 5
Carcinoid syndrome, 316
Cardiovascular effects of renomedullary prostaglandins, 215-23
Cardiovascular system, 24, 41-47, 51-56
Carotid artery, 223
Carotid circulation, 64
Catecholamines, 45, 49, 82
Cell receptor thesis, 215
Cellular mechanisms, 29
Cellular source of renomedullary prostaglandins, 212-15
Cerebellum, 67, 70
Cerebral blood vessels, 64, 223
Cerebro-spinal fluid, 67
Chemical properties, 13-14
Chemical stability, 13
Chemical structure, 1
Cholera, 162
Cholera enterotoxin, 298, 299
Cholesterol, 84
Chromatography, 6, 9, 10
Contraception, 167, 172
Coronary arterial system, 58, 222
Corpua luteum, 37-41
Cyclic-AMP, 24, 29, 39, 76, 77, 82-84, 88, 90-92, 94, 95, 151-65, 276, 278, 299, 310, 311, 312, 314
  biological role, 156
  formation, 161
  in control of metabolism, 161
  in disease, 161
  intracellular concentrations of 152-56, 158
    control of, 155-56
    effects of prostaglandins in various tissues, 159

Cyclic-AMP–*cont.*
  mechanism, 153-55
  metabolism, 151, 152, 162
  prostaglandins in, 158
  production of, 152-54, 156
  role of, 151, 156
  second messenger, 29, 82, 156-62
Cyclohexane analogues, 13, 16
Cyclopentane ring variations, 26

D

Dehydration, 1, 10
Deoxyprostaglandins, 5
Depressor action, 27, 28, 45, 74, 240, 241
  prolonged, 217-20
Dialysis, 6
Diarrhoea, 314-17
Distribution, 125
Dixon-Brodie method, 262
DMPP, 313
DOCA-salt, 202, 203, 239
Drugs, 162, 279, 292
Duodenal ulcers, 305, 316
Dysmenorrhoea, 172

E

Electrolyte transport, 297-99
Electrolytes, 29
Endocrine system, 24, 86-92
Endometrium, 316
Enzyme system, 6, 136
Essential fatty acid deficiency, 99
Extraction, 5, 125, 142
Extremity circulation, 65
Eye, 24, 95-97

F

Fallopian tubes, 35-37
  *in vitro*, 35
  *in vivo*, 36
Fat cells, 78, 157, 160
Fatty aldehydes from ANRL, 238
Fertility, ix, 33, 40, 172

First messenger, 156
Flushing, 97
Foetus, intrauterine death, 191-95
Forced expiratory volume in 1 s (FEV$_1$), 266-70
Free fatty acids, 78-82

### G

Gastric circulation, 62
Gastric secretion, 62
  animal studies, 300-5
  in humans, 305-11
    oral administration, 305-6
    parenteral administration, 306-8
    mechanism of action on, 308-11
Gastric ulcers, 304, 316
Gastrin, 310
Gastro-intestinal irritation, 316
Gastro-intestinal motility, 315
  and transit, 295-96
  in humans, mechanism of action on, 297
  *in vitro*, 287-92
  *in vivo*, 292-97
    animal studies, 292-93
    in humans, 294-96
Gastro-intestinal smooth muscle, 317
  for biological assay, 287-89
  *in vitro*, 291
  longitudinal, *in vitro*, 289
Gastro-intestinal system, 24, 287-323
  pathological role in, 314-16, 317
  peptic ulcers, 312
  physiological role in, 312-14, 317
  therapeutic application, 316-17
Glucose, 86
Glycogen, 84-86
Goldblatt hypertension, one-kidney, 206, 232
  two-kidney, 202, 232
Gorgonian, 5

### H

Haematological system, 24, 92-95
Heart rate, 50

Heparin, 84
Hepatic circulation, 61
Histamine, 258, 261, 262, 264, 265, 303-9
Hydatidiform mole, 192-95
Hydrogenation, 13
Hydroxyl groups, 3
$\omega$-Hydroxylation, 139
15-Hydroxyprostaglandin dehydrogenase, 136
Hyperglycemia, 85-86, 92
Hypertension, 75, 77, 78, 201
  arterial, 233
  Golblatt and Page types of, 229
  one-kidney Goldblatt, 206, 232
  renal, 77, 227, 230
  renomedullary prostaglandins in, 227-33
    interpretations of action of, 230-33
  renoprival, 78, 203, 206, 209, 227, 230, 242
  renovascular, 202, 227, 232
  two-kidney Goldblatt, 202, 232
  use of prostaglandins in, 230
  *see also* Antihypertensive function
Hypotensive action, 27, 43, 45
Hypothalamus, 70, 86, 88

### I

Indomethacin, 313, 317
Induction, of labour, ix, 167, 186-89, 270, 294
  double blind trial of prostaglandins and oxytocin, 189-91
  of therapeutic abortion, ix
Inflammatory processes, 99
Inhibitors, 28, 100-2
Inotropic action, 54, 55
Insulin, 92
Intestinal water, 297-99
Intraocular pressure, 96-97
Intrauterine death of foetus, 191-95
Irin, 127
Isomerization, 226
Isoprenaline, 262-67, 270. 274

## K

Kidney, antihypertensive function of, 201, 202-3, 242
medulla of, *see* Renal medulla
transplantation, 203
Konsett-Rössler method, 259, 262

## L

Labour, induction of, ix, 167, 186-89, 270, 294
double blind trial of prostaglandins and oxytocin, 189-91
missed, 192
Lipid metabolism, 78
Lipolysis, 160
antilipolytic action, 82-84
*in vitro*, 78-81
*in vivo*, 81-82
Lipoprotein lipase, 84
Lung resistance, 269, 271
Lung tissue, 274
Lungs, 162, 253, 257, 259, 271, 276, 277, 278
*see also* Respiratory system
Luteinizing hormone, 161

## M

Mechanism of action, 151
Medullin, 210
Menstrual fluid, 126
Menstrual stimulants, 170, 172
Menstruation, 31, 170-72, 316
Mesenteric vessels, 222
Metabolism, 24, 133-42, 161
action of prostaglandins on, 78-86
carbohydrate, 84-86
cyclic AMP, 151, 152, 162
lipid, 78
protein, 86
*in vitro*, 137-39
*in vivo*, 139-42
Methyl substituents, 11
Methyl xanthines, 160
Microcirculation, 47
Missed abortion, 191, 192-95

Missed labour, 192
Myocardial contractility, 51-56
Myocardial metabolism, 58
Myometrium, 30, 31, 32
non-pregnant, 169

## N

Nasal circulation, 24, 66
Negative feed back, 29
inhibition of, 314
Nephrectomy bilateral, 202, 209
Nervous system, 24, 37, 67-73, 126, 131, 314
Nomenclature, 1-5
Noradrenaline, 309

## O

*Ophiobolus graminis*, 7
Optically active forms, 3
Ovarian circulation, 63
Ovaries, 37-40, 161
Oxaprostaglandins, 5
$\beta$-Oxidation, 136, 140-41
$\omega$-Oxidation, 136, 140
Oxytocin, 33, 170, 173, 174, 178, 189-91, 192

## P

Pain, 73
Pancreatic secretion, 92, 311-12
mechanism of action on, 312
Pancreozymin, 312
Parathyroid, 91
Pathological role, 277
in gastro-intestinal tract, 314-16, 317
Pentagastrin, 295, 303, 305, 306, 309, 314
Peptic ulcers, 316
Peristalsis, 290
Peroneal nerve, 73
Phaechromocytoma, 315
Pharmacological activity, 14, 23-123, 142, 167
Phenoxybenzamine, 258
Phlebitis, 175

Phosphodiesterase (PDase), 153-55, 160
   and adenyl cyclase relationship, 155
Physiological role, 129, 277
   in gastro-intestinal tract, 312-14, 317
Pituitary gland, 86, 87
Placenta, 34
Placental circulation, 63
Platelet adhesiveness, 94
Platelet aggregation, 25, 27, 94, 95
*Plexaura homomalla*, 5
Polyphloretin phosphate, 96, 101, 280
Portal circulation, 61
Prednisolone, 305
Pregnancy, *see* Uterus
Pressor action, 27
Progesterone, 37-38, 41
Propranolol, 258
Prostaglandin metabolites, 11
Prostaglandin synthetases, 134
Prostaglandins
   A series 1, 2, 3
     dehydration, 10
     pharmacological actions, 24
     structure-activity relationships, 16
     vasodilator, 26
   $A_1$, action on cardiovascular system, 43
     derivatives, 7
     19-hydroxy, action on cardio-vascular system, 44
     intraluminal administration, 303
     metabolism, 139
     synthesis, 10
   $A_2$, action on cardiovascular system, 43
     inactivation, 135
     intraluminal administration, 303
     15-R, action on cardiovascular system, 44
   alkyl side chain variations, 28
   B series 1, 2, 3
     structure-activity relationships, 16
     synthesis, 10-11
   $B_1$, 11
     conversion to C-16 and C-18 homologues, 139
   $B_2$, 15-hydroxy, action on cardio-vascular system, 44

Prostaglandins—*cont.*
   $B_3$, 3
   biosynthesis, 5-8, 133
   breakdown, 135-37
   C series, 1, 16
   C-9 keto, 137
   C-15 hydroxyl group, 137
   carboxyl side chain variations, 25
   cellular mechanisms, 29
   chemical properties, 13-14
   chemical stability, 13
   chemistry, structure and availability, 1
   classification, 1
   cyclopentane ring variations, 26
   $\Delta^{13}$ reductase, 135, 136, 137, 141
   11-deoxyprostaglandins, 12, 13, 16
   dienoic, 13
   15-dehydroprostaglandins, 11
   13, 14-dihydroprostaglandins, 11, 16
   E series 1, 4
     $\alpha$-homo, 15
     $\alpha$-nor, 15
     biosynthesis, 7
     chemical properties, 14
     compounds, 13, 14
     derivatives, 7
     pharmacological actions, 24
     sources of supply, 6
     unnatural stereoisomers, 10
     vasodilator action, 26, 310
   $E_1$, 3, 4, 253, 293
     action on cardiovascular system, 41
     aerosol administration, 265
     biosynthesis, 6
     bronchodilator effect, 270, 274
     chemical properties, 13
     conversion to C-16 and C-18 homologues, 139
     dihydro, 137, 138
     dihydro, action on cardiovascular system, 44
     effect on cyclic AMP levels, 158
     in fat cells, 160-61
     intraluminal administration, 299, 303

Prostaglandins—*cont.*
15-keto, 137, 138
  action on cardiovascular system, 44
15-keto-dihydro, 138
metabolism, 133, 137, 139, 140
occurrence, 125, 126, 127
pharmacological actions, 24
15-R, action on cardiovascular system, 44
release, 132, 133
removal from circulation, 135, 139
side chain variants, 4
stereochemical variants, 3
structure-activity relationships, 14, 15
synthesis, 10, 11, 12
vasodilator, 26
$E_2$, 3, 127, 129, 143, 253
  action on cardiovascular system, 41
aerosol administration, 265
biosynthesis, 6
bronchodilator effect, 270, 274
chemical properties, 13
deterioration in storage, 14
inactivation, 135
intra-amniotic injection, 179
intravenous administration, 271
metabolism, 133, 134, 137, 139, 140, 141
occurrence, 125, 126
pharmacological actions, 24
release, 129, 131, 132
removal from circulation, 135
structure-activity relationships, 14-15
synthesis, 10, 134
unnatural stereoisomer, 10
$E_3$, 3, 253
  action on cardiovascular system, 41
biosynthesis, 6
metabolism, 133, 137
occurrence, 125
structure-activity relationships, 14
synthesis, 9, 10

Prostaglandins—*cont.*
'ent' compounds, 9
15-*epi*, 5
F series, 1, 4
  chemical properties, 13, 14
compounds, synthesis, 10
pharmacological actions, 24
unnatural stereoisomers, 10
$F_\alpha$ compounds, 4
  biosynthesis, 4, 6
chemical properties, 14
structure-activity relationships, 15
synthesis, 10
$F_\beta$ compounds, 4
  structure-activity relationships, 15-16
synthesis, 10
$F_1$, synthesis, 10
$F_{1\alpha}$, 4, 7, 26
  action on cardiovascular system, 45
chemical properties, 13
conversion to C-16 and C-18 homologues, 139
metabolism, 140
occurrence, 125, 126, 127
release, 132, 133
removal from circulation, 139
synthesis, 10, 12
$F_{1\beta}$, 4
  conversion to C-16 and C-18 homologues, 139
synthesis, 12
$F_2$, synthesis, 10
$F_{2\alpha}$, 26, 129, 143
  action on cardiovascular system, 45
aerosol administration, 271
chemical properties, 13
inactivation, 135
intra-amniotic injection, 179
intravenous administration, 271
metabolism, 134, 140, 141
occurrence, 125, 126, 127
pharmacological actions, 24
release, 129, 131, 132, 133, 143
removal from circulation, 135
synthesis, 10, 13, 134

Prostaglandins—*cont.*
  $F_{3\alpha}$, synthesis, 10
  function of, 161, 162
  *homo,* 7
  15-hydroxyprostaglandin   dehydro-
    genase, 138
  in disease, 161
  8-iso-PGE, 7
  metabolism, *in vitro,* 137-39
  metabolism, *in vivo,* 139-42
  15-methylprostaglandins, 11, 16
  monoenoic, 13
  natural, 1, 2, 4, 9
    derivatives and structural variants
      of, 4
  nomenclature, 1-5
  *nor,* 7
  novel synthetic, 11
  occurrence, 133
  optically active forms, 3
  oxaprostaglandins, 16
  3-oxaprostaglandins, 11
  7-oxaprostaglandins, 12
  pharmacological actions of, 23-123
  possible therapeutic applications, ix
  primary, *see* Prostaglandins, E and F
    series
  quantitative  and  qualitative  dif-
    ferences, 288
  racemic mixtures, 9
  relative potency, 288
  release by various stimuli, 129-33
  removal from circulation, 134
  renomedullary, *see* Renomedullary
    prostaglandins
  solutions, 13
  stereochemical variants, 3-4
  stereoisomers, 9
  structure-activity relationships,
    14-16, 25-29, 288, 289
  subcellular mechanisms, 29, 76
  supply sources, 5-13
    direct extraction from tissues, 5
    extraction, 125, 142
    total chemical synthesis, 8-13
  synthesis, 8-13, 133, 142, 278
  synthetic stereoisomers, 15
  trienoic, 13

Prostanoic acid, 1, 4
Protein metabolism, 86
Pulmonary circulation, 57-58
Pulmonary function, 277
Pulmonary tissues, 277-78
Pulmonary vasculature, 223
Purkinje cells, 70

R

Release by various stimuli, 129-33
Renal autoexplantation, 205, 225
Renal autotransplantation, 206
Renal function, effect of renomedullary
  prostaglandins, 224-26
Renal hypertension, 77, 227, 230
Renal medulla, 74
  antihypertensive function, 203-10
  vasodepressor lipid of, 210-11
Renal system, 24, 63, 74-78
Renal vasculature, effect of renomedullary prostaglandins, 224-26
Renal  venous  effluent,  release  of
  renomedullary prostaglandins into,
  226-27
Renomedullary interstitial cells, 239
Renomedullary lipid, antihypertensive
  neutral (ANRL), 233-40
Renomedullary prostaglandins, 211-12
  cardiovascular effects, 215-23
  cellular source, 212-15
  dose response to, 216
  effect on cerebral vasculature, 223
  effect on coronary arterial system,
    222
  effect on mesenteric and splenic
    beds, 222
  effect on pulmonary vasculature, 223
  effect on renal vasculature and renal
    function, 224-26
  effect on various vascular beds, 220
  effect on vascular bed of extremities,
    222
  in hypertension, 227-33
    interpretations  of  action  of,
      230-33
  *in vitro* arterial effect, 222
  release into renal venous effluent,
    226-27

Renoprival hypertension, 78, 203, 206, 209, 227, 230, 242
Renovascular hypertension, 202, 227, 232
Reproductive system, 24, 30, 167-99
Respiratory disease, therapeutic application, 280
Respiratory smooth muscle, 24, 253-85
  aerosol administration, 274
  animal studies, 253-56
  human studies, 257-59
  isolated effects on, 253-59
  mechanism of action on, 275-77
  physiological and pathological involvement, 277-80
  potency in relation to route of administration, 274
  therapeutic possibilities, 280-82
Respiratory system, irritant effect, 268, 270, 281
Rubin's test, 36

S

Sciatic nerve section, 71
Second messenger system, 29, 82, 156-62
Secretin, 309, 312
Seminal fluid, 33, 125, 167, 168, 172
Shay ulcers, 304
Side effects, 172, 174, 176, 177, 178, 181, 182, 183, 185, 186, 287, 307, 308
Skin, 24, 97-99, 132
  of chicken, 100
  of frog, 99
Smooth muscle, 15, 16, 25, 27, 28, 101, 170
  active principle, 215
  see also under specific systems
Solubility, 13
Solvent extraction, 6
Spinal cord, 67, 73
Splanchnic circulation, 61
Spleen, 62, 162
Splenic circulation, 61, 62, 222
SRS-A, 257, 258, 262
Stereochemistry, 3-4

Storage, 13
Structure, chemical, 1
Structure-activity relationships, 14-16, 25-29, 288, 289
Subcellular mechanisms, 29, 76
Supply sources, see under Prostaglandins
Synthesis, 8-13, 133, 142, 278
Systemic actions, 30
Systemic venous return, 56

T

Tachyphylaxis, 170
Testicle, 90
Theophylline, 83, 314
Therapeutic abortion, ix, 270, 271, 274
Therapeutic applications, 167
  cardiovascular, 240
  gastro-intestinal tract, 316-17
  reproductive system, 167
  respiratory disease, 280
Third messenger, 156
Thyroid, 28, 89
Thyroid stimulating-hormone (TSH), 87, 89, 90
Tracheal muscle, 254, 25, 260, 275
Transplantation, kidney, 203
Tumours, 315

U

Ulcer, formation in rats, 304
Umbilical cord, 34
Uterine circulation, 63
Uterus, 30-34
  early pregnant, 172-85
    in vitro studies, 172-85
    in vivo studies, 173
    in vivo studies, intra-amniotic route, 179
    in vivo studies, intramuscular route, 179
    in vivo studies, intrauterine route, 182
    in vivo studies, intravaginal route, 181

Uterus—*cont.*

    *in vivo* studies, intravenous route, 173

    *in vivo* studies, oral route, 184

    *in vivo* studies, subcutaneous route, 179

  *in vivo,* 33

  mid-pregnant, 169

  non-pregnant, 167-72

    cyclic variation in sensitivity, 170

    *in vitro* studies, 167-68

    *in vivo* studies, 168-70

  pregnant, 33

  pregnant at term, 185-91

    double blind trial for induction of labour, 189-91

    induction of labour, oral and vaginal route, 191

Uterus—*cont.*

  *in vitro* studies, 185

  *in vivo* studies, 186

**V**

Vascular beds, effect of renomedullary prostaglandins on, 220-23

  of extremities, 222

Vascular effects, 201-50

  constrictor, 27, 64, 66, 102, 223

  dilator, 26, 27, 28, 64, 65, 215, 223, 226, 310

Vasodepressor action, 27, 28, 45, 74, 217-20, 240, 241

Vasodepressor lipid, 224, 226, 227, 232, 233, 235

  renal medulla, 210-11

Vasopressin, 76-77, 170

/RMbbb.P857(87>C1/

/RMbbb.P857(87>C1/